Pediatric Vascular Neurosurgery

Guest Editors

PAUL KLIMO Jr, MD, MPH, Maj, USAF
CORMAC O. MAHER, MD
EDWARD R. SMITH, MD

NEUROSURGERY
CLINICS OF NORTH AMERICA

www.neurosurgery.theclinics.com

Consulting Editors
ANDREW T. PARSA, MD, PhD
PAUL C. McCORMICK, MD, MPH

July 2010 • Volume 21 • Number 3

SAUNDERS an imprint of ELSEVIER, Inc.

W.B. SAUNDERS COMPANY
A Division of Elsevier Inc.

1600 John F. Kennedy Blvd. • Suite 1800 • Philadelphia, PA 19103-2899

http://www.theclinics.com

NEUROSURGERY CLINICS OF NORTH AMERICA Volume 21, Number 3
July 2010 ISSN 1042-3680, ISBN-13: 978-1-4377-1840-9

Editor: Ruth Malwitz
Developmental Editor: Donald Mumford

Neurosurgery Clinics of North America (ISSN 1042-3680) is published quarterly by Elsevier Inc., 360 Park Avenue South, New York, NY 10010-1710. Months of issue are January, April, July, and October. Business and Editorial Offices: 1600 John F. Kennedy Blvd., Suite 1800, Philadelphia, PA 19103-2899. Customer Service Office: 11830 Westline Industrial Drive, St. Louis, MO 63146. Periodicals postage paid at New York, NY, and additional mailing offices. Subscription prices are $296.00 per year (US individuals), $447.00 per year (US institutions), $324.00 per year (Canadian individuals), $546.00 per year (Canadian institutions), $414.00 per year (international individuals), $546.00 per year (international institutions), $149.00 per year (US students), and $204.00 per year (international students). International air speed delivery is included in all *Clinics* subscription prices. All prices are subject to change without notice. **POSTMASTER:** Send address changes to *Neurosurgery Clinics of North America*, Elsevier Periodicals Customer Service, 11830 Westline Industrial Drive, St. Louis, MO 63146. **Customer Service: 1-800-654-2452 (US and Canada). From outside the US and Canada, call: 1-314-453-7041. Fax: 1-314-453-5170. E-mail: JournalsCustomerService-usa@elsevier.com (for print support) and journalsonlinesupport-usa@elsevier.com (for online support).**

Reprints. For copies of 100 or more, of articles in this publication, please contact the Commercial Reprints Department, Elsevier Inc., 360 Park Avenue South, New York, NY 10010-1710. Tel. (212) 633-3812; Fax: (212) 462-1935; E-mail: reprints@elsevier.com.

Neurosurgery Clinics of North America is covered in *MEDLINE/PubMed (Index Medicus), EMBASE/Excerpta Medica, and Current Contents/Clinical Medicine (CC/CM).*

Printed and bound in the United Kingdom
Transferred to Digital Print 2011

Contributors

CONSULTING EDITORS

ANDREW T. PARSA, MD, PhD
Associate Professor; Principal Investigator, Brain Tumor Research Center; Reza and Georgianna Khatib Endowed Chair in Skull Base Tumor Surgery, Department of Neurological Surgery, University of California, San Francisco, San Francisco, California

PAUL C. MCCORMICK, MD, MPH, FACS
Herbert & Linda Gallen Professor of Neurological Surgery, Department of Neurological Surgery, Columbia University Medical Center, New York, New York

GUEST EDITORS

PAUL KLIMO Jr, MD, MPH, Maj, USAF
Chief, Neurosurgery, Wright-Patterson Air Force Base, Ohio

CORMAC O. MAHER, MD
Assistant Professor, Department of Neurosurgery, University of Michigan, Ann Arbor, Michigan

EDWARD R. SMITH, MD
Director, Pediatric Cerebrovascular Surgery, Department of Neurosurgery, Children's Hospital Boston, Harvard Medical School, Boston, Massachusetts

AUTHORS

RICHARD C.E. ANDERSON, MD
Assistant Professor of Neurosurgery and Pediatric Neurosurgery, Columbia University Medical Center; Director, Pediatric Neurosurgery, St Joseph's Children's Hospital, New York, New York

LORI BILLINGHURST, MD, MSc, FRCPC
Division of Neurology, Hospital for Sick Children, Toronto, Ontario, Canada

ROUKOZ B. CHAMOUN, MD
Division of Pediatric Neurosurgery, Department of Neurosurgery, Texas Children's Hospital, Baylor College of Medicine, Houston, Texas

NOMAZULU DLAMINI, MBBS, MRCPCH, MSc
Division of Neurology, Hospital for Sick Children, Toronto, Ontario, Canada; Neurosciences Unit, UCL Institute of Child Health, London, United Kingdom

DANIEL K. FAHIM, MD
Resident, Department of Neurosurgery, Baylor College of Medicine, Houston, Texas

ANDREW B. FOY, MD
Chief Resident Associate, Department of Neurologic Surgery, Mayo Clinic and Foundation, Rochester, Minnesota

HUGH J.L. GARTON, MD, MHSc
Associate Professor, Department of Neurosurgery, University of Michigan, Ann Arbor, Michigan

SASIKHAN GEIBPRASERT, MD
Department of Diagnostic Radiology, The Hospital for Sick Children, University of Toronto, Toronto, Ontario, Canada; Department of Radiology, Ramathibodi Hospital, Mahidol University, Bangkok, Thailand

NALIN GUPTA, MD, PhD
Associate Professor, Chief, Pediatric Neurosurgery, Department of Neurological Surgery, University of California, San Francisco, San Francisco, California

RAPHAEL GUZMAN, MD
Assistant Professor of Neurosurgery, Bechtel Foundation Faculty Scholar in Pediatric Translational Medicine, Division of Pediatric Neurosurgery, Lucile Packard Children's Hospital, Stanford University School of Medicine, Stanford, California

SHAWN L. HERVEY-JUMPER, MD
Resident, Department of Neurosurgery, University of Michigan, Ann Arbor, Michigan

STEVEN W. HETTS, MD
Assistant Professor, Department of Radiology, University of California, San Francisco, San Francisco, California

ANDREW JEA, MD
Assistant Professor, Division of Pediatric Neurosurgery, Department of Neurosurgery, Texas Children's Hospital, Baylor College of Medicine, Houston, Texas

BRIAN J. JIAN, MD, PhD
Resident, Department of Neurological Surgery, University of California, San Francisco, San Francisco, California

FENELLA KIRKHAM, MD, FRCPCH
Neurosciences Unit, UCL Institute of Child Health, London, United Kingdom

PAUL KLIMO Jr, MD, MPH, Maj, USAF
Chief, Neurosurgery, Wright-Patterson Air Force Base, Ohio

TIMO KRINGS, MD, PhD, FRCP(C)
Division of Neuroradiology, Department of Medical Imaging, Toronto Western Hospital, University of Toronto, Toronto, Ontario, Canada; Department of Neuroradiology, University Hospital Aachen, Aachen, Germany; Service de Neuroradiologie Diagnostique et Therapeutique, CHU Le-Kremlin-Bicetre, Paris, France

MICHAEL T. LAWTON, MD
Professor, Department of Neurological Surgery, University of California, San Francisco, San Francisco, California

CORMAC O. MAHER, MD
Assistant Professor, Department of Neurosurgery, University of Michigan, Ann Arbor, Michigan

FRANCESCO T. MANGANO, DO
Assistant Professor of Neurosurgery and Pediatrics Director, Pediatric Epilepsy Surgery Program, University of Cincinnati, Department of Neurosurgery, Division of Pediatric Neurosurgery, Cincinnati Children's Hospital Medical Center, Cincinnati, Ohio

TOBA N. NIAZI, MD
Department of Neurosurgery, Primary Children's Medical Center, University of Utah, Salt Lake City, Utah

NEIL N. PATEL, DO, MBA
Fellow, Pediatric Neurosurgery, Cincinnati Childrens Hospital Medical Center, Cincinnati, Ohio

BRUCE E. POLLOCK, MD
Professor, Department of Neurologic Surgery, Mayo Clinic and Foundation; Department of Radiation Oncology, Mayo Clinic and Foundation, Rochester, Minnesota

COREY RAFFEL, MD, PhD
Chief, Section of Pediatric Neurosurgery, Nationwide Children's Hospital; Vice-Chair, Department of Neurological Surgery, The Ohio State University College of Medicine, Columbus, Ohio

CHARLES RAYBAUD, MD
Hospital for Sick Children, Toronto, Ontario, Canada

R. MICHAEL SCOTT, MD
Department of Neurosurgery, Children's Hospital Boston, Harvard Medical School, Boston, Massachusetts

EDWARD R. SMITH, MD
Director, Pediatric Cerebrovascular Surgery, Department of Neurosurgery, Children's Hospital Boston, Harvard Medical School, Boston, Massachusetts

DEBBIE SONG, MD
Chief Resident, Department of Neurosurgery, University of Michigan, Ann Arbor, Michigan

GARY K. STEINBERG, MD, PhD
Bernard and Ronni Lacroute-William Randolph Hearst Professor of Neurosurgery and the Neurosciences; Chairman, Department of Neurosurgery, Stanford University School of Medicine, Stanford, California

KAREL TERBRUGGE, MD, FRCP(C)
Division of Neuroradiology, Department of Medical Imaging, Toronto Western Hospital, University of Toronto, Toronto, Ontario, Canada

MONIQUE J. VANAMAN, MD
Resident, Department of Neurosurgery, University of Michigan, Ann Arbor, Michigan

NICHOLAS WETJEN, MD
Assistant Professor of Neurologic Surgery, Department of Neurologic Surgery, Mayo Clinic and Foundation, Rochester, Minnesota

Contents

The brain vascular system develops in such a way that it continuously adapts the supply of oxygen and other nutrients to the needs of the parenchyma. To accompany the developing brain vesicles, it evolves in several steps: superficial meningeal network first; intraventricular choroid plexuses which determine the arterial pattern; penetrating capillaries from the surface to the ventricular germinal matrix forming simple transcerebral arteriovenous loops; cortical capillaries last, mainly in the last trimester. The venous return becomes connected to both the surface and to the choroidal veins, so forming distinct meningeal and subependymal venous drainage systems, while the arteries are on the surface only. While the arterial system was determined early (week 8), the venous system is continuously remodeled by the morphological changes of the base of the skull and the expansion of the brain vesicles. Until late in gestation, the vascular system is made of simple endothelial channels in which the arterial or venous fate is determined primarily by the direction of flow.

Pediatric and inherited neurovascular syndromes have diverse presentations and treatments. Although many of these diseases are uncommon, they must be included in the differential diagnosis for children with strokes or hemorrhages. In neurosurgical practice, familial cavernous malformations, hereditary hemorrhagic telangiectasia (HHT), and moyamoya are the most frequently encountered of these diseases. In this article, we will discuss familial cavernomas and HHT, as well as more unusual entities such as PHACE(S) syndrome, Klippel-Trenaunay syndrome, Wyburn-Mason syndrome, sinus pericranii, radiation-induced vasculopathy, and blue rubber bleb nevus (BRBN) syndrome. Moyamoya disease is covered in several other articles in this volume.

Arteriovenous malformation (AVM) is the most common cause of spontaneous intraparenchymal hemorrhage in children, excluding hemorrhages of prematurity and early infancy. Because most children diagnosed with an AVM undergo initial treatment emergently, the natural history of AVMs in the pediatric population is not well understood. Most pediatric AVMs do not come to clinical attention unless they hemorrhage. Therefore, their optimal management remains controversial. Children with intracranial AVMs represent a special challenge in that they harbor unacceptable lifelong risks of hemorrhage and potential neurologic deficits. Patients should be evaluated on a case-by-case basis to determine the best multidisciplinary treatment regimen that can be used to preserve neurologic function and eradicate

should be considered for surgical resection. Close follow-up after diagnosis and treatment is helpful to identify lesion progression or recurrence.

Pediatric Intracranial Aneurysms 491

Brian J. Jian, Steven W. Hetts, Michael T. Lawton, and Nalin Gupta

Intracranial pediatric aneurysms arising in children are rare. The treatment of these lesions requires both an understanding of their unique features as well as surgical, interventional, and pediatric critical care expertise offered through a multidisciplinary setting. The patient population, clinical presentation, complications, and trends in treatments are discussed in this article.

Spinal Cord Vascular Malformations in Children 503

Debbie Song, Hugh J.L. Garton, Daniel K. Fahim, and Cormac O. Maher

Spinal vascular malformations comprise a diverse group of abnormalities, including arteriovenous malformations (AVMs), cavernous malformations, dural arteriovenous fistulas (AVFs), and capillary telangiectasias. These conditions each have distinct causes, presentations, radiologic appearances, and natural histories. This article explores the presentation, natural history, investigation, and treatment of spinal AVMs, spinal AVFs, and spinal cavernous malformations.

Cerebral Venous Sinus (Sinovenous) Thrombosis in Children 511

Nomazulu Dlamini, Lori Billinghurst, and Fenella J. Kirkham

Cerebral venous sinus (sinovenous) thrombosis (CSVT) in childhood is a rare, but underrecognized, disorder, typically of multifactorial etiology, with neurologic sequelae apparent in up to 40% of survivors and mortality approaching 10%. There is an expanding spectrum of perinatal brain injury associated with neonatal CSVT. Although there is considerable overlap in risk factors for CSVT in neonates and older infants and children, specific differences exist between the groups. Clinical symptoms are frequently nonspecific, which may obscure the diagnosis and delay treatment. While morbidity and mortality are significant, CSVT recurs less commonly than arterial ischemic stroke in children. Appropriate management may reduce the risk of recurrence and improve outcome, however there are no randomized controlled trials to support the use of anticoagulation in children. Although commonly employed in many centers, this practice remains controversial, highlighting the continued need for high-quality studies. This article reviews the literature pertaining to pediatric venous sinus thrombosis.

Traumatic Intracranial and Extracranial Vascular Injuries in Children 529

Roukoz B. Chamoun and Andrew Jea

Trauma continues to be the leading cause of death in children older than 1 year of age. Although vascular injuries are uncommon, they contribute significantly to the mortality and morbidity related to traumatic injuries in the pediatric age group. In a recently reported large series of children, the head and neck location constituted 19.4% of all pediatric vascular injuries and accounted for most of the mortality observed. Catheter angiography is still considered as the gold standard diagnostic modality. However, because of its invasive nature, other techniques such as computed tomography angiography and magnetic resonance angiography are emerging as alternative diagnostic screening tools. Traumatic vascular injuries can involve the carotid as well as the vertebral arteries. They can be extracranial or intracranial. As a result, traumatic vascular injuries are a heterogeneous group of entities with potential significant implication on the natural history and prognosis. The optimal management of these injuries remains unclear and current practice is largely individualized. This report reviews the available literature regarding the current trends in diagnosis and management of pediatric traumatic vascular injuries.

Moyamoya: Epidemiology, Presentation, and Diagnosis **543**

Edward R. Smith and R. Michael Scott

Moyamoya syndrome is an increasingly recognized arteriopathy associated with cerebral ischemia and has been associated with approximately 6% of childhood strokes. It is characterized by chronic progressive stenosis at the apices of the intracranial internal carotid arteries, including the proximal anterior cerebral arteries and middle cerebral arteries and ultimately results in decreased cerebral blood flow with an increased resultant risk of stroke. This article discusses the epidemiology, presentation, and diagnosis of this condition in children.

Indirect Revascularization Techniques for Treating Moyamoya Disease **553**

Neil N. Patel, Francesco T. Mangano, and Paul Klimo Jr

There have been many indirect revascularization techniques described by surgeons for the treatment of moyamoya disease. These surgical procedures are typically used more commonly in pediatric, than in adults', cases. Some of the techniques include: cervical sympathectomy, omental transplantation, multiple burr holes, encephalo-myo-synangiosis (EMS), encephalo-arterio-synangiosis (EAS), encephalo-duro-synangiosis (EDS), encephalo-myo-arterio-synangiosis (EMAS), encephalo-duro-arterio-synangiosis (EDAS), encephalo-duro-arterio-myo-synangiosis (EDAMS), encephalo-duro-galeo (periosteal)-synangiosis (EDGS), and combinations of all the above. This chapter will detail the technical aspects of many of these procedures and some of the reported clinical outcomes.

Direct Bypass Techniques for the Treatment of Pediatric Moyamoya Disease **565**

Raphael Guzman and Gary Steinberg

Moyamoya is an increasingly recognized cause of stroke in children and adults. Identification of the disease early in its course with prompt institution of therapy is critical to providing the best outcome for patients. Revascularization surgery seems to be effective in preventing stroke in moyamoya, with direct techniques providing durable protection when performed at experienced centers.

Index **575**

Neurosurgery Clinics of North America

FORTHCOMING ISSUES

October 2010

Minimally-Invasive Intracranial Surgery
Michael Sughrue, MD, and Charles Teo, MD, *Guest Editors*

January 2011

Management of Brain Metastases
Ganesh Rao, MD, and
Anthony D'Ambrosio, MD, *Guest Editors*

April 2011

Functional Imaging
Peter Black, MD, PhD, and
Alexandra Golby, MD, BWH, *Guest Editors*

RECENT ISSUES

April 2010

Aneurysmal Subarachnoid Hemorrhage
Paul Nyquist, MD, MPH, Neeraj Naval, MD, and Rafael J. Tamargo, MD, *Guest Editors*

January 2010

Immunotherapy
Issac Yang, MD, and Michael Lim, MD, *Guest Editors*

October 2009

Neuroendovascular Management: Cranial/Spinal Disorders
Robert H. Rosenwasser, MD, and
Pascal M. Jabbour, MD, *Guest Editors*

Preface
Introduction to Pediatric Vascular Neurosurgery

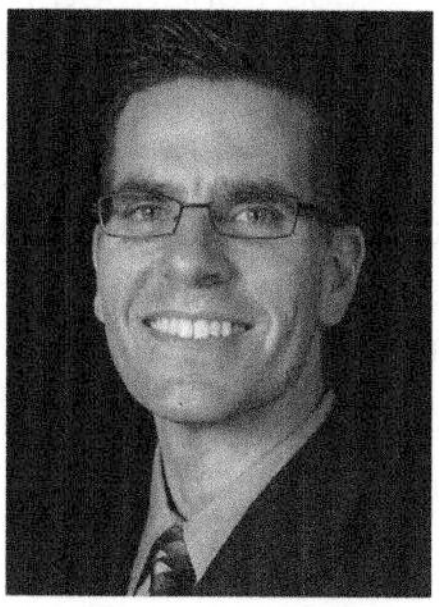
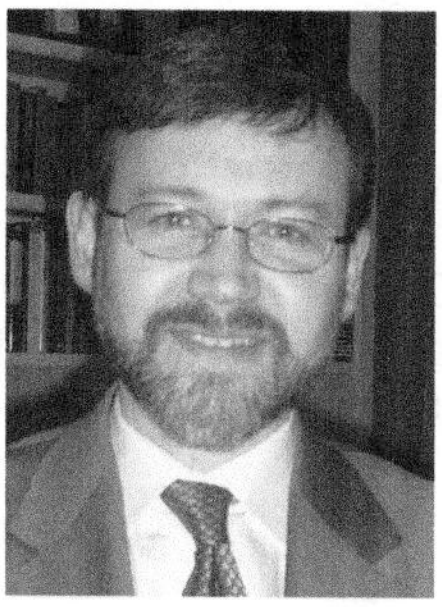
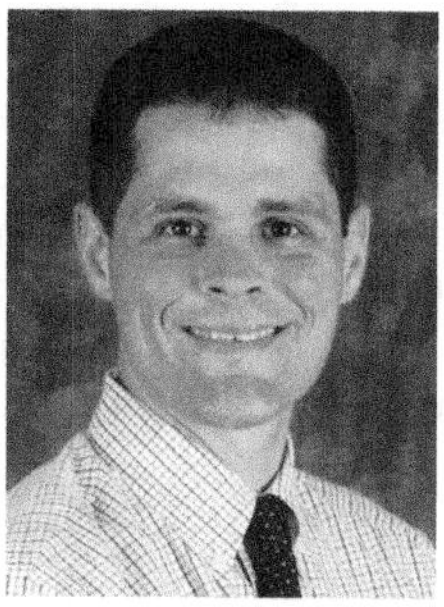

Paul Klimo Jr, MD, MPH, Maj, USAF   Cormac O. Maher, MD   Edward R. Smith, MD
Guest Editors

Children afflicted with neurovascular diseases can pose formidable diagnostic and therapeutic challenges to neurosurgeons. Recent technologic advancements in neuroimaging, endovascular therapies, radiosurgery, and intraoperative capabilities have provided new tools to help overcome many of these challenges. Increasingly, the use of multidisciplinary teams in the management of these conditions has markedly improved the ability of clinicians to achieve optimal outcomes. As guest editors of this issue of *Neurosurgery Clinics of North America,* we are proud to have assembled a series of articles on these topics from a distinguished group of specialists in this field.

Pediatric cerebrovascular disease is a broad topic that encompasses several distinct pathologies. Neurovascular disease in children differs from adult neurovascular disease in many important ways. For example, certain conditions are nearly unique to the pediatric age group; diagnosis and management can be more challenging with young children who have yet to develop the communication skills taken for granted in adults; and theraputic decisions need to be made within the context of the expected long lifespan of a child. The topics in this issue were selected for their practical relevance to practitioners.

The issue begins with a discussion on the normal and abnormal development of the intracranial vasculature and transitions to an article on congenital and inheritable vascular diseases. Subsequently, experts discuss the management of pediatric arteriovenous malformations, including surgical, radiosurgical, and endovascular viewpoints. The fascinating disease of moyamoya is the subject of several articles, including ones that provide technical details and outcomes for the indirect and direct bypass techniques. Other topics covered in this book include cavernous malformations, spinal vascular malformations, traumatic intracranial and extracranial vascular injuries, sinovenous thrombosis, and intracranial aneurysms.

Our goal in putting this project together was to present the major issues in pediatric vascular neurosurgery in a comprehensive, up-to-date, and accessible format. It is our hope that this issue of *Neurosurgery Clinics of North America* is valuable not only to neurosurgeons but also our colleagues in allied specialties, such as neuroradiology, radiation oncology, neurology, pediatrics, and interventional neuroradiology. We are honored to have convened an outstanding group of authors to write this issue and we have benefited greatly from their expertise. We hope that readers enjoy

Neurosurg Clin N Am 21 (2010) xiii–xiv
doi:10.1016/j.nec.2010.03.014

reading and learning from these articles as much as we enjoyed assembling them.

Paul Klimo Jr, MD, MPH, Maj, USAF
88th Medical Group, SGOS/SGCXN
4881 Sugar Maple Drive
Wright-Patterson Air Force Base, OH 45433, USA

Cormac O. Maher, MD
Department of Neurosurgery
University of Michigan Health System
1500 East Medical Center Drive
Room 3552 Taubman Center
Ann Arbor, MI 48109-5338, USA

Edward R. Smith, MD
Pediatric Cerebrovascular Surgery
Department of Neurosurgery
Children's Hospital Boston
Harvard Medical School
300 Longwood Avenue
Boston, MA 02115, USA

E-mail addresses:
atomkpnk@yahoo.com (P. Klimo)
cmaher@med.umich.edu (C.O. Maher)
Edward.Smith@childrens.harvard.edu
(E.R. Smith)

Normal and Abnormal Embryology and Development of the Intracranial Vascular System

Charles Raybaud, MD

KEYWORDS

- Embryological development • Brain morphology
- Vascular system • Angiogenesis

The development of the blood-vessels of the head demonstrate[s] the embryologic principle of what may be termed integrative development. [The vascular apparatus] reacts continuously in a most sensitive way to the factors of its environment, the pattern in the adult being the result of the sum of the environmental influences that have played upon it throughout the embryonic period. [...] This apparatus is continuously adequate and complete for the structures as they exist at any particular stage; as the environmental structures progressively change, the vascular apparatus also changes and thereby is always adapted to the newer condition. [...] For each stage it is an efficient and complete going-mechanism, apparently uninfluenced by the nature of its subsequent morphology.

George L. Streeter, 1918

Oxygen cannot diffuse beyond 150 to 200 μm in a living tissue at 37°C. As a consequence, the vascular system develops in such a way that it continuously adapts the supply of oxygen and other nutrients to the needs and the morphology of the evolving brain. Schematically, 4 overlapping consecutive steps can be described.

1. Initially (weeks 2–4) the exposed neural plate and groove and the open neural tube are simply fed by diffusion from the amniotic fluid (**Fig. 1**).[1]
2. After closure (week 4) the neural tube is surrounded by a dense connective tissue, the meninx primitiva (weeks 5–8) (for review, see Ref.[2]). This meninx primitiva contains primitive vascular loops (meningeal meshwork)[3] developed by vasculogenesis from the primitive dorsal aorta and cardinal veins, and through them connected with the primordial vascular organ initially developed over the yolk sac (**Fig. 2**).[4,5]
3. As the cephalic portion of the neural tube grows and expands to form the 3 primary brain vesicles (rhombencephalic, mesencephalic, and prosencephalic vesicles), the meninx primitiva further evolves and to better supply the neural tissue invaginates into the roofs of the prosencephalic and rhombencephalic vesicles, forming the primordia of the choroid plexuses (weeks 5–7).[1] At this stage, diffusion of nutrients to the neural tissue is both peripheral from the meninx primitiva and ventricular from the developing choroid plexuses.[1] From the point of view of the morphogenesis of the cerebral vasculature, this plexular differentiation is crucial: it leads to the early differentiation of specific choroid feeders within the meningeal vascular meshwork from which all brain arteries eventually evolve (for review, see Ref.[6]): from that stage, the final arterial pattern is already recognizable.[7] By contrast, the venous outflow that is specifically adapted to the choroid stage is only transitory and the veins will continue to adapt passively to local circulatory factors until after birth, even though

The Hospital for Sick Children, 555 University Avenue, Toronto, ON M5G 1X8, Canada
E-mail address: Charles.raybaud@sickkids.ca

Neurosurg Clin N Am 21 (2010) 399–426
doi:10.1016/j.nec.2010.03.011
1042-3680/10/$ – see front matter

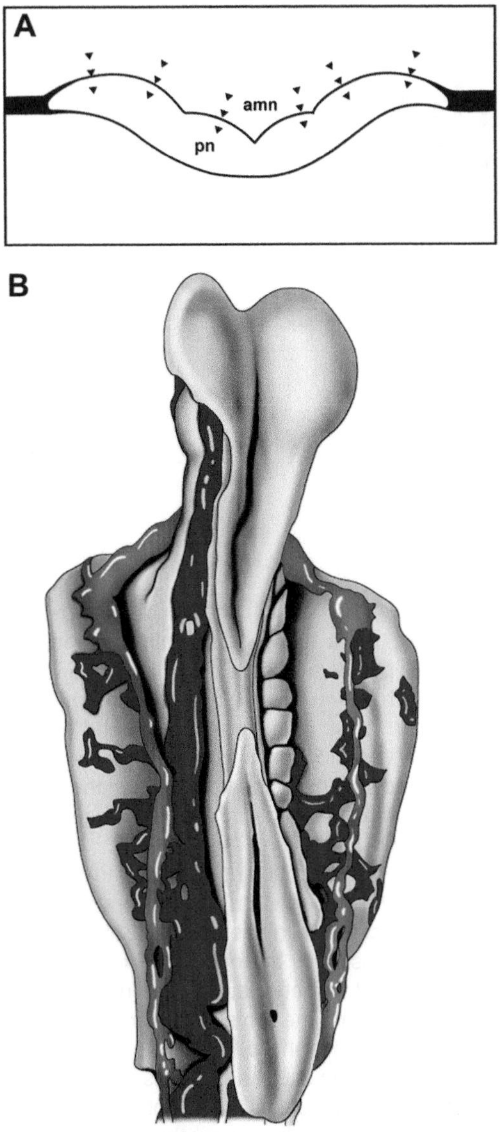

Fig. 1. Week 4. The neural tube is not closed yet, and the neural plate (pn) receives oxygen and nutrients from the surrounding amniotic fluid (amn) (*A*). Endothelial vasculogenesis is building up the cardiovascular organ system that already extends toward the cephalic extremity of the embryo (*B*).

the gross venous pattern can be recognized at the end of the first trimester.[6,8]

4. When the neural tube becomes too thick to be nourished by extrinsic diffusion alone, intrinsic capillaries develop by sprouting (angiogenesis) from the vessels of the meninx primitiva covering the brain surface. According to the same principles, they will supply the most demanding areas: first the ventricular-subventricular proliferative germinal zone already at the second month, then much later in the last trimester the developing cortex when it becomes widely connected and functional.[1,9] Together with the development of the early intrinsic vasculature, the meninx primitiva undergoes progressive changes resulting in the fluid-filled leptomeninges and the dense dural coverings and reflections,[10] as well as the opening of the fourth ventricular outlets.

THE PRIMITIVE PERINEURAL VASCULAR MESHWORK

Shortly after its closure (week 4), the neural tube becomes embedded in a solid mesenchyme that forms the meninx primitiva (see **Fig. 2**). This meninx primitiva of the forebrain (anterior neural plate) derives from the neural crest of the more caudal posterior diencephalic and mesencephalic segments.[2,11] The meninx primitiva of the developing spinal cord, hindbrain, midbrain, and posterior diencephalon derives from the somitic mesoderm.[2]

Vasculogenesis produces the vascular organ system and the first blood cells; it extends to the meninx primitiva and forms the first arteriovenous loops.

The vascular system as an organ system derives from a differentiation of lateral and posterior mesodermal cells that migrate toward the yolk sac and form blood islands or hemangioblastic aggregates.[4,5] These aggregates differentiate into peripheral endothelial cells and central hematopoietic cells.[12,13] Endothelial cells form vascular cords that canalize and become interconnected in a plexular network that extends into the embryo, building the cardiovascular system, the first organ system of the embryo.[4,5,12,13] This process is under the control of, among others, the vascular endothelial growth factor VEGF and its receptor VEGFR2.[13] Vasculogenesis proceeds cranially and invades the meninx primitiva to form a vascular meshwork around the primitive cephalic central nervous system.[14] The vascular lumen forms by vacuolization of the endothelial cords (a truly intracellular lumen). These primordial vessels connect together to form an indistinct meshwork without clear preferential channels (hence its name of primary head *plexus*)[3] and it is impossible at the beginning to differentiate between arteries and veins.[3] This early process was not studied in human embryos but in chick embryos between the stages of 9 and 16 somites; this would correspond to day 28 in human, that is, just before and at the time of the closure of the neuropores (for developmental staging, see Ref.[15]).

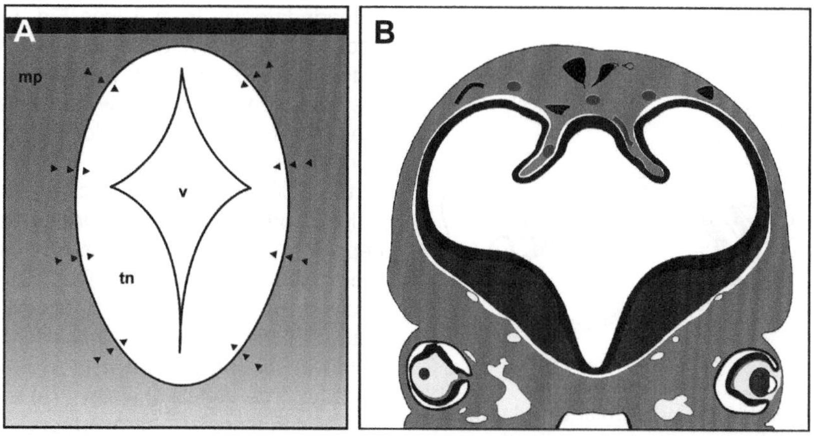

Fig. 2. Week 5. The neural tube is embedded into a dense connective tissue, the meninx primitiva (mp) (*A, B*) that contains vascular loops (*B*) connected to the dorsal aortae and cardinal veins. They are forming the primordial brain vascular meshwork, from which oxygen and nutrients diffuse to the neural tissue.

Over the next day or so, an active proliferation of endothelial channels takes place between the cranial ectoderm and the neural surface. This proliferation starts early around the forebrain and the midbrain, and later around the hindbrain; it also proceeds from the ventral aspect of the brain vesicles to its dorsal aspect.[3] At the same time the meninx primitiva begins to undergo the dramatic changes that will result in the formation of the calvarium, dura, and fluid-filled leptomeninges, to the development of the choroid plexuses and to the opening of the fourth ventricular outlets. The perineural vascular meshwork follows this meningeal reorganization.[3] The deeper vascular endothelium that covers the wall of the neural tube flattens and takes the appearance of a capillary network. The superficial vascular layer takes the appearance of larger and more continuous channels that form clear connections with the paired dorsal aorta and cardinal veins, and will eventually become the major brain arteries and veins. Between these deep and superficial vascular layers, a few communications persist and become the branches of the arteries and the tributaries of the veins[3]: arterial supply and venous drainage channels become selected from this initial meningeal meshwork as they respond to the evolving and species-specific needs and morphology of the developing brain.

The morphogenetic alterations that result in the adult pattern of brain arteries has been described in great detail by Padget,[7] while the morphogenesis of the veins has been mostly described by both Streeter[3] and Padget.[16,17]

MORPHOGENESIS OF THE BRAIN ARTERIES

Padget[7] studied the development of the cerebral arteries by using a method of graphic reconstruction from 22 sectioned embryos of the Carnegie Collection ranging in age from 24 to 52 days (4–43 mm). Her outstanding contribution therefore rests on a relatively limited number of specimens. Based on the evolution of the cardiovascular system, especially the aortic and pulmonary arches, Padget identified, defined, and illustrated 7 steps or stages in the development of the brain arteries, from an early undifferentiated pattern to the essentially adult pattern.

At stage 1, the primitive carotid artery supplies the forebrain as well as the hindbrain through the transient carotid-vertebrobasilar connections (4–5 mm, 28–29-day embryo).

The internal carotid artery (ICA) can already be recognized at this stage. The ICA supplies the 3 forebrain, midbrain, and hindbrain vesicles. Rostrally when reaching the forebrain, it divides into an anterior olfactory branch (future anterior cerebral artery, ACA) that passes dorsal to the optic vesicle, and a posterior branch that resolves into a plexus around the midbrain without reaching the hindbrain. The ICA also connects with the contralateral ICA behind the Rathke pouch, so forming the posterior segment of the future circle of Willis.

More proximally, the hindbrain instead is fed by 3 presegmental and 1 intersegmental arterial channels. Two originate from the proximal ICA: the trigeminal artery at the level of the trigeminal ganglion, and the otic artery at the level of the otic vesicle. Two originate from the paired dorsal aorta: the hypoglossal artery along the hypoglossal nerve, and the proatlantal artery (first intersegmental cervical C1 artery) along the first cervical nerve (**Fig. 3**). These trunks supply the paired ventral bilateral longitudinal neural arteries that feed the hindbrain on either side at this stage

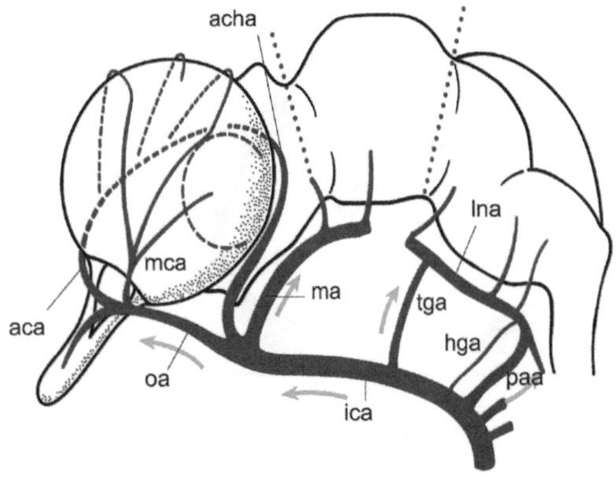

Fig. 3. Week 5. Within the primordial vascular meshwork, the ICA can be recognized. It supplies the forebrain and the midbrain via its terminal branches, the olfactory artery (oa) and the mesencephalic artery (ma). The olfactory gives off the early ACA cranially and the ACHA caudally around the neck of the growing hemisphere; the MCA appears as a lateral branch of the ACA. More caudally, the ICA and the primitive aorta send three branches that supply the hindbrain via the longitudinal neural artery (lna); these branches are named after their accompanying nerves/location: craniocaudally the trigeminal (tga), hypoglossal (hga) and proatlantal (paa) arteries.

(**Fig. 4**A). The trunks eventually regress, after the bilateral longitudinal neural arteries have fused on the midline, and connected cranially with the caudal division of the ICA and caudally with the longitudinal paravertebral anastomosis that will become the vertebral artery. The channels actually exist for a very short time of 4, at most 8 days (for the trigeminal and proatlantal arteries) before vanishing at about stage 3.[7] Uncommonly they may persist and be functional as anatomic variants/malformations in clinical settings.

At stage 2 the posterior communicating artery forms (5–6 mm, 29-day embryo).

The caudal divisions of the ICAs extend caudally and join the bilateral longitudinal neural arteries to form the true posterior communicating arteries (PCOMs). Consequently, the trigeminal arteries are dwindling at their carotid origin, as well as the hypoglossal arteries. The longitudinal neural arteries tend to unite along the midline to form the basilar artery (BA) (see **Fig. 4**B). At this stage they still remain largely dependent on the proatlantal (first intersegmental) arteries for their caudal supply.

At stage 3 the forebrain arteries can be recognized; the basilar and vertebral arteries are completed (7–12 mm, 32 days).

Within the primitive meshwork, the trunk of the ACA develops rostrally around the neck of the growing hemispheric vesicle, and the early stem of the future middle cerebral artery (MCA) extends laterally from it (see **Fig. 5**). Behind the neck of the growing hemisphere, the primitive anterior choroidal artery (ACHA) courses toward the diencephalon; it is now the largest branch of the ICA. The ICA also provides a primitive dorsal ophthalmic artery. Caudally, from the caudal end of the PCOM 2 dorsal branches emerge, 1 posterior choroidal artery (PCHA) toward the diencephalon and 1 mesencephalic artery toward the midbrain (**Fig. 6**A). The BA has further evolved by midline fusion of the longitudinal neural arteries; the trigeminal artery may still be found at this stage, but it is usually interrupted already.[7] The vertebral artery (VA) is now forming as a longitudinal paravertebral anastomosis between the intersegmental cervical arteries from C7 to C1[7]; (see also Fig. 1 in Ref.[18]). Over the rhombencephalon the anterior superior cerebellar artery (ASCA) becomes distinguishable.

At stage 4 the mature pattern becomes apparent (12–14 mm, 35 days).

The anterior division of the ICA now provides clearly recognizable although still plexiform branches: the ACA with a medial branch that approaches the midline to form the anterior communicating artery (ACOM), the early MCA, dorsal and ventral primitive ophthalmic branches, the prominent ACHA, as well as the PCHA and the mesencephalic arteries. The BA and the VA show further development, and early rhombencephalic branches can be recognized.

At stage 5, which can be called the choroid stage, the adult pattern has become obvious (16–18 mm, 40-day embryo).

Klosovskii[1] stressed the role the choroid plexuses play in supporting the early brain tissue. During weeks 5 to 7, these projections of the meninx primitiva develop into the fourth, third, and lateral ventricles (**Fig. 5**A, B).[19,20] Because they become extremely active from a metabolic point of view, they induce a clear selection of their arterial feeders: the ACA anteriorly,[7,21] the ACHA inferiorly, and the PCHA posteriorly (see **Fig. 5**C). (Although the adult ACA is separated from the tela choroidea by the callosal and hippocampal commissures, it is originally a choroidal artery. Its subfornical branch still reaches the foramen of Monro in the human fetus,[7,16] the adult chimpanzee,[22] and in injected adult human anatomic specimens [personal data]). The MCA grows as a lateral branch, primarily striatal at this stage, of the proximal ACA. The mesencephalic artery also is now prominent and forms a rich plexiform network over the tectal plate. This specific pattern at this stage—choroidal arteries including the ACA, and mesencephalic arteries—corresponds to the anatomy of the

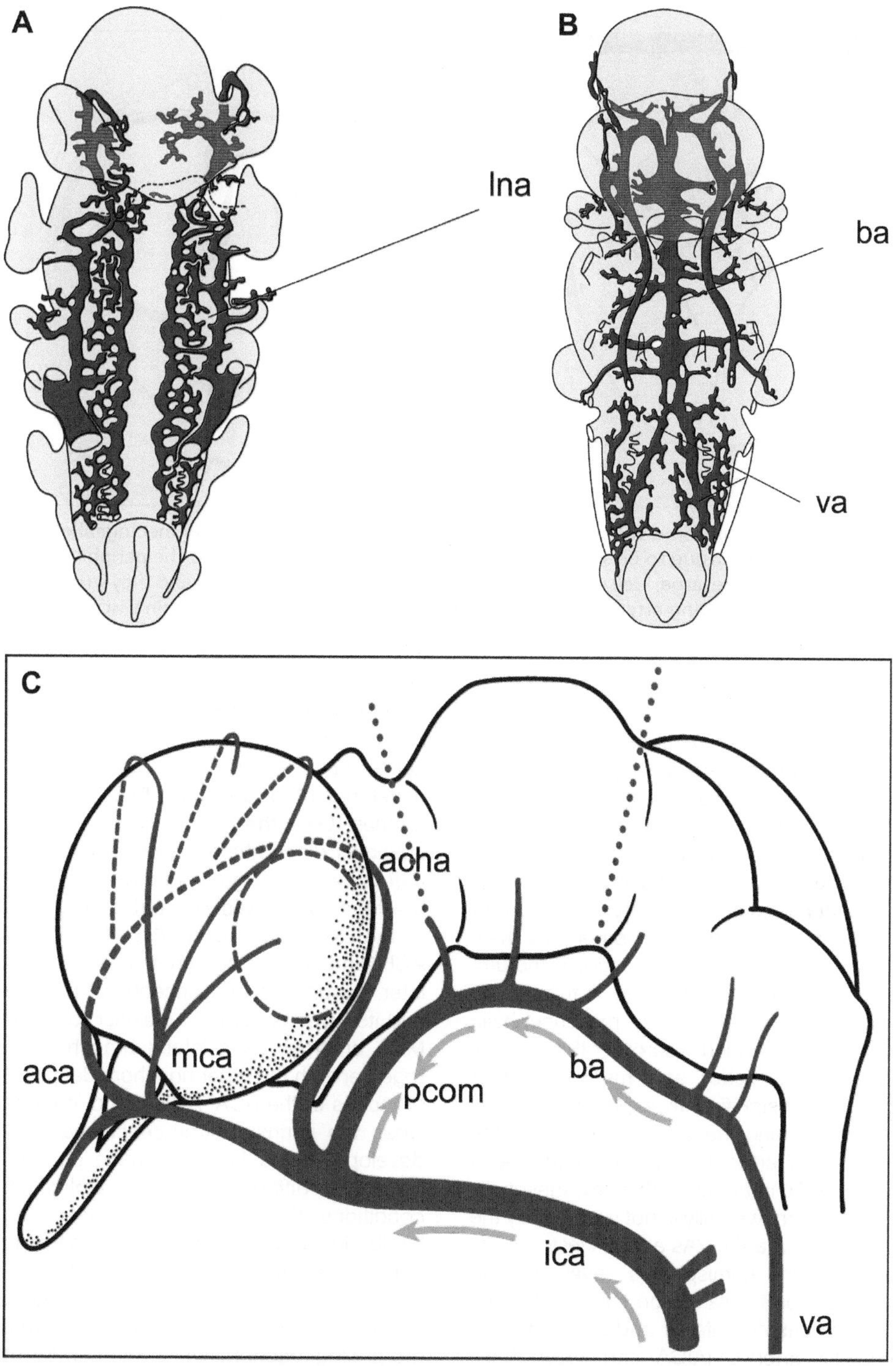

Fig. 4. Week 5. The paired longitudinal neural arteries (lna) extend along either sides of the hindbrain; at this stage, all brain arteries are plexular (*A*). They tend to unite by fusion along the midline, to form the BA (*B*). Simultaneously they become connected cranially with the mesencephalic artery via the PCOMs, and caudally with the forming intersegmental anastomotic VAs (*C*). This new blood supply results in the regression of the trigeminal, hypoglossal and proatlantal arteries.

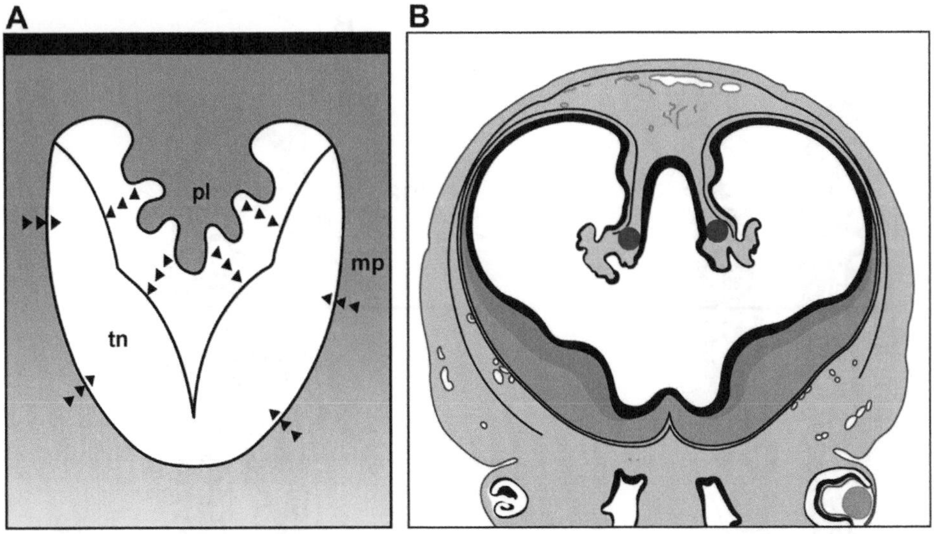

Fig. 5. Week 6. The meninx primitiva forms the choroid plexuses (pl), intraventricular meningeal extensions that allow the growing neural tissue to be supplied by the ventricular CSF in addition to the peripheral meninge (*A, B*). The choroid plexuses are large, well vascularized structures loaded with glycogen and they strongly determine the prominence of their feeding arteries: ACA, ACHA, PCHA, from which the whole brain vasculature originates.

arterial feeders of the vein of Galen arteriovenous malformations.[6]

At stages 6 (20–24 mm, 44 days) and 7 (40 mm, 52 days), the mature pattern is completed with the circle of Willis and the capture by the posterior hemispheres of the vertebrobasilar blood supply.

A completed, still plexiform ACOM sends a branch to the anterior corpus callosum. A prominent perforant (intracerebral) artery, the recurrent artery of Heubner is already apparent as well, coursing from the ACA toward the medial striatum. The MCA, striatal also at this stage, is fully developed. Dorsal branches of the mesencephalic arteries have extended across the dorsal meninges to the inferior and medial-posterior portion of the now significantly expanded cerebral hemispheres, forming the cortical territory of the posterior cerebral artery (PCA) at the expense of the ACHA (**Fig. 6**). In addition, this new mesencephalic-PCA territory typically is not supplied by the ICA any more but via the VAs and BA instead: the now huge cerebral hemispheres have captured part of the vertebrobasilar blood supply. Besides the ASCA, the anterior inferior and posterior inferior cerebellar arteries (AICA and PICA) have become more apparent in the plexus that still covers the caudal hindbrain (**Fig. 6**).

In summary, the arterial system of the brain evolves within and from an initially undifferentiated vascular meshwork, always in a precisely adapted response to the evolving metabolic requirements of the expanding neural tissue.[3] Initially, the ICA feeds the fore- and the midbrain through its anterior and posterior terminal divisions, while the hindbrain is fed by presegmental/intersegmental branches from the ICA and the paired aorta: these transient branches regress with the development of the final PCOM and vertebral arteries. Over the brain surface, specific arterial channels differentiate, which at the early stages correspond to the growing zone (neck) of the cerebral hemispheric vesicles and to the differentiation of the choroid plexuses: the ACA anteriorly, the ACHA posteriorly; together with the PCHA, they later supply the prosencephalic tela choroidea and its glycogen-loaded plexular formations. The MCA emerges as a lateral branch of the ACA, together with the other nonchoroidal parenchymal branches of the ACA, ACHA, and (captured) PCA when the intrinsic intraparenchymal vasculature develops at the late embryonic and early fetal period. In a different way because of different local conditions, the vasculature of the midbrain and hindbrain evolve according to the same hemodynamic (ie, metabolic) rules. The conditions in which the initial meshwork consolidates into discrete arteries explain most of the many variants and morphologic abnormalities that can be observed in later life. As the metabolically defined territories are species-specific and essentially constant, distal arterial distribution is fairly constant and most variations are found in the proximal segments of the feeders, where different hemodynamic "solutions" may become selected in the initial meshwork (resulting in a "variations on a theme" anatomy).

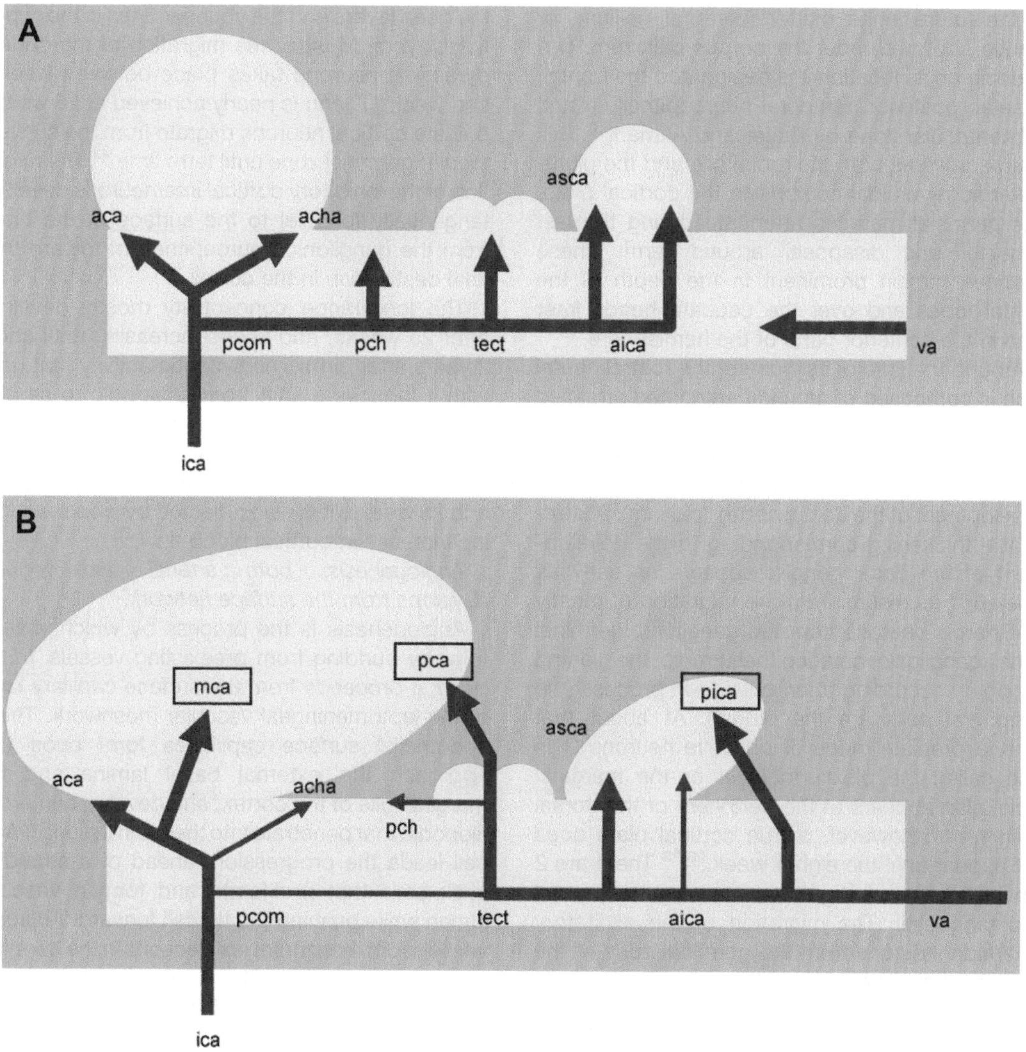

Fig. 6. Weeks 7–8. The initial arterial vasculature responds to the segmentation of the brain into the telencephalon, diencephalon, mesencephalon, metencephalon and myelencephalon (*A*). However the hugely expanding cerebral hemispheres and the cerebellum capture the territories of normally more caudal arteries: the PCA, branch of the mesencephalic arteries for the cerebral hemispheres, and the PICA, initially a branch of the medulla oblongata, for the cerebellum (*B*) (to do that arteries must cross the meningeal spaces, which is possible because at this stage the dorsal meninx primitiva is still compact). This also results in the capture of the vertebral blood by the cerebral cortex.

ANGIOGENESIS: THE INTRINSIC VASCULARITY OF THE BRAIN

The 2 main steps in the development of the forebrain (using it as a model of the whole brain) are firstly the cellular proliferation (in the germinal matrices or neuroepithelia) and migration, and then the energy-avid intracortical organization. Cellular proliferation and migration mainly occur before week 20, while cerebral connectivity becomes significant in the last trimester of gestation until well after birth. Accordingly, the brain vasculature develops in 2 separate episodes: the first, within the periventricular germinal zone, mostly before week 20, fading progressively toward the end of gestation, and the second in the cortical plate, mostly after week 27.

Two discrete kinds of germinal matrices exist in the forebrain. One overlays the central gray matter (ganglionic eminence), and is designated the striatal neuroepithelium and subventricular zone by Bayer and Altman.[20] In addition to glial cells, it provides mostly GABAergic cells, both to the underlying basal ganglia (local migration) and distantly to the cerebral cortex (tangential migration). The other germinal matrix sits in the depth of the future white matter (cerebral pallium, or mantle), but not under the corpus callosum. Depending on its location it is designated the frontal, parietal, posterior, temporal neuroepithelium and subventricular zone by Bayer and Altman.[20] This matrix provides both the radial glia and the glutamatergic pyramidal neurons to the cortical plate. The germinal matrices attenuate during the last trimester and disappear around term. These matrices remain prominent in the depth of the frontal lobes and over the caudate heads later than in the posterior parts of the hemisphere.

Around the time of its closure, the rostral neural tube is composed of an undifferentiated stratified epithelium surrounding a ventricular lumen. In the 2 following weeks, the development of the ventral ganglionic gray matter (subpallium) antecedes the development of the dorsal cortex (pallium). A laterobasal thickening corresponding to the development of the basal ganglia appears as early as week 6[20]; its results from the migration of mostly GABAergic neurons from the ganglionic germinal zone (ganglionic neuroepithelium) to the ventral periphery according to an outside-in process (the peripheral cells are the oldest). At about that time, a preplate made of primitive neurons (it is also called the plexiform layer or the marginal zone) also appears at the periphery of the dorsal pallium[20,23]; however, a true cortical plate does not appear until the eighth week.[20,23] There are 2 types of neuronal migrations to the cortex, radial and tangential. The migration of the excitatory pyramidal neurons from the germinal zone of the pallium (cortical neuroepithelium) develops radially in an inside-out fashion, the older neurons sitting in the deep layers and the younger ones in the superficial layers. Most of the migration of the cortical pyramidal neurons takes place between week 8 and week 17, and is nearly achieved at 20 weeks, but late cortical neurons migrate from the subventricular germinal zone until term time.[24] The migration of the inhibitory cortical interneurons develops tangentially (parallel to the surface of the brain) from the ganglionic neuroepithelium toward their final destination in the cortex.[25]

The long-range connectivity mostly develops after 25 weeks, and keeps increasing until about 2 years after birth. The synaptic activity that goes with it induces a shift from anaerobic to aerobic cortical metabolism, which is supported by a shift of the angiogenetic activity from the (fading) germinal zone to the cortical plate between 20 and 25 weeks. It is also reflected by a corresponding increase in cortical blood flow.[26]

Angiogenesis, both arterial and venous, develops from the surface network.

Angiogenesis is the process by which vessels form by budding from preexisting vessels. In the brain, it proceeds from the surface capillary layer of the leptomeningeal vascular meshwork. These endothelial surface capillaries form buds that approach the external basal lamina and the marginal glia of the cortex, and develop numerous filopodia that penetrate into the brain tissue.[1,9] A tip cell leads the progression, ahead of a strand of stalk cells that proliferate and form a vascular lumen while pushing the tip cell forward. Adjacent vessels form horizontal connections in the germinal zone so that a flow with incoming ("arterial") and outgoing ("venous") blood is constituted (**Fig. 7**A,

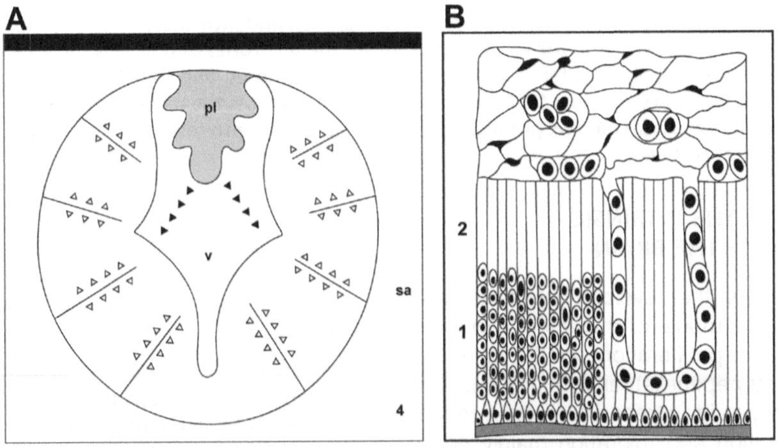

Fig. 7. Week 6 onward. When the neural tissue becomes too thick to be fed by extrinsic diffusion alone and while the germinal matrix develops, the intrinsic vascularization appears (*A*), while the meninx primitiva becomes the subarachnoid space (sa). Intrinsic vessels form by angiogenesis: capillaries grow from the surface and extend toward the periventricular germinal zone where they connect together to form primitive arterio-venous loops (*B*). The cortex itself is not significantly vascularized until well after mid gestation.

B). Oxygen concentration obviously is a potent regulator of angiogenesis. From the genetic point of view, *VEGF-A* (vascular epithelial growth factor) is the main actor in the angiogenetic process through the receptor *VEGFR-2* and the coreceptor *Neuropilin-1*; *VEGF-A* is highly expressed in the subventricular zone first, then later in the neurons of the cortical plate, then after vascular remodeling is completed, in the glial cells.[14] *VEGFR-2* is expressed in the endothelial cells of the perineural vascular plexus and in the capillary sprouts.[14] The *Dll4/Notch* signaling pathway further regulates the number/density of vessels within the parenchyma, as well as the *Slit2/Robo4* signaling pathway: both prevent endothelial stalk cells from acquiring the tip cell phenotype.[14] *Integrins* are cell adhesion receptors involved in cell-to-cell and cell-to-matrix interaction; they help to regulate angiogenesis by maintaining the endothelial cell communication with the neuroepithelium.[14] *Wnt7a* and *Wnt7b* also appear to be critical in the regulation of central nervous system (CNS) angiogenesis, and their expression is required in the neuroepithelium during the angiogenetic process.[14] After migration into the CNS, the blood vessels need maturation, remodeling, and pruning, together with the recruitment of vascular smooth muscle cells (VSMC): this involves the *Pdgfb/Pdgfrβ* pathway.[14] The *TGFβ* signaling pathway is important for endothelial cell proliferation and differentiation, and for recruitment of VSMC; it involves *endoglins* and *alk1,* whose mutations cause hereditary hemorrhagic telangiectasia (HHT).[14] A last pathway crucial to CNS angiogenesis is the *Angiopoietin/Tie2* signaling pathway: deficient mice present with immature vessels lacking branching, organization in large and small vessels, and VSMC.[14] Finally, a last interesting point to mention is that the tip cells of the endothelial channels behave like the growth cones of the axons: in the processes of remodeling and vessel navigation, they respond to the influence of the same guidance molecules. For example, *ephrinB2* (arterial) and *EphB4* (venous) are repulsive and are required for establishing and maintaining the arterial-venous interface; *netrins* are mostly repulsive (mostly attractant for axons); *Slit/Robo* are involved also, as mentioned above, as well as the *Semaphorin3E-PlexinD1* signaling pathways (see Ref.[27] for review).

Intrinsic vascularity develops from ventral (ganglionic) to dorsal (pallial) and in the germinal zone long before the cortex.

From a morphologic point of view, endothelial cell proliferate, canalize, approach, and connect with the neighboring channels to form simple arteriovenous loops into the deep germinal matrix first, and much later in the cortex: early branching does not appear in the cortical layers until week 20.[1,9] At the early stages the vessels are not yet differentiated, their arterial or venous function being determined by the direction of the blood flow only (see **Fig. 7**). However, the vascular pattern becomes more elaborate as the cerebral mantle thickness and complexity increase, with a multiplication of intermediate small-caliber arteriovenous connections that become true capillaries (<2 red cells), and enlarging feeding and draining trunks (up to 10 red cells) that behave like true arterioles and venules.[28] Only in the germinal zone do the primitive "sinusoid" capillaries remain undifferentiated until the germinal zone disappears at term. Because the perforators originate from the surface to feed the most active layer in the deep ventricular zone first, all arterial perforators are transcerebral.[28–30]

- At 5 weeks, intrinsic vessels are seen entering the medulla and pons to ramify in the ventricular zone; this process becomes more prominent at 6 weeks, with other vessels entering the cerebellar rudiment as well as the rhombencephalic tela choroidea.[29] In the following weeks the vasculature of the cerebellum expands to the territory of the 3 future cerebellar arteries.[29] The development of the cerebellar cortex is significantly different in its modalities from the development of the cerebrum; however, to the best of the author's knowledge, no specific description of the cerebellar angiogenesis is found in the literature.
- The early vascularization of the midbrain develops in a similar fashion, very dense from the early stage (5 weeks), first in the ventricular area, and later more diffusely.[29] The vasculature of the diencephalon is also dense. Both start ventrally from the PCOMs, with longer feeders extending to the dorsal diencephalon (tela choroidea), and from the midbrain further toward the posterior and medial part of the cerebral hemispheres after 9 weeks,[29] thus establishing the distal hemispheric territory of the PCA. At the same time, these distal branches of the PCOMs become supplied by the vertebrobasilar arteries.
- In the telencephalon, the first striatal branches appear at 5 weeks and become more numerous at week 6. These branches develop from the olfactory artery, future ACA (forming the artery of Heubner), and from the stem of the future MCA.[29] The ACHA also gives branches to the basal diencephalon as well as to the

posteromedial part of the hemisphere: the later contribution, however, regresses as that of the PCA expands, so that the ACHA comes to supply mostly the choroid plexus of the forebrain (and the temporal uncus).[29]

- The cortex itself does not demonstrate any endothelial structure at 5 weeks.[29] At 6 weeks a few endothelial strands without apparent lumen and without apparent connection with the surface network have been noted,[29] suggesting that endothelial channels could originate de novo also in the parenchyma. By week 7 these channels seem to establish links with the leptomeningeal plexus while becoming canalized.[29] By 12 to 15 weeks, radial, likely arterial vessels connected to the meningeal plexus course toward the germinal zone where they form a subventricular plexus, still without giving off any ramification to the cortical plate.[28–30] Only by 20 weeks do horizontal intracortical branches start to arise in the deep cortical layers, with few recurrent branches directed to the more superficial cortex.[30] These horizontal branches and their associated recurrent collaterals become more numerous from 20 to 27 weeks while new horizontal branches develop in the superficial layers of the cortex.[30] From 27 weeks to term, new superficial radial branches develop from the superficial network.[30] After birth the cortical vasculature becomes much denser, especially in the intermediate cortical layers.[30] It seems that in response to the predominantly peripheral brain growth, shorter vessels develop in between the longer ones[28]; in the rat brain this has been described as forming a system of hexagonally packed vascular supply units that would provide and maintain an even distribution of the perfusion.[31]

Similar findings were reported, obtained by using microradiography (radiopaque vascular injections) in brain specimens of neonates ranging in age from 23 to 40 weeks' gestation. An abundant arteriolar network fed by the transcerebral arterial perforators was demonstrated in the ventricular and subventricular zone in preterms from 23 to 30 weeks. After 34 weeks this deep network progressively fades away to disappear toward the time of term. Note that the absence of any centrifugal arterial pattern and of any deep arterial border zone is specifically mentioned in the anatomic literature of the last decades,[28,32] especially when using stereoscopic analysis.[28]

The vascular fate (arteries, capillaries, veins) depends primarily on flow.

In the early fetal period all vessels are simple endothelial channels, and it is impossible to identify morphologically what is arterial, capillary, or venous. Because of their very simple hollow structure they are designated as "sinusoid" channels or "sinusoid" capillaries (this undifferentiated appearance is reproduced in undifferentiated tumors such as the glioblastoma multiforme). The arterial versus venous function is defined by the direction of flow only, not by the vascular structure. In addition, the arterial or venous fate of the vessels may change over time depending on the local metabolic conditions. However, most horizontal connections between the perforators are likely to represent the early capillary network.

- By tracking the course of the perforators, Allsopp and Gamble[29] were able to identify transcerebral perforators from the germinal zone that seemed to connect with the venous plexus on the brain surface in a 5-week embryo, suggesting that the pattern of transcerebral medullary vein could be present early in the development. In the same developmental period they also noted vessels lining the third ventricular ependyma, possibly forming early subependymal collectors.[29]
- Kuban and Gilles[28] noted that while all channels in the germinal zone are sinusoid capillaries devoid of media and adventitia, larger channels with the characteristics of veins are identified at 27 weeks at the interface between the germinal tissue and the caudate, as well as at the angles of the lateral ventricles, so forming the early subependymal veins.
- A muscularis appears at midgestation (20 weeks) in the striatal vessels, giving them their arterial appearance. Development of this muscularis extends from the pial vessels toward the putamen (24 weeks) and the caudate (26 weeks), but does not extend into the germinal tissue.[28]
- The extrastriatal parenchymal vessels remain sinusoid channels without a muscularis until the end of the gestation. At 24 weeks, they are relatively small (10–25 μm); they may divide into 5- to 15-μm capillaries, or converge to form 20- to 40-μm vessels at the ventricular surface, presumably venous. Toward the end of gestation, transcerebral trunks measure 20 to 40 μm and the collecting vessels 50 to 120 μm[28]: a clear arteriovenous differentiation in the pallium therefore appears in the last weeks of gestation only.[28]

For all observers, the arterial, venous, or capillary fate of the primary vessels appears to depend mainly on the flow. Still, specific signaling molecules have been identified that label the channels as arterial or venous at very early stages (see Ref.[13] for review): *ephrin-B2*, *neuropilin-1*, *notch3*, *Dll4*, and *gridlock* for arteries; *EphB4*, receptor for ephrin-B2, and *neuropilin-2* for veins. However, experiments in which the flow pattern was artificially modified could reverse the arterial or venous character of the channels, and even change the expression of the markers, suggesting that it is the hemodynamics that plays the major role in arteriovenous specification and patterning of the intrinsic brain vessels.[13]

The cranial neural crest cells give the forebrain arteries their identity.

A last point that should be mentioned regarding the brain arteries concerns the origin of their smooth muscle cells and pericytes (cells that mediate vasoconstriction and form part of the blood-brain barrier). Like that of the meninx primitiva, this origin is different in the cord, hindbrain, and midbrain vessels on the one hand, and in the forebrain vessels on the other hand. In the caudal parts of the brain and in the cord the arterial media and the pericytes derive from the mesoderm like the endothelial cells. By contrast, in the forebrain they originate from the neural crest (or mesectoderm[33]). The forebrain itself originates from the anterior neural plate, which forms an expansion of the neural tube rostral to and beyond the anterior end of the notochord. As mentioned earlier, the skeleton of the face and anterior skull base (maxillary, nasal, orbital regions, paranasal sinuses) as well as the coverings of the brain (meninges, calvarium, scalp, dermis) cannot have a somitic origin, and instead are produced by the neural crest. As the anterior neural plate itself is also devoid of neural crest, the midfacial skeleton and the coverings of the forebrain are made by neural crest cells that migrate from the posterior diencephalic and the mesencephalic portions of the neural tube.[33] In a similar way, the same groups of neural crest cells form the muscular media and the pericytes of the forebrain arteries as well.[34] The limit between the neural crest-associated forebrain arteries and the classic endothelium-associated mid- and hindbrain arteries is clearly demarcated at the level of the circle of Willis.[34] Such a difference in origin might explain why arterial pathologies may be different in the forebrain from the more posterior segments: not only Stürge-Weber disease or meningo-angiomatosis,[34] but also Moya-Moya disease and syndromes that characteristically affect the arterial supply to the forebrain only.

MORPHOGENESIS OF THE BRAIN VENOUS SYSTEM

Unlike the arterial supply (from the periphery to the ventricle), there is dual venous drainage of the brain: the deep white matter veins drain into the subependymal venous system toward the vein of Galen, while the cortex and superficial white matter veins drain into the superficial, meningeal venous system. As for the arteries, the shaping of the venous system follows chronologically the development of the brain metabolism.

Before the intrinsic vasculature develops, the venous drainage is strictly meningeal and choroidal; transient vein of Markowski.

As Streeter described it, the vascular system in weeks 5 and 6 is confined to the meninx primitiva.[3] The pericerebral meshwork divides into a deep (future pial) layer over the brain surface and a superficial (future dural) layer. The deep layer is a simple capillary layer. In the superficial layer channels become continuous and connect with the paired aorta and the cardinal veins, to form early arterial and venous trunks. Connections between the superficial layer and the deep capillary layer become the arterial feeders and the venous draining channels (early form of bridging veins).

During weeks 6 to 8, the tela choroidea becomes specialized and, to better support the brain tissue, develops the intraventricular choroid plexus.[1,6,7,20] Specific feeding and draining channels develop accordingly. The feeding channels are the ACA, ACHA, and PCHA (see earlier discussion). The venous drainage has been shown to run successively through a ventral diencephalic vein toward the primitive transverse sinus and then, more importantly, through prominent bilateral dorsal choroid veins.[17] The main collector of the superior choroid veins is a single, median dorsal vein called the vena mediana prosencephali or median prosencephalic vein (**Fig. 8**). First described by Markowski in 1911,[8] then by Hochstetter in 1938,[35] it was later described by Padget who called it the "primitive internal cerebral vein," recognizing however that such a term was confusing, as both the tributaries and the course of this single median meningeal vein are different from those of the later true, paired, choroidal internal cerebral veins.[17] The vein of Markowski is a single, median, dorsal prosencephalic vein that is not contained within the tela choroidea, but instead stretches as a true bridging vein across the would-be arachnoid space to the dorsal dura. It originates at the level of the paraphysis where it receives both superior choroid veins, and runs dorsally to the dorsal interhemispheric marginal venous sinus.[8,17,35] (The paraphysis is a transient evagination at the anterior fold of the

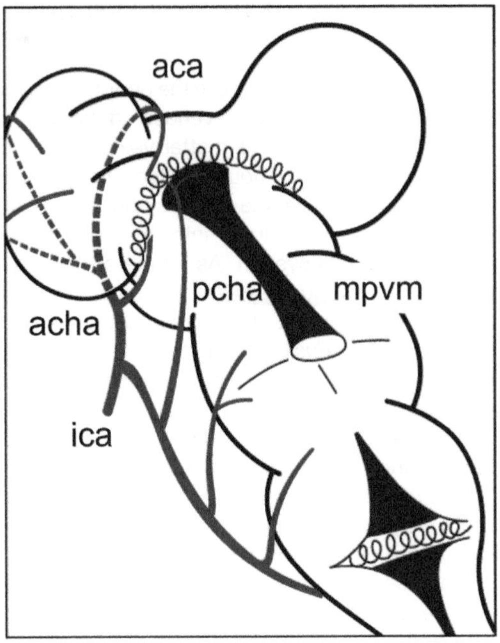

Fig. 8. Weeks 6–11. The choroid stage. The ACA cranially, the ACHA caudally encircle the neck of the hemispheres toward the tela choroidea and the plexuses, together with the PCHA, branch of the midbrain arteries. The tela choroidea and plexuses are drained by a single, median dorsal bridging vein (median prosencephalic vein of Markowski) (mpvm) that antecedes the development of the internal cerebral veins and vein of Galen.

tela choroidea, located between the interventricular foramina of Monro.) The vein of Markowski is a specific drainage vein of the choroid plexuses, found as soon as the choroid arteries are identified (week 6). It regresses and disappears after week 11, at the end of the choroid stage, replaced by the vein of Galen when the subependymal drainage appears following the development of the intrinsic vasculature of the marginal zones.[35]

The subependymal venous system develops de novo from subependymal anastomoses extending to the tela choroidea.

As mentioned above, at the early stages all intrinsic vessels develop centripetally by sprouting from the initial surface capillary meshwork and extend to the metabolically active germinal zone, where they form simple vascular loops in which some trunks act as arteries and others as veins. Therefore in principle, and apparently at the beginning at least (5 weeks),[29] the veins draining the germinal zone empty into the surface meningeal veins and are therefore true transcerebral veins (see **Fig. 7**B). The shift of the dorsal drainage from a purely choroid one into the vein of Markowski to a common choroid and parenchymal drainage through the vein of Galen around week 11 means that it is about that time that connections have become established between the veins draining the germinal zone and those in the tela choroidea, providing the subependymal veins with a dorsal outlet. The first deep vein noted to join the Galenic system is a vein of the anterior nucleus of the thalamus that is seen joining the superior choroid vein at the foramen of Monro about week 9.[17] But to the best of the author's knowledge, no description is found in the literature of how the vasculature of the germinal zone secondarily forms subependymal collectors, nor how these collectors connect to the dorsal dural veins.

For the former question, it is logical to assume that as the deep vasculature of the germinal zone forms a richly interconnected capillary network, draining channels may become selected within that network that would flow under the ventricular surface. Although the process is not specifically analyzed, the location of such channels, at the interface between the germinal tissue and the caudate (for the ganglionic eminence) and under the ependyma (for the pallium) has been described, though only at 26 to 27 weeks, a relatively late stage.[28,32] For the second question, on how the subependymal veins become connected to the system of the vein of Galen, there is no description either. It is logical again to assume that the venous anastomoses may extend from the deep white matter neuroepithelium to the neuroepithelium of the basal ganglia, and from there to the veins of the tela choroidea. As a matter of fact, Padget mentioned the vein of the anterior nucleus of the thalamus as being the first to do so at 9 weeks, joining the superior choroid vein at the level of the foramen of Monro, presumably via the insertion line of the tela choroidea on the surface of the thalamus. This pattern for the veins in the tela choroidea of draining both the choroid and the basal ganglia (and by anastomotic extension the deep white matter) is similar to there being a common arterial supply to both the choroid structures and the deep gray nuclei; however, no arterial anastomosis with the white matter arteries has ever been convincingly documented,[28,32] while the subependymal system drains both the gray and the white matters. In any case, the importance of the drainage from the dorsal thalamus and dorsal basal ganglia would explain the prominence of the intrachoroidal channels that become the internal cerebral veins and therefore, the importance of the vein of Galen and straight sinus. On the contrary, the contribution of the choroid plexus becomes relatively small and can not maintain the patency of the vein of Markowski.

The intracerebral venous anatomy is affected by the cerebral development.

Anatomically, the intracerebral veins can now be differentiated into 3 groups (**Fig. 9**)[36,37]:

- Deep medullary veins and dorsal nuclear veins draining into the subependymal system
- Cortical-subcortical medullary veins and ventral nuclear veins draining into the leptomeningeal system
- A few transcerebral veins connecting the surface network with the subependymal network; although their existence has been controversial,[16] it is now well documented.[16,38,39]

It can be inferred from the embryology that the first veins to develop are the transcerebral veins, which are followed by the subependymal veins, then by the cortical-subcortical veins. Indeed, as the first vascular trunks originate from the brain surface capillaries and form loops in the marginal zone about week 6, the trunks that function as veins return to the surface and therefore form true transcerebral veins.[16,29] The drainage of the deep vascular network forms later: at least some drainage toward the vein of Galen is attested at about 9 to 11 weeks.[17,35] Last to develop, the cortical venous drainage likely becomes apparent in the third trimester only, as the cortical metabolism and vascularization do not become significant until 27 weeks.[28] In injected specimens of premature neonatal brains, a dense periventricular venous network contrasting with a sparse drainage of the cortical ribbon has been documented (26 and 29 weeks), as well as the relatively early presence of transcerebral veins (25 weeks)[32]; at term, the venous channels appeared much more evenly distributed from the depth to the surface.[32] In adult brains studied in a similar fashion, the venous density appears much higher in the cortex, the subcortical white matter, and the basal ganglia than in the periventricular white matter.[36,37] Because of the precedence in development of the transcerebral veins and of their relative rarity in mature brains, it has been hypothesized that most of them would attenuate or

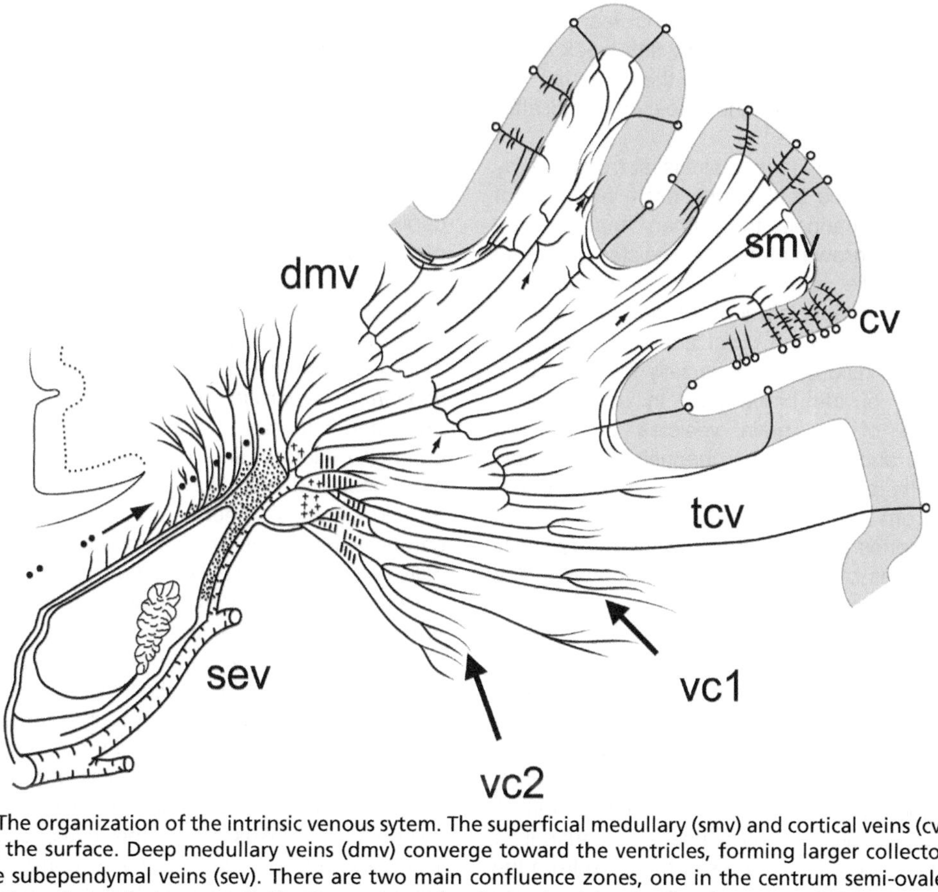

Fig. 9. The organization of the intrinsic venous sytem. The superficial medullary (smv) and cortical veins (cv) drain toward the surface. Deep medullary veins (dmv) converge toward the ventricles, forming larger collectors that join the subependymal veins (sev). There are two main confluence zones, one in the centrum semi-ovale (vc1), one in the subventricular zone (vc2), that seem to be determined by the development of the white matter. (*Data from* Okudera T, Huang YP, Fukusumi A, et al. Micro-angiographical studies of the medullary venous system of the cerebral hemispheres. Neuropathology 1999;19:93–111.[37])

become discontinuous during the period of mostly peripheral expansion of the hemispheres.[37]

Analyzing the collaterals of the medullary veins, Okudera and colleagues[37] made the observation that the mode of branching of the veins and the location of the venous confluence zones reflected in some way the organization of the white matter, especially its predominantly peripheral expansion during the second half of gestation (see **Fig. 9**). These investigators also noticed that certain bundles at least could be identified by the location of the lines of confluence: optic radiations and arcuate subcortical fibers.[37]

The morphogenesis of the extracerebral venous system is affected by the morphologic development of both the brain and the skull.

The development of the extracerebral veins is complex,[3,16,17] evolving according to the increasing cerebral vascularity, the changes in the skull base in large part, and the changes in the brain morphology itself reflected by the changes in the calvarium. The development has been divided into 7 stages by Padget,[17] covering the period between just after the closure of the neural tube and the time when the adult pattern is clearly established, that is, between the early fifth week to the 11th to 12th week. However, the fact that the venous arrangement continues to evolve until after birth must be stressed.[16]

Simply put, the early brain is surrounded by a vascular plexus that drains itself in a pair of ventrolateral channels, the primary head sinuses (**Fig. 10**). The growth of the otic vesicles interrupts the flow in the ventral primary head sinus and results in the development of dorsal collateral channels that may be dural and, depending on the local conditions and especially the increasing vascularity of the brain, pial. In addition, the expansion of the brain vesicles pushes the meninges and the venous channels they contain toward the periphery, so that the flow is transferred from some channels in the plexus to adjacent ones that are better protected, typically at the edges of the brain vesicles: between the cerebral hemispheres and the vault (forming the superior sagittal sinus), between the cerebral hemispheres, the cerebellum, and the vault (forming the transverse sinuses), and between the cerebral hemispheres and the tentorium (forming the straight sinus). In fetuses, sinuses may still be found anywhere within the falx or the tentorium, which therefore retain their plexular pattern.[40] However, as dural venous sinuses with a triangular section are more likely to resist pressure from the surrounding cerebrospinal fluid than sinuses with parallel walls, they are the ones that remain patent throughout adult life.

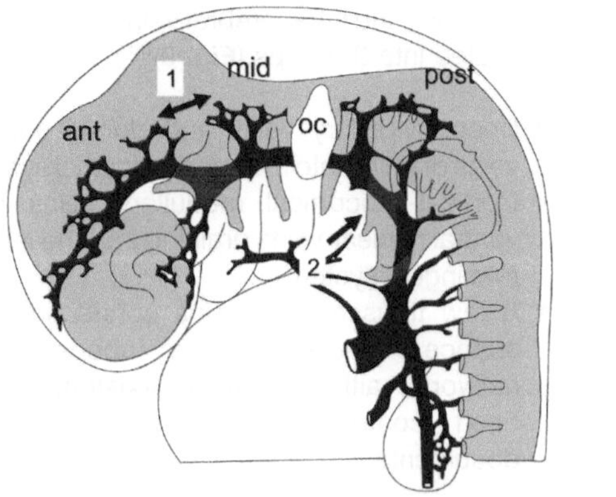

Fig. 10. Week 6, early. Early venous drainage system. Three venous plexuses (ant, mid, post) drain the neural tube via three venous stems into a ventrolateral primary head sinus. This head sinus also receives a maxillary vein cranially. It passes ventral to the otic capsule (oc). The major event is the growth of the otic capsule that will induce a dorsal collateralization, notably between the anterior and middle plexuses (**1**). The head sinus also passes medial to the trigeminal ganglion and vagus nerve (**2**).

At the time of closure of the neuropores, the first endothelial channels surround the brain, but blood is not yet circulating.[3] Shortly after, however, as described earlier, the meningeal stratification begins, together with a corresponding stratification of the vascular meshwork into a "pial" meshwork of capillary on the neural surface, a "dural" meshwork of larger vessels connected to the paired aorta and the cardinal veins, and an intermediate layer of "arachnoid" connections between the 2, which allows for the formation of arteriovenous loops.

This corresponds to *Padget stage 2 (early week 5; 5 mm)*. The carotid artery then supplies the forebrain and midbrain rostrally through its terminal anterior olfactory and posterior mesencephalic branches, and more caudally the hindbrain and the longitudinal neural arteries through the carotid-vertebrobasilar anastomoses. Schematically on each side, the venous plexuses that surround the laterodorsal aspect of the brain are drained by 3 venous stems into a lateroventral channel: the primary head sinus, which is continuous caudally with the cardinal veins. The venous plexuses are divided into 3 groups: the anterior plexus covers the forebrain and the midbrain (not unlike the rostral territory of the ICA at this stage), the middle plexus covers the metencephalon, and the posterior plexus covers the myelencephalon. The plexuses are drained by 3 corresponding venous stems: the anterior stem runs just rostral to the trigeminal ganglion, the middle stem between the trigeminal ganglion and the otic vesicle, and the posterior stem caudal to the vagus nerve. The primary head sinus receives the primitive maxillary vein, a rostral tributary that also drains the optic vesicle, then the anterior stem; it passes medial to the trigeminal ganglion (in the location of the future cavernous sinus) and receives the middle stem; then it passes lateral to the otic vesicle and surrounds the vagus nerve (by way of a lateral anastomosis), and receives the posterior stem while becoming the cardinal vein (see **Fig. 10**).

At *stage 3* (*week 6, 10 mm*) the main brain arteries are forming: the ACA, MCA, ACHA, PCOM, BA, and early VA. The anterior venous plexus expands over the forebrain and midbrain; it receives an early telencephalic (actually striatal) vein and caudally establishes dorsal anastomoses with the middle plexus (eventually this anastomosis will be the transverse sinus) (**Fig. 11**). The primary head sinus has now migrated through its lateral anastomosis in a position lateral to the vagus nerve (see **Fig. 11**) (the medial channel will remain as the inferior petrosal sinus) and, as a consequence, the cardinal vein can now be called a true internal jugular vein. This vein evolves further at *stage 4* (*week 7, 10–16 mm)*, when pial-arachnoid and dural channels are better individualized with now obvious telencephalic, diencephalic, mesencephalic, mesencephalic, and myelencephalic pial veins, mostly on the ventral aspect of the brain. This architecture reflects the early vascularization of the germinal matrix and the early development of the basal structures (especially the striatum).

Stage 5 (*late week 7 to early week 8, 16–21 mm*) corresponds to the development of the choroid plexuses and therefore of the choroid arteries (ACA, ACHA, PCHA). The first drainage of the choroid plexuses of the forebrain is through the ventral pial diencephalic vein. The telencephalic vein is now fully individualized; as it is still partly intradural, it is called the tentorial sinus (**Fig. 12**). Because of the continuous expansion of the otic vesicle (now the otocyst) a large dural anastomosis develops between the middle and the posterior plexuses; together, the anastomosis and the posterior stem form the sigmoid sinus (see **Fig. 12**). As a consequence; the stem of the middle dural plexus is dwindling but remains connected to the anterior segment of the primary head sinus; together they form the pro-otic sinus, the future cavernous sinus. The channels of the anterior part of the anterior plexus gather in between the growing hemispheres to form the sagittal plexus, and over the midbrain, between the forebrain and the hindbrain, to form the tentorial plexus.

Stage 6 (*week 8, 18–26 mm*) is the full-fledged choroid stage. The choroid plexuses of the forebrain are now drained by a specific choroid vein, the median prosencephalic vein of Markowski (identified as the "primitive internal cerebral" vein by Padget, who however mentions how such a name can be confusing[17]) (**Fig. 13**). This vein posteriorly defines the early straight sinus within the tentorial plexus, which suggests that the vein of Galen would integrate at least part of the vein of Markowski.[35] The continuous expansion of the otocyst completely effaces the corresponding segment of the primary head sinus, and its flow of blood instead is conveyed by the now achieved collateral that with the stem of the posterior plexus forms the sigmoid sinus (see **Fig. 13**). The stem of

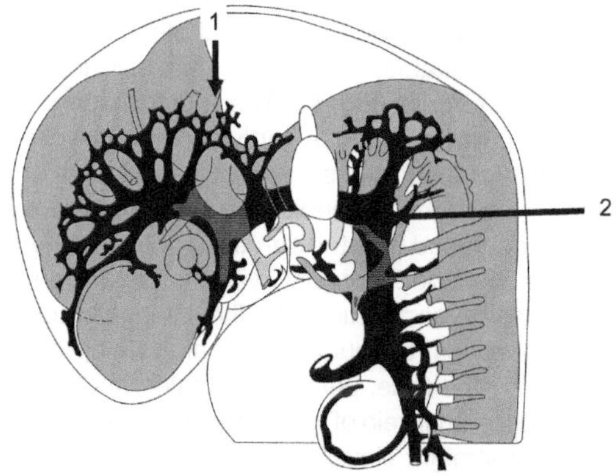

Fig. 11. Week 7. The dorsal collateralization develops (**1**). Via a lateral anastomosis, the primary head sinus passes lateral to the vagus nerve: by this translation, it becomes the jugular vein (**2**).

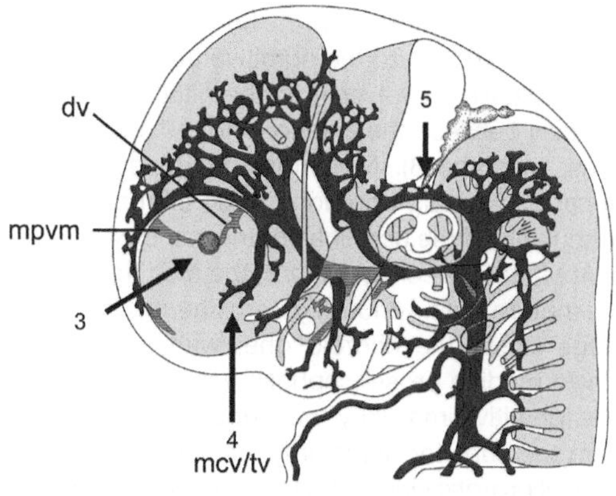

Fig. 12. Week 8. The choroid plexus develops (**3**), drained ventrally (diencephalic vein, dv) and soon dorsally (vein of Markowski, mpvm). A telencephalic vein drains the lateral aspect of the hemisphere (future middle cerebral vein and tentorial sinus) (mcv/tv) (**4**). The growth of the otic vesicle progressively obliterates the primary head sinus and a collateral develop dorsal to the otic vesicle between the middle and the posterior plexuses (**5**).

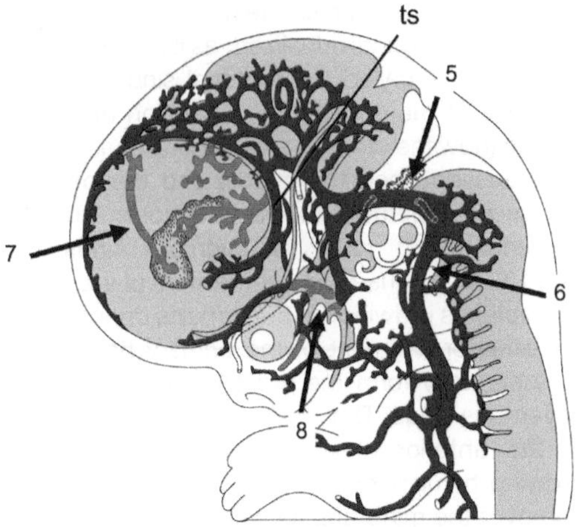

Fig. 13. Week 9. The primary head sinus has become obliterated by the otic capsule, and replaced by a dorsal collateral (**5**); together with the posterior stem (**6**), this collateral forms the complete sigmoid sinus. The initial anastomosis between the anterior and middle plexuses now is pushed caudally by the growth of the hemispheres and forms the transverse sinus (ts). The vein of Markowski is now the main choroidal vein (**7**). The middle stem forms the pro-otic sinus (**8**); it drains anteriorly into the remaining anterior segment of the primary head sinus.

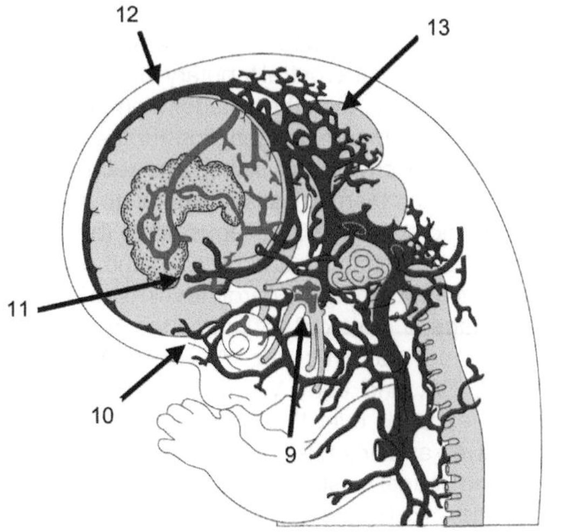

Fig. 14. Month 3, early. The anterior portion of the pro-otic sinus medial to the trigeminal ganglion forms the cavernous sinus (**9**). It receives the facial/maxillary vein and the superior ophtlamic vein (**10**). The middle cerebral vein is well apparent (**11**). The consolidation of the dorsal dural plexuses forms the superior sagittal sinus (**12**). More posteriorly, the tentorial plexus is still primitive (**13**).

the middle plexus joins the primary head sinus in front of the otocyst and forms the pro-otic sinus (see **Fig. 13**). The pro-otic sinus remains connected cranially to the primitive maxillary vein and the primitive supraorbital vein, and thus forms the primitive cavernous sinus. At the same time the stem of the anterior plexus that drained the forebrain regresses and disappears while on the contrary, the tentorial sinus expands, prolonging the now apparent middle cerebral vein toward the primitive transverse sinus (which itself has evolved from the initial dorsal anastomosis between the anterior and the middle plexuses, at stage 3). More pial tributaries become apparent ventrally and dorsally on the brain as the vascularity of the germinal matrices increases.

At *stage 7* (*week 9, 40 mm*) the main features of the mature brain venous system are apparent. This stage is still the choroid one, with a prominent single median prosencephalic vein of Markowski. The primitive maxillary vein now has evolved to form the superior ophthalmic vein; it is drained by the still pro-otic sinus, located medial to the trigeminal ganglion and forming the cavernous sinus (**Fig. 14**). Due to the hemispheric expansion, the superior sagittal sinus has resulted from the "concentration" of the sagittal plexus and the tentorial sinus has elongated, becoming parallel to the transverse sinus. Finally, the veins of the superficial tissues that were initially drained by the intracranial plexus and secondarily became tributaries of the external jugular system become embedded in the chondrification of the occipital bone and form the anterior, lateral, and posterior condylar, the mastoid, and the occipital emissary veins.[16,17,41,42] Because the vascularization of the scalp develops much later than that of the meninges, no emissary vein exists at the level of the calvarium except, inconstantly, in the parietal squamae.[16,17]

At the last developmental stage, identified by Padget as *stage 7a* (*third month, 12 weeks, 60–80 mm*), the expansion of the brain has further accentuated the mature appearance of the venous system. Posteriorly the remains of the conglomerate of channels that formed the tentorial plexus result in the usually variable, asymmetric, plexular appearance of the torcular (**Fig. 15**). The anterior expansion pulls the partly arachnoid, partly dural middle cerebral vein-tentorial sinus toward the edge of the lesser wing of the sphenoid (see **Fig. 15**), where it is often confused with the so-called sphenoparietal sinus of Breschet. Dorsally, with the expansion of the intrinsic vasculature into the intensely active germinal zones, the subependymal system now is drained by the (true, paired, final) internal cerebral veins via the final vein of Galen into the now well-established straight sinus (see **Fig. 15**). The internal cerebral veins are joined dorsally by the basal veins (of Rosenthal), a relatively new anastomotic channel that links, from ventral to dorsal, a tributary of the telencephalic vein, part of the ventral diencephalic

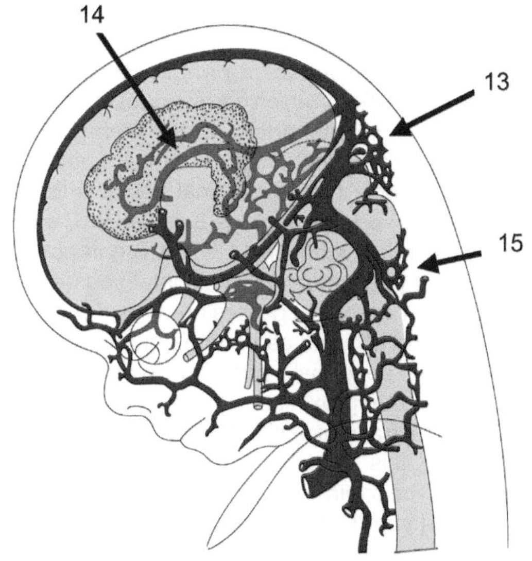

Fig. 15. Month 3, late. Condensation of the tentorial plexus results in the plexular appearance of the torcular (**13**). Shortly after the shift from the choroid stage to the intrinsic vasculature stage, the final internal cerebral veins are formed together with the final vein of Galen and straight sinus (**14**). The posterior dural plexus persists until after term (**15**).

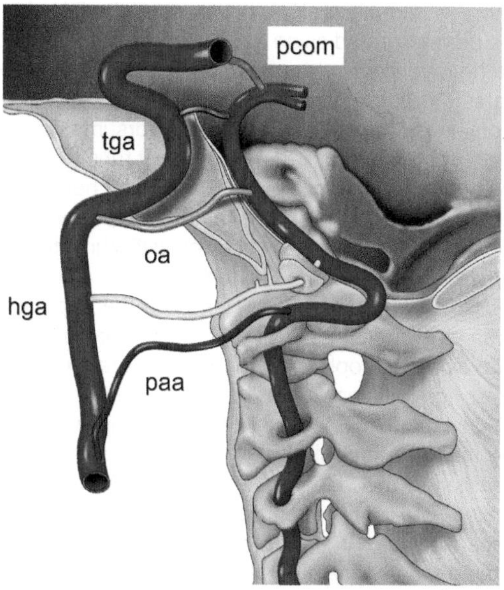

Fig. 16. Persistent vestigial arteries: trigeminal, between the proximal carotid siphon and mid BA (tga); otic, between the proximal intrapetrous segment and the inferior third of the BA via the IAM (it probably doesn't actually exist) (oa); hypoglossal, between the extracranial IAC and the intracranial VA at the origin of the PICA (hga); proatlantal, between the extracranial ICA and the occipitovertebral segment of the VA (paa).

vein, the mesencephalic vein, and the dorsal diencephalic vein.[17,43] The possible drainage pathways of the basal vein result from this multisegmental structure: mainly but not only posterior toward the vein of Galen via the dorsal diencephalic vein; laterally to the superior petrosal sinus via the mesencephalic vein[17,43] and to the superior petrosal sinus via the ventral diencephalic-peduncular segment; anteriorly to the cavernous sinus-sphenoparietal sinus or the tentorial sinuses-transverse sinus via the telencephalic segment.[43]

VARIANTS, DOUBTS, AND MALFORMATIONS

Persistent Vestigial Carotid-Vertebrobasilar Anastomoses

These are occasional angiographic findings, identified as the persistent trigeminal, otic, hypoglossal, and pro-atlantal arteries, felt to reflect the homonymous embryonal (rather than fetal) arterial supply to the hindbrain (see **Fig. 3; Fig. 16**). It should be remembered that this embryonal (not fetal) pattern concerns tiny capillaries, lasts a few days only, and was identified in a very small number of specimens. This is likely the oldest brain vascular abnormality that can be clinically observed, as this arterial arrangement occurs immediately after the closure of the neural tube. The persistent vestigial arteries can hardly be called malformations as they have essentially no impact on the life. These arteries are commonly found in association with vascular diseases, mostly aneurysms, but this association is biased by the fact that the pathology leads to the vascular investigation. No explanation is found in the literature for their persistence. Usually a normally transient embryonal vessel may persist in development when a flow is abnormally maintained in its lumen; because this vestigial vessel is maintained and hemodynamically significant, the normal later-appearing vessels are typically altered. However, in this instance it is hard to assume that it is an initial hemodynamic disorder that would have induced the abnormality: those embryonic arteries are present at a stage when flow is quantitatively close to zero, occurring in purely endothelial channels that can become reversibly either arterial or venous.[3,17] So it is more logical to assume that the persistence of the embryonal vessels is due to either a defect of the inhibition processes, or a defect of induction of the normally later-appearing vascular changes (eg, PCOM connection, VA connection).

The *persistent trigeminal artery* (*PTA*) (the most common vestigial artery observed, which usually regresses at week 5, before stage 3) has been extensively described.[44–52] The PTA extends from the ICA when it enters the cavernous sinus, to the midportion of the basilar BA; it may originate more proximally on ICA, however, and might then be misinterpreted as an otic artery. The PTA is said to be medial when it runs into the sella and perforates the dura in a groove lateral to the clivus, or sometimes apparently through the dorsum sellae itself[46]; and it is said be lateral when it runs together with the sensory roots of the trigeminal nerve and exits at the Meckel's cave, below the petroclinoid ligament. PTAs have also been classified in different types depending on the territory they supply.[44] Saltzman type I is when it supplies the upper BA with the paired ASCAs and PCAs; the proximal BA is typically hypoplastic and the ipsilateral PCOM is missing. Saltzman type II is when it supplies the BAs with the ASCAs only, both PCAs being supplied by the ICAs through the PCOMs; the first segment (basilar) of the PCAs is then missing. A third type, called PTA variant (or Saltzman III) is when the trigeminal artery joins a remnant of the primitive paired longitudinal neural artery and supplies one ipsilateral cerebellar artery only, mostly AICA, sometimes PICA or ASCA, without joining the BA.

Multiple associations have been mentioned: arterial aneurysms obviously, either because of unusual weakness points in the arterial system, or flow related but possibly also because of a diagnostic bias[53]; arteriovenous malformations, with the same possible explanation as the aneurysms; mechanical complications, mostly tic douloureux but also pituitary disorders and oculomotor deficits; and even such a bizarre association as a hemangioblastoma.[54]

The *persistent otic artery* (*POA*) has been exceedingly rarely reported, with apparently only 8 cases published with this diagnosis.[45,48,55–58] In fact its very existence is denied by many. To be a real otic artery, it must arise from the lateralmost portion of the petrous segment of the ICA (proximal to the caroticotympanic artery), travel through the internal auditory meatus, and join the BAs at its caudal end. Apparently, none of the rarely reported cases displayed those features convincingly.[56] This finding makes one wonder whether such an anastomosis actually exists even in the embryo (apparently only described by Padget as "remnants of highly transitory presegmental branches" from 1 illustrated specimen, and possibly 2 more not illustrated, at stage 1 only, in early week 5[7]).

The *persistent hypoglossal artery* (*PHA*) is the second most common persistent vestigial artery, though much less common than PTA. It is normally short-lived, regressing before stage 2, in week 5. The vessel leaves the ICA at the C1 to C3 level, enters the skull through the anterior condylar (hypoglossal) canal where it courses posteromedially to form the terminal segment of the VA that gives off the PICA and the BA itself, as typically both VAs are absent or hypoplastic, the contralateral one terminating in the contralateral PICA.[50,59–63]

The last is the *persistent pro-atlantal intersegmental artery* (*PPIA*), which corresponds to the first spinal intersegmental artery. In the embryo it is, besides the trigeminal artery, the most important vessel to supply the longitudinal neural arteries. The PPIA disappears at stage 3, in week 6, when the VA becomes functional.[7,64–66] Even in normal anatomy, it persists as the horizontal segment of the vertebral artery that passes between the occipital bone and C1, and as portions of the occipital artery.[67] The abnormally persistent vestigial artery actually is the proximal segment that extends from the extracranial ICA (initially the primitive aorta) to this horizontal interoccipito-atlantal segment. The origin is usually in the lower segment of the ICA (type I PPIA); it less commonly originates from the external carotid artery (ECA) (type II PPIA), and rarely from the common carotid artery (CCA). (A distinction also is made sometimes between the type I as a true proatlantal artery and type II as a simple persistent primitive first cervical intersegmental artery,[66] but the consequences of this distinction are not clear.) A PPIA may rarely be bilateral.[65] The VAs commonly are absent or hypoplastic, uni- or bilaterally. Other major associated vascular abnormalities may affect the aortic arch,[66] the CCA and its bifurcation,[66] or the ECA.[64]

Segmental agenesis/hypoplasia of the vertebrobasilar junction. The agenesis or hypoplasia of the terminal segments of the vertebral arteries may represent the reverse situation from the persistent lower vestigial arteries. This situation is extremely common when it is unilateral, but it is extremely rarely bilateral.[68] A globally hypoplastic VA may supply an ipsilateral PICA only, and the missing segment is then between the PICA and the BA, or the VA is totally absent and the PICA is supplied by the BA. It may be speculated that this would correspond to a failure to form the distal hypoglossal artery for the former and the proatlantal/intersegmental artery for the latter.

Variations of the Leptomeningeal Segments of the Brain Arteries

It is beyond the scope of this review to present the variations and malformations of the extradural ICA (for reviews, see Refs.[69,70]) or VA. The many variations of the cisternal segments of the brain arteries have been associated with an increased incidence of aneurysms.

The circle of Willis is extremely variable. It is composed of the ACOM, proximal ACA, the end of the carotid siphon (segment 8 of the ICA for Gailloud and colleagues[70]), the PCOM, the proximal PCA and the BA bifurcation. This BA bifurcation may be classic, between the PCAs, or more caudal at the level of the ASCA. Asymmetry and hypoplasia of one or several segments of the circle of Willis are extremely common and likely reflect the hemodynamic balance of a specific individual. This balance may even change over time, and the circle of Willis may be accordingly remodeled.[71] One proximal ACA may be larger than the other one, and supply the ipsilateral hemisphere and most of the contralateral one. One PCOM may be large and supply the distal PCA territory; this carotid origin of the PCA is erroneously described as a "fetal" PCA—if anything, it would be an "embryonal" PCA. It is as a rule associated with a hypoplasia of the proximal (basilar) segment of the PCA, and often with a hypoplastic A1 segment of the ipsilateral ACA. A PCA with carotid origin (ACHA is identified) should not be confused with the hyperplastic ACHA (then a usual tiny ACHA is not identified): this is the retention of the early embryonic pattern of distribution (see later discussion).

Fenestration of the different segments may occur, reflecting the original plexiform arrangement from which the arterial trunks became selected by preferential flow.

Whereas hypoplasia of any of the various segments of the circle of Willis is common, complete aplasia is less common and may suggest a true malformation rather than an anatomic variant. Complete aplasia certainly may compromise collateral flow in case of disease (or even of positional arterial compression); it also may alter the even distribution of the perfusion pressure in normal conditions.

The anterior cerebral artery. The azygos ACA describes a condition in which the first segments of the ACA join each other on the midline to form a single median trunk that runs for some distance before sending branches to both cerebral hemispheres. It can be considered a midline fusion of normally paired trunks, or as an extended form of ACOM. It is a primarily vascular abnormality, which is different from the azygos ACA seen in holoprosencephalies, when a single ACA attached to a single telencephalic vesicle. Another, more common variation of the ACA is the bihemispheric pattern in which one ACA supplies both hemispheres, using the ACOM as a bifurcation, while the contralateral A1 segment is hypoplastic.

In the rare case of persistent primitive olfactory artery (PPOA), the ACA runs ventrally along the olfactory bulb into the anterior cranial fossa before turning back abruptly (hairpin turn) to join its distal cortical territory, or form the ethmoidal artery.[72] This could be thought to simply represent an extreme form of variation within the primordial network. However, it is associated with the absence of the striatal artery of Heubner (presumably compensated for by striatal branches of the MCA) and also by the absence of an ACOM[72]; this latter feature can be considered a true malformation.

The last malformation is the infraoptic origin of the ACA,[73] which has also been called carotid-anterior cerebral artery anastomosis (**Fig. 17**).[74,75] The ACA originates, oddly, at the level of the ophthalmic artery (or even proximal to it[76]) and runs under the optic nerve (or may pierce it, or the chiasm[76]) to join its distal territory at the level of the ACOM. It may be strictly infraoptic or, together with a "normal" A1, form a ring about the optic nerve.[73,76] This malformation seems to result from the initially plexular ACA together with the complex development of the primitive maxillary, transient ventral, and dorsal ophthalmic arteries (for review see Ref.[73]).

The middle cerebral artery. Three types of abnormality can be observed to affect the MCA: fenestration, duplication, and accessory MCA. Although they have fed much controversy, these abnormalities seem relatively simple to understand from an embryologic point of view. A fenestration is a focal remnant of the plexular pattern that is the rule at the beginning of the development; it is no different from the fenestrations of other brain arteries. The simplest definition of the other MCA variants is that of Teal and colleagues[77]:

- The duplicated MCA is the early origin from the ICA of one of the MCA trunks.
- The accessory MCA originates from the ACA; it can be considered a cortical extension of the medial striatal artery of Heubner into the cortical territory of the MCA.[78–80]

From the early vascular embryogenesis, it is known that 2 forebrain arteries initially emerge from the ICA around the neck of the hemispheric

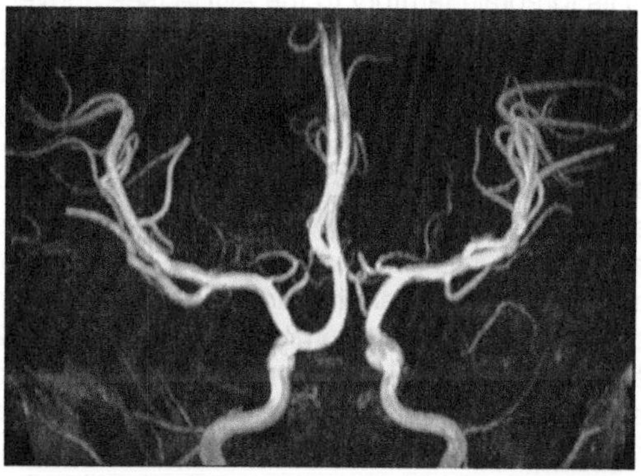

Fig. 17. Infraoptic ACA (or carotid-ACA anastomosis). The right ACA originates from the ICA at the level of the ophthalmic artery and runs medially under the optic nerve toward the ACOM.

vesicle and toward the tela choroidea: the ACA anteriorly (primitive olfactory at this stage) and the ACHA posteriorly. Both the artery of Heubner and the MCA develop as basal striatal branches of the primitive ACA. Normally, only the MCA is to develop later laterodorsal branches toward the cerebral mantle, but it is not abnormal for the artery of Heubner to do so. Typically and logically, the cortical branches of the artery of Heubner supply the frontobasal cortex adjacent to the medial striatum, and the more proximal (ie, caudal) duplicate MCA supplies the temporal territory of the MCA.[81]

The anterior choroidal artery. One of the 2 oldest and prominent brain arteries in the embryo, the ACHA in the mature brain territory is typically restricted to: (1) a temporal choroid branch to the choroid glomus, where it is in balance with the posterolateral choroidal artery; (2) deep perforators to the optic tract, posterior limb of the internal capsule and deep white matter, and variable portions of the adjacent medial globus pallidus and lateral thalamus, in balance with the MCA and PCA territories; (3) anterior hippocampal, parahippocampal, and uncal cortices with the amygdala, again in balance with the PCA through multiple surface anastomoses.

Embryologically, the inferior temporo-occipital and medially the occipital cortices should have belonged to the ACHA; however, they became supplied by the PCA. The rare cases of hypertrophic ACHA are cases in which this artery supplies the whole hemispheric territory of the PCA. Cases of "duplicate" PCAs are cases in which the ACHA supplies the inferior temporal cortex and the PCA supplies the medial temporo-occipital cortex.

The posterior cerebral artery is the most variable. Very commonly, it may originate hemodynamically from the carotid arteries ("embryonic" pattern) or from the BAs (classic pattern), or differently on each side. Uncommonly, it may leave part or all of its forebrain territory to the ACHA (see above).

The vertebrobasilar system. The BAs results from the midline fusion of the paired longitudinal neural arteries. The fusion is said to be craniocaudal by most investigators,[82–85] in reference to Goldstein and colleagues[83] and Padget,[7] but also caudocranial[86] in reference to Goldstein and colleagues.[83] The author was unable to find any comment in Padget about a craniocaudal or caudacranial progression of the fusion: the only comment is that at stage 2 and from a single specimen, the fusion islands would be present in all parts of the BA but more in the caudal end.[7] The fusion has been subdivided into 2 processes, which have been named a "longitudinal" fusion (midline fusion of the 2 longitudinal neural arteries) and an "axial" fusion (fusion of the initially discrete craniocaudal segments of the BA: trigeminal segment first, joined by a carotid segment and by a vertebral segment).[85]

- The so-called longitudinal nonfusion[82] is usually segmental and is commonly designated fenestration of the BA: only a small segment of the artery is duplicated. The BA is the most common fenestrated site among the cerebral arteries. Fenestrations are usually, but not always located in the caudal part of the artery. Fenestrations reflect the description by Padget at stage 2 of multiple midline fusion areas (or "islands") that become secondarily continuous.[7] Intraluminal septations are likely mild forms of fenestrations.[87] Complete or near-complete nonfusion (or extreme fenestration) of the BA is exceptional but can be observed in clinical settings,[83–85] mostly in association with pituitary duplication (**Fig. 18**).[84,86]
- In the so-called axial nonfusion, the 3 segments that are constitutive of the BAs remain discontinuous: a caudal "vertebral" segment that supplies the PICAs only; an intermediate "trigeminal" segment that supplies the AICA, ASCA, and the pontine perforators; and a cranial "carotid" segment that supplies the PCAs.[85] Accordingly, the PTA Saltzman type II, or the bilateral terminal segmental agenesis of the vertebral arteries[68] are variants of this so-called axial nonfusion. Of note, the 2 processes can be mingled when only the proximal/caudal/vertebral, or only the distal/cranial/carotid segments remain unfused on the midline.

(It should be mentioned that these terms are confusing. The "longitudinal" nonfusion would be better named "midline [or median] nonfusion" [holoprosencephaly often is described as a *midline fusion* of the hemispheres, with *midline fusion* of the thalami, of the caudates]. The longitudinal discontinuity between the caudal, middle, and cranial segments of the BAs could then be named "longitudinal nonfusion.")

Finally, the lateromedullary duplication of the terminal VA is caused by the persistence of a normal, typically transient parallel anastomotic artery that runs parallel to the terminal vertebral artery between CN VII and CN XI.[7]

The Aneurysm of the Vein of Galen as a Model

The development of the endovascular approach to treat intracranial arteriovenous malformations and fistulae in the last decades has generated much

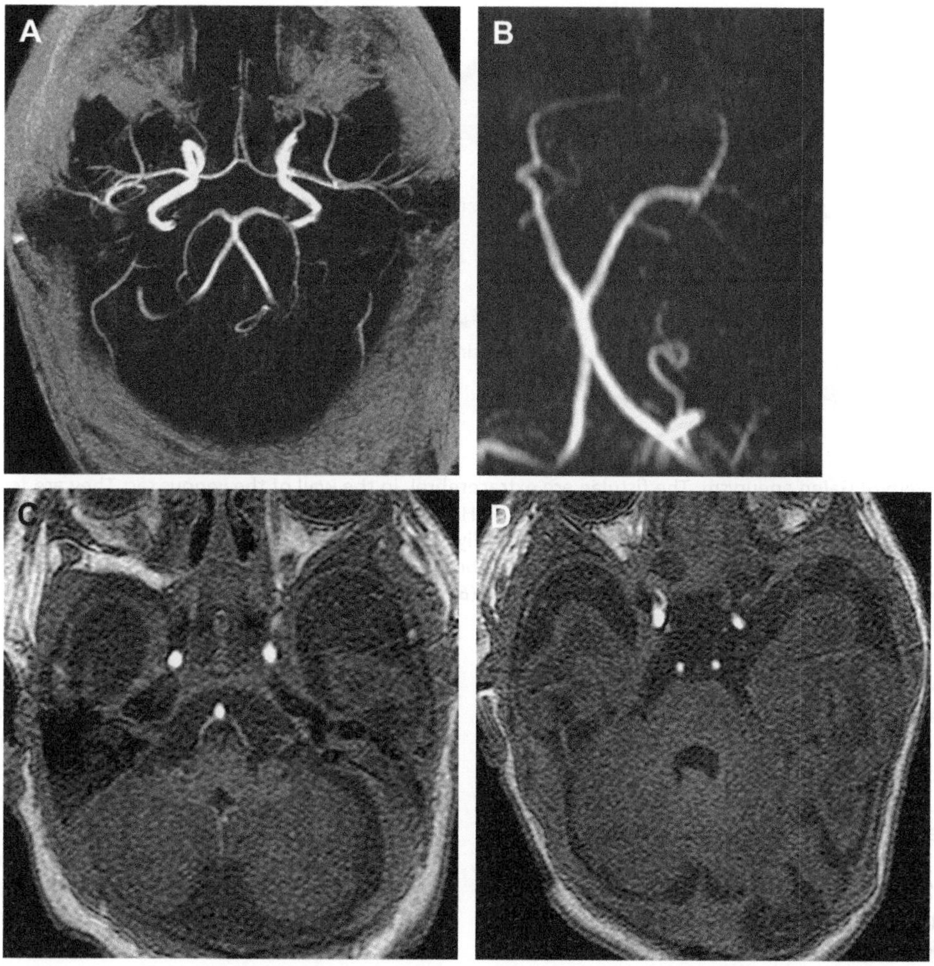

Fig. 18. Midline non-fusion of the BA. Patient with cleft palate, nasal dermoid and pituitary duplication. The BA is divided except for its low ponto-medullary segment. The PCOMs are absent (*A*). The left PICA has a low origin (*B*). AICAs originate at the level of the ponto-medullary sulcus, where the BA is fused (*C*). BA is widely divided at the pontine level (*D*).

interest in the so-called vein of Galen aneurysms (for review, see Refs.[6,88]). This renewed interest in the vascular anatomy of the malformation has cast new light on the embryology.

The first point to consider is the malformation is supplied by the ACA, ACHA, and PCHA anteriorly, and the dorsal midbrain arterial plexus more posteriorly (**Fig. 19**). The choroid afferents point to the tela choroidea; the normal drainage of the tela choroidea is through the paired internal cerebral veins toward the vein of Galen: a double drainage pattern therefore could be expected. Instead, the venous sac is always single. Therefore it could be identified not as a vein of Galen, but as the dorsal prosencephalic vein (of Markowski)[8,35] (see **Figs. 8, 12,** and **19**) (described by Padget as the primitive internal cerebral vein[17]). This vein is not identified before week 8, and not after week 11. This finding brought a better understanding of the malformation. As a purely choroidal vein, it fits the purely choroidal arterial pattern of the malformation. It also fits the dorsal midbrain arterial supply, which is described as dense at this stage of development.[7,29] Anatomically, it points to an extraparenchymal, that is, a meningeal fistula in what is going to be the velum interpositum and the ambient cistern. It can therefore be related to the congenital dural arteriovenous fistulae that involve the torcular and transverse sinus; embryologically the tentorial plexus and meningeal arteries often contribute to the fistulae of the vein of Galen aneurysm.[6]

Chronologically, the malformation points to the choroid stage of Klosovskii,[1] the relatively short period in which the meninges and choroid plexuses represent the main structures feeding the neural tissue, with specific and well-defined arteries and veins. This period extends roughly (there is much overlap) from week 8 to week 11. It is therefore logical

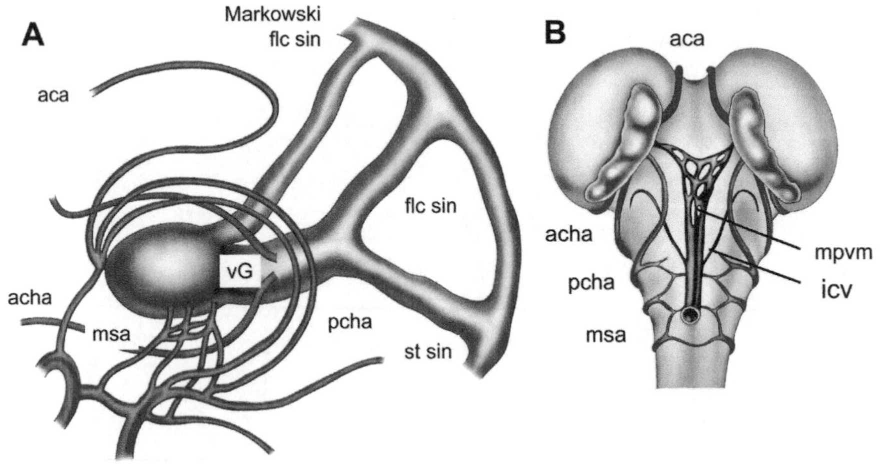

Fig. 19. Vein of Galen aneurysm. The fistulae are extracerebral, in the wall of the venous sac. They are fed by the originally choroidal arteries anteriorly (ACA, ACHA, PCHA) and by the dorsal midbrain arteries posteriorly. The venous sac is single, midline. It may be drained dorsally toward the straight sinus (vein of Galen pattern), or toward a falcine sinus (vein of Markowski pattern), or both (*A*). On the whole, the vascular pattern of the malformation reflects the anatomy at the choroidal stage (*B*).

to assume that the hitting event that generated the fistula(e) occurred about week 8, and that the high flow in the fistula(e) prevents the regression of the vein. However, in medical environments where fetal ultrasound is performed at 12, 22, and 32 weeks, aneurysms of the vein of Galen are commonly reported in the last trimester, and apparently never before 22 weeks.[89] This means that it may be well compensated for over a long time, and the decompensation may be related to the rapid increase of cortical vascularization in the last trimester. Alternatively, it could be that the vein of Markowski does not really disappear and that it could be hemodynamically "reactivated" by the fistula.

The second point concerns the morphogenesis of the vein of Galen. It is implicit from the description of Padget that the "primitive internal cerebral vein" (truly the vein of Markowski according to the accompanying description)[17] is continuous with the straight sinus, meaning that it shares common portions with the final vein of Galen. This point is mentioned also by Hochstetter, who states that the vein of Galen forms from the caudalmost part of the vein of Markowski, after regression of its rostral part.[35] So a bridging vein drained by the future straight sinus would have 2 successive tributaries, one anterior (from the choroid plexuses to the vein of Markowski) and one posterior (tributaries of the true internal cerebral and basal veins to the vein of Galen). This is not illogical, and would explain why many vein of Galen aneurysms drain "normally" into a normally located straight sinus (complemented or not by a falcine sinus), and further, why some present with normally located internal cerebral veins draining into the aneurysmal sac (see **Fig. 19**).[90,91] However, it is not always so, and there are examples of "vein-of-Galen aneurysms without a vein of Galen" in which the malformation is drained directly into a falcine sinus toward the superior sagittal sinus and then, via another falcine sinus, toward the straight sinus (falcine loop) (**Fig. 20**).[6] Such cases suggest that rather than a partly common Markowski-Galen vein, a separate vein of Markowski may occur that cannot connect with a true vein of Galen. This suggestion is consistent with the general variability of the bridging venous pattern. The clinical implication is that the organization of the venous drainage of the brain may be dramatically different in different patients presenting with a vein of Galen malformation.

It should mentioned that a separate drainage via a falcine sinus, common in the fetus,[40] does persist in atretic parietal cephaloceles[92] (**Fig. 21**) because the path to the straight sinus is interrupted by the dysraphic cleft. It may even also be observed incidentally as an apparently normal variant (**Fig. 22**).

Developmental Venous Anomalies

The so-called venous angiomas have been known for a long time from angiography (caput medusae with dilated transcerebral venous stem).[93] Huang and colleagues[36] proposed the more precise anatomic name of medullary venous malformation, correlating them with the normal intrinsic venous anatomy.[94] The term DVA for *developmental venous anomaly* was introduced by Lasjaunias

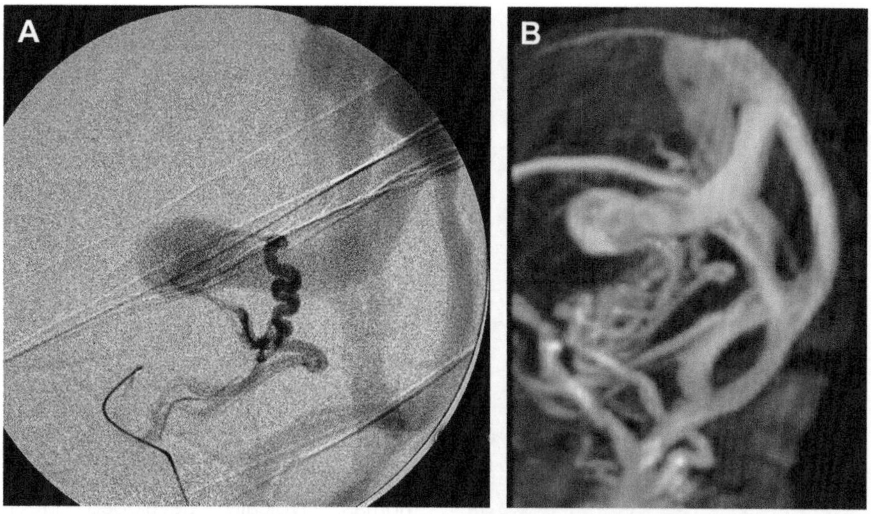

Fig. 20. Vein of Galen aneurysm, falcine loop. On the angiogram the aneurysm drains into a falcine sinus, presumably according to the vein of Markowski pattern, toward the superior sagittal sinus, then through another falcine sinus anteriorly and to the straight sinus. No vein corresponding to the vein of Galen is interposed between the venous sac and the straight sinus (*A*). Similar MR angiographic pattern in another patient; the straight sinus appears to be fed primarily by the falcine loop and inferior sagittal sinus (*B*).

and colleagues[95] in 1986 to stress the fact that in their view, this venous abnormality was not a pathologic condition, only an extreme but normal variant of the brain drainage pattern; besides the white matter, this enlarged vein may be located also in the basal ganglia, thalamus, or brainstem. Thanks to the wide use of brain computed tomography and magnetic resonance imaging, it has become clear that they are the most common vascular malformation found in the brain; however, their significance is still uncertain (for review, see Refs.[96–98]).

The anatomy of DVAs reproduces the normal mature venous parenchymal anatomy.[36,93–100] The histology of DVA is consistent with that of a normal vein. A DVA is composed of a convergent array of collectors that may be subcortical or periventricular (umbrella-like or jellyfish-like, hence caput medusae), and of a single collector that may be subcortical, deep paraventricular, or transcerebral, in any combination.[99] A DVA drains a larger territory than would be expected from any normal collector, and its size is proportionate to the size of the portion of brain tissue it drains. The lesion is considered congenital (ie, developmental) because locally, the area that it drains is devoid of its normal veins.[97,100] However, how this would happen is uncertain.

- An early arrest of venous development has been suggested, that would result in the retention of an assumedly embryonal/fetal

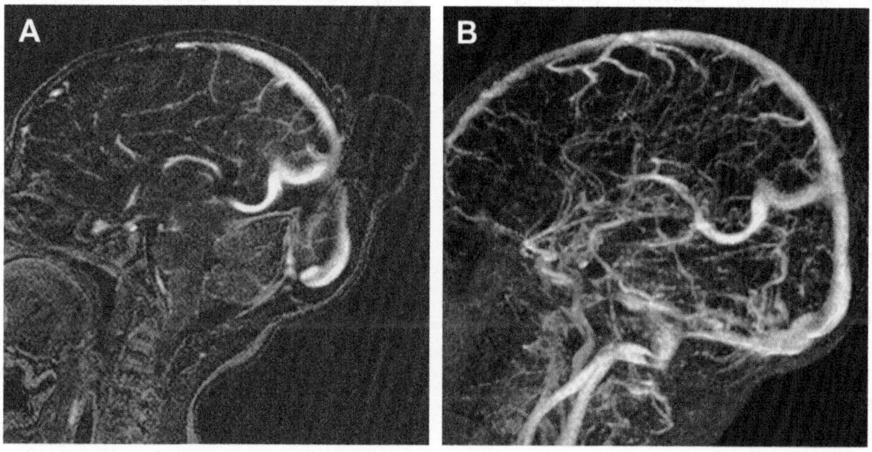

Fig. 21. Parietal cephalocele. The dysraphic cleft separates the diencephalic veins from the tentorium and as a consequence the internal cerebral veins drain into a likely retained vein of Markowski. Source image (*A*) and MIP (*B*).

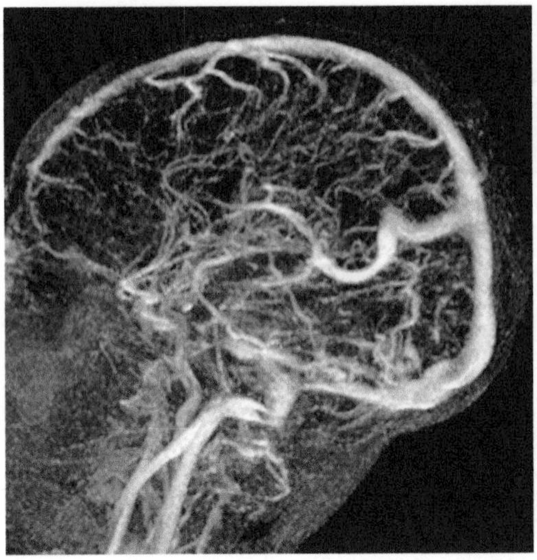

Fig. 22. Incidental finding in a child investigated for arrested hydrocephalus. A pattern similar to that of **Fig. 21** is observed: venous curve around the splenium, perhaps longer and wider than usual (retained vein of Markowski?), falcine sinus, no straight sinus. No associated malformation.

pattern.[96–99] Yet, the anatomy of the malformation reproduces the normal anatomy, not any intermediate pattern.[28,32] Also, if one looks at the principles that rule the arteriovenous differentiation, nothing is likely to arrest the development of a vein: the venous anatomy passively adapts to the arterial hemodynamics, and flow may even change the fate of a channel from artery to vein.[13] At the early stages of gestation, until 20 weeks in the basal ganglia[28] and close to term in the cortex,[28] all vessels are histologically undifferentiated, and only their size and branching pattern (dividing vs converging) tells what they are.[28] Early perforators form simple arteriovenous loops that go to the paraventricular germinal zone, so all the early veins are transcerebral, which is not the case for DVAs. Furthermore, the cortical-subcortical region does not show any vascularization until midgestation (first cortical collaterals) and is not significant before the last trimester. Therefore, in any case, a developmental arrest as the cause of DVA would occur late, and from the data of embryology, it is hard to conceive when and how it would happen.

- A second somewhat related suggestion was made that DVA would result, again as an embryonal/fetal structure, from the reactivation of dormant embryonal sinusoid channels as an adaptation to a lesion affecting the surrounding veins.[94]
- The last hypothesis is that the DVA would have simply been a preexisting medullary vein that would have been used as a collateral channel to compensate for the loss of adjacent veins; it would therefore be an acquired lesion.[97–99]

However, circumstantial evidence suggests the likelihood of a truly developmental, dysplastic lesion. DVAs may be part of more diffuse vascular pathologic entities such as the Blue Rubber Bleb Nevus (BRBN) syndrome, possibly HHT (personal data), sinus pericranii, head and neck superficial venous[101] or venolymphatic[98] malformations. DVAs are known for being associated with cavernomas, typically developed in the caput medusae[98]; it is assumed that some microbleeds from the DVA would induce a neoangiogenesis, but the possibility that both the cavernoma and the DVA would be expressions of the same defect cannot be ruled out. Besides, because the morphogenetic paths are few, DVAs might represent a single, common morphologic end result of various pathogenetic processes. By comparison, polymicrogyria may be clearly familial or genetic on the one hand and obviously environmental on the other hand (fetal cytomegalovirus infection), besides being, most of the time, idiopathic.

Or else DVA might be a capillary disease. All real vascular malformations of the brain involve the capillary bed: arteriovenous malformation or fistula (no interposed capillaries) and telangiectasia (ectatic capillaries), possibly related to cavernomas or angiomas. The arterial "malformations" described above are deviations from the classic anatomic pattern but the arteries themselves are not malformed. The capillary is the primordial vessel that only secondarily becomes differentiated into arteries and veins. It may be speculated that the dilated DVA could result from a hypertrophic malformed capillary bed, for which there are some supportive facts. Some diffuse enhancement may be demonstrated within the field of the DVA, which has been assumed to reflect a venous restriction[96] but might as well be a primary lesion. Hemodynamic studies have demonstrated increased cerebral blood volume in the field of drainage of the DVA[102]; it is assumed to be related to the same venous restriction, but it might reflect an abnormal capillary bed also. De novo development of a telangiectasia or a cavernoma in the caput medusae is well documented, spontaneously[103–106] or after radiotherapy (**Fig. 23**).[107] There are several reports linking DVAs with the development of "arterialized DVAs" and AVMs.[97,108–110] All these secondary, clinically

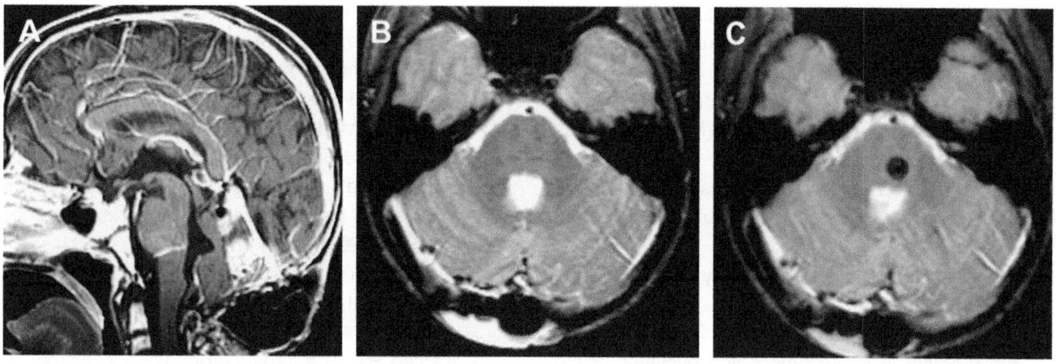

Fig. 23. Medulloblastoma. DVA crosses the brainstem at the lower pons (*A*); otherwise normal axial GET2* appearance of the pons (*B*). Three months later axial GET2* demonstrates the image of a cavernoma adjacent to the DVA (*C*).

significant lesions are assumed to be induced by the DVA, but they might as well represent evolutive forms of a capillary disorder. All this, of course, is speculative and does not say why the (hypothetically) abnormal capillary territory of the DVA would be devoid of normal venous drainage. However, a similarity can be found with Stürge-Weber disease, in which the extensive superficial angioma drains through DVA-like channels toward the subependymal vessels only, without any superficial drainage. Classic embryology does not explain this either.

REFERENCES

1. Klosovskii BN. Fundamental facts concerning the stages and principles of development of the brain and its response to noxious agents. Chapter 1. In: Haigh B, editor. The development of the brain and its disturbance by harmful factors. London: Pergamon Press; 1963. p. 3–43 [in Russian].
2. McLone DG. The subarachnoid space: a review. Childs Brain 1980;6:113–30.
3. Streeter GL. The developmental alterations in the vascular system of the brain of the human embryo. Contrib Embryol 1918;271(24):5–38.
4. Sabin FR. Preliminary note on the differentiation of angioblasts and the method by which they produce blood-vessels, blood-plasma and red blood-cells as seen in the living chick. Anat Rec 1917;13:199–204.
5. Sabin FR. Origin and development of the primitive vessels of the chick and the pig. Contrib Embryol 1917;226(6):61–124.
6. Raybaud CA, Strother CM, Hald JK. Aneurysm of the vein of Galen: embryonic considerations and anatomical features relating to the pathogenesis of the malformation. Neuroradiology 1989;31:109–28.
7. Padget DH. The development of the cranial arteries in the human embryo. Contrib Embryol 1948; 212(32):205–71.
8. Markowski J. Über die Entwicklung der Sinus durae matris und der Hirnvenen bei menschlichen Embryonen 15.5-49 mm. Bulletin de l'Académie des Sciences de Cracovie Série B 1911;590–611 [in German].
9. Marin-Padilla M. Early vascularization of the embryonic cerebral cortex: Golgi and electron microscopic studies. J Comp Neurol 1985;241: 237–49.
10. Osaka K, Handa H, Matsumoto S, et al. Development of the cerebrospinal fluid pathway in the normal and abnormal human embryo. Childs Brain 1980;6:26–38.
11. Couly GF, Le Douarin NM. Mapping of the early neural primordium in quail-chick chimeras. II. The prosencephalic neural plate and neural folds: implication for the genesis of cephalic human congenital abnormalities. Dev Biol 1987;120:198–214.
12. Conway EM, Collen D, Carmeliet P. Molecular mechanisms of blood vessel growth. Cardiovasc Res 2001;49:507–21.
13. Eichmann A, Yuan L, Moyon D, et al. Vascular development: from precursor cells to branched arterial and venous networks. Int J Dev Biol 2005; 49:259–67.
14. Mancuso MH, Kuhnert F, Kuo CJ. Developmental angiogenesis of the central nervous system. Lymphat Res Biol 2008;6:173–80.
15. ten Donkelaar HJ, van der Vliet T. Overview of the development of the human brain and spinal cord. Chapter 1. In: ten Donkelaar HJ, Lammers M, Hori A, editors. Clinical neuroembryology. Berlin: Springer; 2006. p. 1–45.
16. Padget DH. The cranial venous system in man in reference to development, adult configuration, and relation to the arteries. Am J Anat 1956;98: 307–55.
17. Padget DH. The development of the cranial venous system in man from the viewpoint of comparative anatomy. Contrib Embryol 1957;247:81–140.
18. Padget DH. Designation of the embryonic intersegmental arteries in reference to the vertebral artery and subclavian stem. Anat Rec 1954;119:349–56.

19. Dziegielewska KM, Ek J, Habgood MD, et al. Development of the choroid plexus. Microsc Res Tech 2001;52:5–20.
20. Bayer SA, Altman J. Atlas of human central nervous system development. New York (NY): CRC Press Taylor and Francis Group; 2008.
21. Bremer JL. Congenital aneurysms of the cerebral arteries; an embryologic study. Arch Pathol 1943; 35:819–31.
22. Shellshear JL. The arterial supply of the cerebral cortex in the chimpanzee. J Anat 1930;65:45–87.
23. Supèr H, Soriano E, Uylings HB. The functions of the preplate in development and evolution of the neocortex and hippocampus. Brain Res Brain Res Rev 1998;27:40–64.
24. Kriegstein AR, Noctor SC. Patterns of neuronal migration in the embryonic cortex. Trends Neurosci 2004;27:392–9.
25. Zecevic N, Chen Y, Filipovic R. Contributions of cortical subventricular zone to the development of the human cerebral cortex. J Comp Neurol 2005; 491:109–22.
26. Chiron C, Raynaud C, Maziere B, et al. Changes in regional cerebral blood flow during brain maturation in children and adolescents. J Nucl Med 1992;33:696–703.
27. Eichmann A, Makinen T, Alitalo K. Neural guidance molecules regulate vascular remodeling and vessel navigation. Genes Dev 2005;19:1012–21.
28. Kuban KC, Gilles FH. Human telencephalic angiogenesis. Ann Neurol 1985;17:539–48.
29. Allsopp G, Gamble HJ. Light and electron microscopic observations on the development of the blood vascular system of the human brain. J Anat 1979;128:461–77.
30. Norman MG, O'Kusky JR. The growth and development of microvasculature in the human cerebral cortex. J Neuropathol Exp Neurol 1986;45: 222–32.
31. Bär T. The vascular system of the cerebral cortex. Adv Anat Embryol Cell Biol 1980;59:1–65.
32. Nakamura Y, Okudera T, Hashimoto T. Vascular architecture in white matter of neonates: its relationship to periventricular leukomalacia. J Neuropathol Exp Neurol 1994;53:582–9.
33. Le Douarin NM, Kalcheim C. The neural crest. Developmental and cell biology, vol. 36. New York (NY): Cambridge University Press; 1999.
34. Etchevers HC, Vincent C, Le Douarin NM, et al. The cephalic neural crest provides pericytes and smooth muscle cells to all blood vessels of the face and forebrain. Development 2001;128:1059–68.
35. Hochstetter F. Über eine Varietät der Vena cerebralis basialis des Menschen nebst Bemerkungen über die Enwicklung bestimmter Hirnvenen. Z Anat Entwicklungsgesch 1938;108:311–36 [in German].
36. Huang YP, Okudera T, Fukusumi A, et al. Venous architecture of cerebral hemispheric white matter and comments on pathogenesis of medullary venous and other cerebral vascular malformations. Mt Sinai J Med 1997;64:197–206.
37. Okudera T, Huang YP, Fukusumi A, et al. Micro-angiographical studies of the medullary venous system of the cerebral hemispheres. Neuropathology 1999;19:93–111.
38. Schlesinger B. The venous drainage of the brain, with special reference to the Galenic system. Brain 1939;62:274–91.
39. Kaplan HA. The transcerebral venous system. An anatomical study. Arch Neurol 1959;1:148–52.
40. Okudera T, Ohta T, Huang YP. Embryology of the cranial venous system. In: Kapp JP, Schmidek HH, editors. The cerebral venous system and its disorders. Orlando (FL): Grune and Stratton; 1984. p. 93–107.
41. Okudera T, Huang YP, Ohta T, et al. Development of posterior fossa dural sinuses, emissary veins, and jugular bulb: morphological and radiologic study. AJNR Am J Neuroradiol 1994;15:1871–83.
42. San Millán Ruíz D, Gailloud P, Rüfenacht D, et al. The craniocervical venous system in relation to cerebral venous drainage. AJNR Am J Neuroradiol 2002;23:1500–8.
43. Susuki Y, Ikeda H, Shimadu M, et al. Variations of the basal vein: identification using tri-dimensional CT angiography. AJNR Am J Neuroradiol 2001;22:670–6.
44. Saltzman GF. Patent primitive trigeminal artery studied by cerebral angiography. Acta Radiol 1959;51:329–36.
45. Tomsick TA, Lukin RR, Chambers AA. Persistent trigeminal artery: unusual associated abnormalities. Neuroradiology 1979;17:253–7.
46. Meaney JF, Sallomi DF, Miles JB. Transhypophyseal primitive trigeminal artery. Demonstration with MRA. J Comput Assist Tomogr 1994;18:991–4.
47. Uchino A, Mizushima A, Aibe H, et al. MR imaging and MR angiographyof persistent trigeminal artery and its variant. Clin Imaging 1996;20:247–52.
48. Luh GY, Dean BL, Tomsick TA, et al. The persistent fetal carotid-vertebrobasilar anastomoses. AJR Am J Roentgenol 1999;172:1427–32.
49. Uchno A, Kato A, Takase Y, et al. Persistent trigeminal artery variants detected by MR angiography. Eur Radiol 2000;10:1801–4.
50. Okahara M, Kiyosue H, Mori H, et al. Anatomic variations of the cerebral arteries and their embryology: a pictorial review. Eur Radiol 2002;12:2548–61.
51. Uchino A, Sawada A, Takase Y, et al. MR angiography of anomalous branches of the internal carotid artery. AJR Am J Roentgenol 2003;181:1409–14.
52. Tubbs RS, Shoja MM, Salter EG, et al. Cadaveric findings of persistent fetal trigeminal arteries. Clin Anat 2007;20:367–70.

53. Cloft HJ, Razack N, Kallmes DF. Prevalence of cerebral aneurysms in patients with persistent primitive trigeminal artery. J Neurosurg 1999;90:865–7.
54. Murai Y, Kobayashi S, Tateyama K, et al. Persistent trigeminal artery aneurysm associated with cerebellar hemangioblastoma. Neurol Med Chir (Tokyo) 2006;46:143–6.
55. Huber G. Die Arteria primitive otica, eine sehr seltene persistierende primitive Arterie. Fortschrift Röntgenstr 1977;127:350–3 [in German].
56. Reynolds AF, Jorgen S, Turner PT. Persistent otic artery. Surg Neurol 1980;13:115–7.
57. Patel AB, Gandhi CD, Bederson JB. Angiographic documentation of a persistent otic artery. AJNR Am J Neuroradiol 2003;24:124–6 [see comments in: AJNR Am J Neuroradiol 2004, 25:160–2;162; and reply 162].
58. Zhang CW, Xie XD, Yang ZG, et al. Giant cavernous aneurysm associated with a persistent trigeminal artery and persistent otic artery. Korean J Radiol 2009;10:519–22.
59. Anderson RA, Sondheimer FK. Rare carotid-vertebrobasilar anastomoses with notes on the differentiation between proatlantal and hypoglossal arteries. Neuroradiology 1976;11:113–8.
60. Oelerich M, Schuierer G. Primitive hypoglossal artery: demonstration with digital subtraction, MR- and CT angiography. Eur Radiol 1997;7:1492–4.
61. Hähnel S, Hartmann M, Jansen O, et al. Persistent hypoglossal artery: MRI, MRA and digital subtraction angiography. Neuroradiology 2001;43:767–9.
62. Vasović L, Milenković Z, Jovanović R, et al. Hypoglossal artery: a review of normal and pathological features. Neurosurg Rev 2008;31:385–96.
63. Bloch S, Danziger J. Proatlantal intersegmental artery. Neuroradiology 1974;7:5–8.
64. Basekim CC, Silit E, Mutlu H, et al. Type I proatlantal artery with bilateral absence of the external carotid arteries. AJNR Am J Neuroradiol 2004;25:1619–21.
65. Gumus T, Önal B, Ilgit ET. Bilateral persistence of type I proatlantal arteries: report of a case and review of the literature. AJNR Am J Neuroradiol 2004;25:1622–4.
66. Vasović L, Mojsilović M, Anđelković Z, et al. Proatlantal intersegmental artery: a review of normal and pathological features. Childs Nerv Syst 2009;25:411–21.
67. Lasjaunias P, Théron J, Moret J. The occipital artery. Anatomy - normal arteriographic aspects - embryological significance. Neuroradiology 1978; 15:31–7.
68. Burger IM, Siclari F, Gregg L, et al. Bilateral segmental agenesis of the vertebrobasilar junction: developmental and angiographic development. AJNR Am J Neuroradiol 2007;28:2017–22.
69. Lasjaunias P, Santoyo-Vazquez A. Segmental agenesis of the internal carotid artery: angiographic aspects with embryological discussion. Anat Clin 1984;6:133–41.
70. Gailloud P, Clatterbuck RE, Fasel JHD, et al. Segmental agenesis of the internal carotid artery distal to the posterior communicating artery leading to the definition of a new embryologic segment. AJNR Am J Neuroradiol 2004;25:1189–93.
71. Lazorthes G, Gouazé A. [Modeling of the diameter of segments of the Willis polygon (circulus arteriosus cerebri). Role of the movements of the head]. C R Acad Sci Hebd Seances Acad Sci D 1970; 271:1682–5 [in French].
72. Nozaki K, Taki W, Kawakami O, et al. Cerebral aneurysm associated with persistent primitive olfactory artery. Acta Neurochir (Wien) 1998;140: 397–402.
73. Wong ST, Yuen SC, Fok KF, et al. Infraoptic anterior cerebral artery: review, report of two cases and anatomical classification. Acta Neurochir (Wien) 2008;150:1087–96.
74. Nutik S, Dilenge D. Carotid-anterior cerebral artery anastomosis: case report. J Neurosurg 1976;44: 378–82.
75. Kiliç K, Orakdöğen M, Bakirci A, et al. Bilateral internal carotid to anterior cerebral anastomosis with anterior communicating aneurysm: technical case report. Neurosurgery 2005;54(Suppl 4):E400.
76. Given CA, Morris PP. Recognition and importance of an infraoptic anterior cerebral artery: case report. AJNR Am J Neuroradiol 2002;23:452–4.
77. Teal JS, Rumbaugh CL, Bergeron RT, et al. Anomalies of the middle cerebral artery: accessory artery, duplication and early bifurcation. AJR Am J Roentgenol 1973;118:567–75.
78. Handa J, Shimizu Y, Matsuda M, et al. Accessory middle cerebral artery: report of further two cases. Clin Radiol 1970;21:415–6.
79. Abanou A, Lasjaunias P, Manelfe C, et al. The accessory middle cerebral artery (AMCA). Anat Clin 1884;6:305–9.
80. Takahashi S, Hoshino F, Uemura K, et al. Accessory middle cerebral artery: is it a variant of the recurrent artery of Heubner? AJNR Am J Neuroradiol 1989;10:563–8.
81. Komiyama M, Nakajima H, Nishikawa M, et al. Middle cerebral artery variations: duplicated and accessory arteries. AJNR Am J Neuroradiol 1998;19:45–9.
82. Krings T, Baccin CE, Alvarez H, et al. Segmental unfused basilar artery with kissing aneurysms: report of three cases and literature review. Acta Neurochir (Wien) 2007;149:567–74.
83. Goldstein JH, Woodcock R, Do HM, et al. Complete duplication or extreme fenestration of the basilar artery. AJNR Am J Neuroradiol 1999;20:149–50.
84. Uchino A, Sawada A, Takase Y, et al. Extreme fenestration of the basilar artery associated with cleft palate, nasopharyngeal mature teratoma and hypophyseal duplication. Eur Radiol 2002;12: 2087–90.

85. Hoh BL, Rabinov JD, Pryor JC, et al. Persistent nonfused segments of the basilar artery: longitudinal versus axial nonfusion. AJNR Am J Neuroradiol 2004;25:1194–6.
86. Shroff M, Blaser S, Jay V, et al. Basilar duplication associated with pituitary duplication: a new finding. AJNR Am J Neuroradiol 2003;24:956–61.
87. Tubbs RS, Shaffer WA, Loukas M, et al. Intraluminal septation of the basilar artery: incidence and potential significance. Folia Morphol (Warsz) 2008;67:193–5.
88. Lasjaunias PL, Chng SM, Sachet M, et al. The management of vein of Galen aneurysmal malformation. Neurosurgery 2006;59:S184–94.
89. Hartung J, Heiling KS, Rake A, et al. Detection of an aneurysm of the vein of Galen following signs of cardiac overload in a 22-week old fetus. Prenat Diagn 2003;23:901–3.
90. Levrier O, Gailloud P, Souei M, et al. Normal galenic drainage of the deep cerebral venous system in two cases of vein of Galen aneurysmal malformation. Childs Nerv Syst 2004;20:91–7.
91. Gailloud P, O'Riordan DP, Burger I, et al. Confirmation of communication between deep venous drainage and the vein of Galen after treatment of a vein of Galen aneurismal malformation in an infant presenting with severe pulmonary hypertension. AJNR Am J Neuroradiol 2006;27:317–20.
92. Morioka T, Hashigushi K, Samura K, et al. Detailed anatomy of intracranial venous anomalies associated with atretic parietal cephaloceles revealed by high-resolution 3D-CISS and high-field T2-weighted reversed MR images. Childs Nerv Syst 2009;25:309–15.
93. Courville CB. Morphology of small vascular malformations of the brain. J Neuropathol Exp Neurol 1963;22:274–84.
94. Huang PY, Robbins A, Patel SC, et al. Cerebral venous malformations. In: Kapp JP, Schmidek HH, editors. The cerebral venous system and its disorders. New York: Grune & Stratton; 1984. p. 373–474.
95. Lasjaunias P, Burrows P, Plante C. Developmental venous anomalies (DVA): the so-called venous angiomas. Neurosurg Rev 1986;9:233–44.
96. Truwit CL. Venous angioma of the brain: history, significance and imaging findings. AJR Am J Roentgenol 1992;159:1299–307.
97. Rammos SK, Maina R, Lanzino G. Developmental venous anomalies: current concepts and implication for management. Neurosurgery 2009;65:20–30.
98. San Millán Ruíz D, Yilmaz H, Gailloud P. Cerebral developmental venous anomalies: current concepts. Ann Neurol 2009;66:271–83.
99. Lee C, Pennington MA, Kenney CM. MR evaluation of developmental venous anomalies: medullary venous anatomy of venous angiomas. AJNR Am J Neuroradiol 1996;17:61–70.
100. Ikezaki K, Nakamizo A, Amano T, et al. Classification of medullary venous malformations in the temporal lobe: according to location and drainage pathway. Neurol Res 2002;24:505–9.
101. Boukobza M, Enjolras O, Guichard JP, et al. Cerebral developmental venous anomalies associated with head and neck venous malformations. AJNR Am J Neuroradiol 1996;17:987–94.
102. Camacho DL, Smith JK, Grimme JD, et al. Atypical MR imaging perfusion in developmental venous anomalies. AJNR Am J Neuroradiol 2004;25:1549–52.
103. Ciricillo SF, Dillon WP, Fink ME, et al. Progression of multiple cryptic vascular malformations associated with anomalous venous drainage. J Neurosurg 1994;81:477–81.
104. Van Roost D, Kristof R, Wolf HK, et al. Intracerebral capillary telangiectasia and venous malformation: a rare association. Surg Neurol 1997;48:175–83.
105. Campeau NG, Lane IJ. De novo development of a lesion with the appearance of a cavernous malformation adjacent to an existing developmental venous anomaly. AJNR Am J Neuroradiol 2005;26:156–9.
106. Abla A, Wait SD, Uschold T, et al. Developmental venous anomaly, cavernous malformation and capillary telangiectasia: spectrum of a single disease. Acta Neurochir (Wien) 2008;150:487–9.
107. Maeder P, Gudinchet F, Meuli R, et al. Development of a cavernous malformation of the brain. AJNR Am J Neuroradiol 1998;19:1141–3.
108. Nussbaum ES, Heros RC, Madison MT, et al. The pathogenesis of arteriovenous malformations: insights provided by a case of multiple arteriovenous malformations developing in relation to a developmental venous anomaly. Neurosurgery 1998;43:347–51.
109. Agazzi S, Regli L, Uske A, et al. Developmental venous anomaly with an arteriovenous shunt and a thrombotic complication. J Neurosurg 2001;94:533–7.
110. Oran I, Kiroglu Y, Yurt A, et al. Developmental venous anomaly (DVA) with arterial component: a rare cause of intracranial haemorrhage. Neuroradiology 2009;51:25–32.

Pediatric and Inherited Neurovascular Diseases

Monique J. Vanaman, MD, Shawn L. Hervey-Jumper, MD, Cormac O. Maher, MD*

KEYWORDS

- Pediatric neurovascular diseases
- Inherited neurovascular diseases
- Familial cavernous malformations
- Hereditary hemorrhagic telangiectasia

FAMILIAL CAVERNOUS MALFORMATIONS

Cavernous malformations are congenital vascular lesions affecting blood vessels of the central nervous system (CNS), and account for 20% to 25% of CNS vascular malformations in children.[1–4] Histologically they consist of sinusoidal-shaped blood vessels with irregular walls that are lined by a single layer of endothelium.[5] Grossly, cavernomas are collections of sinusoidal vascular channels with an appearance similar to a raspberry and lack intervening brain parenchyma.[6] Cavernous malformations may occur as sporadic isolated lesions or in a familial form with an autosomal dominant inheritance pattern. In the familial form there are often multiple cavernomas that may arise throughout the CNS. Familial inheritance is a risk factor for aggressive clinical behavior. Familial cavernous malformations occur most frequently in patients of Hispanic origin, although they can be found in any ethnic group.[4,7–10]

Based on postmortem studies and magnetic resonance imaging (MRI), cavernous malformations have been estimated to affect 0.3% to 0.7% of the general population and represent 5% to 20% of cerebrovascular malformations in all age groups.[11–13] Reviews of pediatric cavernous malformations estimate that between 3.5% and 26.0% are familial.[1,11,14] According to several single-institution reviews, the familial form is estimated to represent 75% of patients who present with multiple cavernous malformations, although this number is likely influenced by the screening selection bias of Hispanic patients.[4,9,15,16]

Familial cavernous malformations are inherited in an autosomal dominant pattern with incomplete clinical penetrance.[9] Gradient-echo MRI is quite sensitive for detecting these lesions, including small associated subclinical brain hemorrhages. Despite the incomplete clinical penetrance, with gradient-echo MRI the radiologic penetrance is nearly complete.[9] The probability that standard T2-weighted MRI fails to detect a lesion, given that one existed on gradient-echo MRI, is estimated to be 5% (**Fig. 1**).[9]

Labauge and colleagues[9] reported on the largest series of familial cavernomas in collaboration with all 28 neurosurgery centers in France. They analyzed 100 symptomatic patients and 278 at-risk relatives without symptoms from 57 indexed families across France. The mean age at clinical onset was 32.6 years (range, 5–74 years). Most patients with familial cavernous malformations had multiple lesions and there was a correlation between the number of lesions and advancing patient age. Surveillance was done using gradient-

Department of Neurosurgery, University of Michigan, 1500 East Medical Center Drive, Room 3552, Ann Arbor, MI 48109-5338, USA
* Corresponding author.
E-mail address: cmaher@med.umich.edu

Neurosurg Clin N Am 21 (2010) 427–441
doi:10.1016/j.nec.2010.03.001

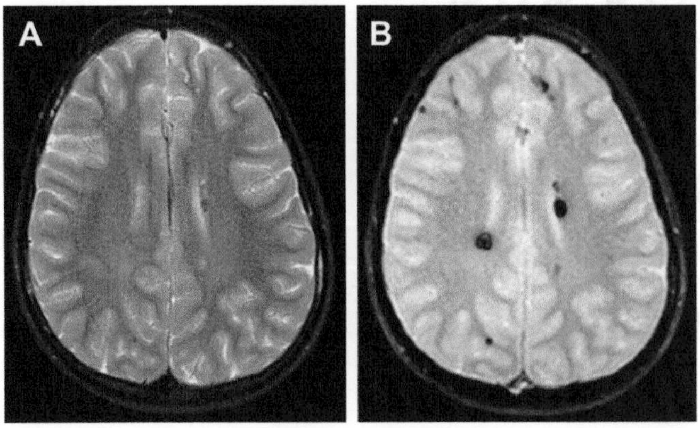

Fig. 1. Axial T2-weighted MRI (*A*) from a patient with familial cavernous malformations. The T2-STAR sequence (*B*) is much more sensitive for detection of these lesions.

echo MRI sequences, which had a higher sensitivity for detection of small lesions. The 2 most common presenting symptoms were seizures (affecting 45 of 100 patients) and cerebral hemorrhage (affecting 41 of 100 patients).[9] Other presenting symptoms included focal sensory and motor neurologic deficits, visual field deficits, and nonmigrainous headaches. The mean age of patients at clinical onset is lower when the initial event is hemorrhage (25.2 years) when compared with all other presenting symptoms (37.8 years).[9]

The natural history of familial cavernous malformations and the optimal radiologic screening protocol has been a topic of debate. Zabramski and colleagues[13] reported their results after prospectively following 59 members of 6 families by serial interviews, physical examinations, and MRI at 6- to 12-month intervals. Both symptomatic and asymptomatic patients were included in the analysis. Sixty-one percent of patients were symptomatic with seizures (39%), headaches (52%), focal neurologic deficits (10%), and visual field deficits (6%). In these patients, 128 individual cavernous malformations were identified and followed for a mean follow-up period of 2.2 years (range, 1 to 5.5 years). Surveillance MRI revealed new lesions in 29.0% of patients, whereas 10.0% of lesions showed some change in radiographic signal appearance, and 3.9% of lesions changed significantly in size.[13] The incidence of symptomatic hemorrhage for familial cavernous malformations was 1.1% per lesion per year in that series.[13] Labauge and colleagues[17] prospectively reviewed the natural history of 33 asymptomatic French patients with relatives diagnosed with familial cavernous malformations. Over a mean period of 2.1 years, 2 patients became symptomatic: 1 with a brainstem hemorrhage, and 1 with a partial seizure. Surveillance MRI found lesion changes in 46% of patients (bleeding in 9.2%, appearance of new lesions in 30.3%, signal intensity changes in 3.0%, and increased lesion size in 9.1%).

Cavernous malformations in children behave differently compared with adults.[18] Cavernous malformations in children occur at a 4 times lower incidence rate than in adults, but have a more aggressive growth pattern and clinical behavior than in adults.[1] The incidence of a symptomatic hemorrhage from cavernous malformations in children is higher than in adults (27%–78% vs 8%–37%, respectively).[1,3,11,19,20] In children, a history of the familial form of disease, craniospinal radiotherapy for CNS tumors, and the existence of venous anomalies predicts worse clinical behavior. The existence of multiple cavernous malformations in children is estimated at 12% of cases, whereas up to 80% of patients harboring multiple cavernous malformations exhibit the familial form of disease.[1,19,21–23] The presence of cavernous malformations with venous anomalies has been reported in as many as 2.1% to 26.0% of patients undergoing surgical treatment.[24,25] Overall, although much is left to be answered, it is generally agreed that the natural history of cavernous malformations is more aggressive in children than in adults, given their higher hemorrhage rate.

Familial cerebral cavernous malformations are inherited in an autosomal dominant pattern with incomplete clinical penetrance. Linkage analysis of several Hispanic families identified the CCM1 gene on chromosome 7 from q11 to q22 with mutations in KRIT1, which is responsible for familial cavernous malformations.[26–28] The homogeneity at the CCM1 locus, however, did not represent the expressive phenotype of familial cavernous malformations in patients of non-Hispanic ethnicity. The CCM2 gene on chromosome 7p13-15 (with MGC4607 or malcavernin mutations) and CCM3 gene at 3q25.2-27 were found after investigation of 20 non-Hispanic white families.[26,28–31] A fourth CCM locus (CCM4) was identified in 3q26.3-27.2, representing a mutation of PDCD10.[26,32] The CCM1 protein, KRIT1, participates in regulation of cell adhesion and migration via its interaction with beta-1 integrin.[26,33,34] This interaction may control endothelial cell behavior. The CCM3 gene (PDCD10) induces apoptosis through modulation of the cell cycle.[35] It has therefore been proposed that aberrant apoptosis, by altering the balance between endothelial and neural crest cells within the neurovascular unit, may lead to cavernoma formation. Identification of these and other molecular defects allows clinicians to better screen at-risk families.[36] Screening of relatives with multiple or sporadic cavernous malformations continues to be a topic of debate. This question has not yet been convincingly answered by the existing clinical data, although it is generally recommended that first-degree relatives of patients with known familial cavernous malformations have a surveillance brain MRI.

Management of familial cavernous malformations differs from sporadic malformations. Although large multicenter trials have not been performed, many single-center studies show that microsurgery can be performed without significant postsurgical complications to prevent recurrent hemorrhage and control seizure disorders in these patients.[37,38] The treatment of choice for symptomatic solitary cavernous malformations is often microsurgery; however, for multiple cavernous malformations, as is the case for many patients with familial cavernous malformations, the decision to offer surgery should be entertained with greater caution.[37,38]

HEREDITARY HEMORRHAGIC TELANGIECTASIA

HHT is an autosomal dominant disorder characterized by arteriovenous malformations (AVMs) of multiple solid organs and telangiectases of the mucous membranes and dermis.[39] In the past, this disease has also been referred to as Rendu-Osler-Weber syndrome or Osler-Weber-Rendu syndrome. It is a disease of high penetrance but variable expressivity.[40] The incidence rate is approximately 1 to 2 individuals per 10,000, with no major ethnic or geographic differences.[41]

HHT is classically caused by one of many possible mutations in either endoglin (ENG) or an activin receptorlike kinase 1 (ALK1). ENG is located on chromosome 9 and causes HHT1, whereas ALK1 is located on chromosome 12 and causes HHT2.[41,42] Both ENG and ALK1 mutations encode receptor proteins in the transforming growth factor-β (TGF-β) family. ALK1 encodes a type 1 receptor, which is expressed in endothelial cells and highly vascularized tissues. Thus, the ALK1 gene is a positive regulator of angiogenesis. ENG encodes endoglin, which is expressed in endothelial cells, activated monocytes, and tissue macrophages. ENG increases the relative amount of ALK1 in endothelial cells. Therefore, mutations in either ALK1 or ENG will produce a similar phenotype.

Epistaxis is the most common presenting complaint among patients with HHT (**Fig. 2**). Half of patients report significant epistaxis by 10 years of age and 90% report epistaxis by 21 years of age.[43] Gastrointestinal bleeding is the second most common presentation of HHT.[44] Patients may also present with dermal telangiectasias, but these typically do not appear until later in life. Telangiectases may be found on the oral and nasal mucosa, tongue, lips, nose, fingertips, trunk, arms, nail beds, or conjunctivae.[45]

AVMs of the CNS, lungs, liver, and upper gastrointestinal tract may present at any age. These lesions may present following hemorrhage or as the result of abnormal shunting.[41] Approximately 20% to 30% of patients with HHT harbor pulmonary AVMs. These often present with exercise intolerance, cyanosis, or pulmonary hemorrhage. However, it is critical to note that 30% to 40% of pulmonary AVMs present with thrombotic or embolic events of the CNS such as stroke, transient ischemic attacks, and abscesses. Abscesses have been reported to occur in 5% to

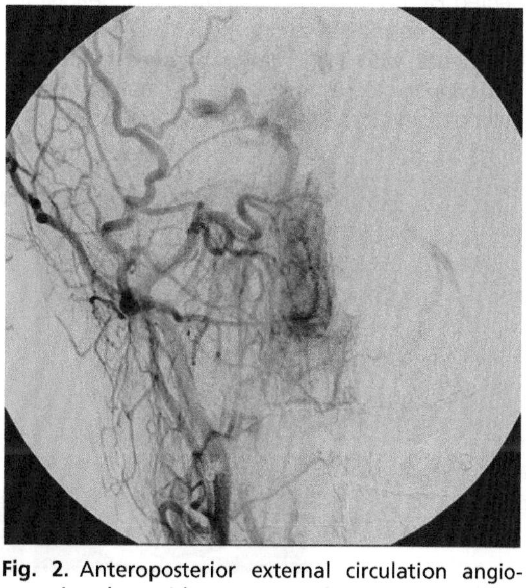

Fig. 2. Anteroposterior external circulation angiogram in a boy with HHT. A nasal vascular malformation is seen. This child presented with epistaxis.

9% of patients with HHT with pulmonary AVMs.[46] In general, cerebral embolic complications are rare in young children, but become increasingly common in the fourth through sixth decades.[46] Hepatic AVMs can present with high-output cardiac failure, portal hypertension, biliary disease, or hepatic encephalopathy. Although rare, AVMs have also been described in the spleen, urinary tract, vagina, coronary arteries, or vessels of the eye.

Clinical evaluation along with molecular and DNA testing are currently used when diagnosing HHT. Clinical diagnostic criteria for HHT are as follows[47]:

1. Spontaneous, recurrent epistaxis, especially if nocturnal.
2. Mucocutaneous telangiectasias, especially on the tongue, lips, oral cavity, fingers, or nose.
3. Internal AVMs; commonly pulmonary, cerebral, spinal, hepatic, or gastrointestinal.
4. First-degree relative with HHT (almost all patients have a positive family history).

Three of these criteria are needed to diagnose HHT. The diagnosis is considered "possible" in the presence of 2 criteria, whereas the diagnosis is unlikely when only 1 criterion is present. Molecular diagnosis is available for HHT. If the molecular test is positive, DNA testing is available for further confirmation. Some authors suggest that patients with symptoms strongly suggestive of HHT, as well as those who are asymptomatic with an affected first-degree relative, should be offered molecular genetic diagnosis.[41] A patient with suspected HHT should be referred to a geneticist for a family-based evaluation.

Patients with HHT are at increased risk for harboring cerebrovascular malformations. Fulbright and colleagues[48] found AVMs in 4.9% of HHT patients. Maher and colleagues[46] found in their study of 321 patients with HHT that 3.7% of patients harbored a cerebral AVM, although asymptomatic patients were not screened. In contrast, Willemse and colleagues[49] reported that 11% of patients with HHT had a cerebral AVM. Differences in AVM incidence among these studies may be attributed to the various screening protocols that were used at those institutions.

These lesions, like AVMs not associated with HHT, may present with hemorrhage, seizures, or other neurologic symptoms. Spinal AVMs occur in 1% of patients with HHT and can present with progressive myelopathy or even radicular pain.[50] Although AVMs are the most classic CNS lesions associated with HHT, cavernous malformations, dural arteriovenous fistulae, or aneurysms have all been reported in these patients.[46]

The risk of hemorrhage from cerebral AVMs associated with HHT is controversial. The risk of hemorrhage in an unruptured, nonsyndromic AVM is 2% to 4% per year[51–53]; however, this rate may not be applicable to AVMs in the HHT population for the following reasons. First, pulmonary and gastrointestinal AVMs in patients with HHT grow and change over time; it is possible that cerebral AVMs in these patients behave similarly. Second, most AVMs described in the HHT literature are smaller than 25 mm in diameter (**Fig. 3**). Although some studies suggest an increased risk of hemorrhage in small AVMs among the general population, this has never been demonstrated in patients with HHT.[46,54] Last, patients with HHT are more likely than the general population to have multiple AVMs and low-flow telangiectasias, which would influence their annual risk of hemorrhage.[55–57] In a study of 321 patients with HHT, Maher and colleagues[46] found the likelihood of a patient with HHT presenting with intracerebral hemorrhage from an

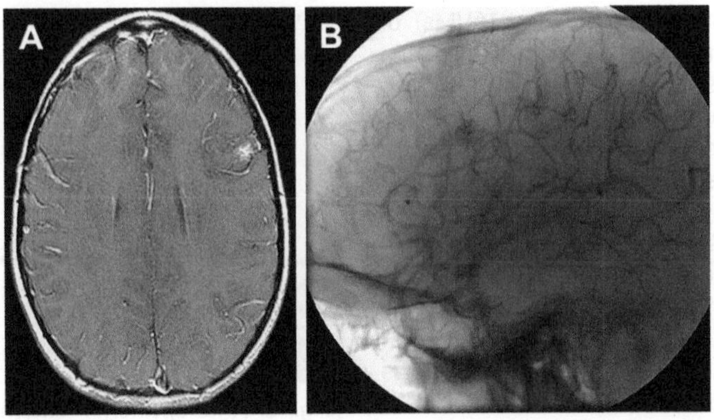

Fig. 3. Axial T1-weighted MRI (*A*) following contrast administration shows a small AVM that is typical of lesions found in patients with HHT. A follow-up cerebral angiogram (*B*) shows 3 small AVMs in this patient.

intracranial AVM was very low, occurring in only 2.1% of patients in that large series. This finding is similar to that of Fulbright and colleagues[48] (0% hemorrhage) and Willemse and colleagues[49] (1.5% hemorrhage). Taken together, these studies suggest that the natural history of AVMs associated with HHTs is more favorable than that of sporadic cerebral AVMs.

In contrast to the common perception, cerebral AVMs are not the most common cause of neurologic symptoms in patients with HHT. In their study, Roman and colleagues[58] found that only 36% of 215 patients with neurologic manifestations harbored a cerebrovascular lesion. Most of these lesions were cavernous malformations or venous angiomas; only 7.9% were AVMs. Emboli passing through a pulmonary arteriovenous fistula may result in cerebral abscess or strokes. Untreated or incompletely treated pulmonary fistulas were the most frequent cause of neurologic morbidity in one large series, causing significantly greater morbidity than cerebral AVMs.[46]

Once a patient is diagnosed with HHT, he or she should undergo a multisystem evaluation. An MRI of the brain with and without gadolinium is appropriate for evaluation of cerebral AVMs. Because small AVMs are sometimes difficult to detect on MRI, one may consider a conventional angiogram if the degree of clinical suspicion is high. Patients with HHT should also be evaluated for occult gastrointestinal bleeding. These patients should also be evaluated for the presence of pulmonary AVMs, given that these lesions are a cause of significantly more neurologic morbidity and mortality than cerebral AVMs in patients with HHT. A pulmonary angiogram is the most sensitive test for detection of pulmonary AVMs. A contrast echocardiogram may also be indicated to evaluate for pulmonary shunting. Pulmonary AVMs are usually treated with embolization. The substantial neurologic risk posed by pulmonary AVMs should be taken into account when making treatment decisions regarding these lesions. Treatments for CNS AVMs include surgical resection or stereotactic radiosurgery. In fact, the small size of most AVMs associated with HHT can make them particularly good candidates for radiosurgery. Symptomatic hepatic AVMs are best treated with liver transplantation.[59] Given the increased risk of bleeding from solid organ AVMs, patients with HHT are generally advised to avoid anticoagulants, including aspirin.

PHACE(S) SYNDROME

PHACE(S) is a neurocutaneous disorder of unknown etiology characterized by posterior fossa malformations (P), facial hemangiomas (H), arterial and cerebrovascular abnormalities (A), cardiovascular abnormalities (C), and eye abnormalities (E). An "S" is sometimes added for those patients who exhibit ventral congenital defects such as sternal clefting or a supraumbilical raphe.[60,61] The syndrome has a strong female predominance, but no familial tendency has been demonstrated.[62] Strict diagnostic criteria for PHACE(S) do not exist. In general, patients are diagnosed with the syndrome if they exhibit the classic cervicofacial hemangioma, as well as at least one extracutaneous anomaly.

Most patients present as infants with large cervicofacial hemangiomas that are not restricted to cutaneous distribution of the trigeminal nerve. These lesions demonstrate a characteristic pattern of rapid neonatal growth, followed by a slow regression.[63] A child who presents with a large cervicofacial hemangioma should be evaluated for the extracutaneous manifestations of PHACE(S). The work-up generally includes an echocardiogram to evaluate for cardiac anomalies, as well as an MRI and magnetic resonance angiography (MRA) with and without gadolinium to detect abnormalities of the CNS. If indicated by clinical examination or MRI findings, a conventional angiogram may be considered.

Children with PHACE(S) may harbor congenital malformations of the cerebrum, cerebellum, or cerebral vasculature, including progressive stenosis and occlusion of cerebral arteries. The most common intracranial abnormalities diagnosed in patients with PHACE(S) are posterior fossa lesions ranging from cerebellar hypoplasia to the Dandy-Walker syndrome (**Fig. 4**). Approximately 43% to 81% of children diagnosed with PHACE(S) have posterior fossa abnormalities.[60,63] Focal cerebellar lesions tend to occur ipsilateral to the facial hemangioma.[63] Poetke and colleagues[64] found that 81% of patients diagnosed with PHACE(S) also had Dandy-Walker syndrome. Interestingly, another study found that as many as 10% of patients with Dandy-Walker syndrome have a history of infantile hemangiomas, and that 73% of children with both Dandy-Walker syndrome and facial hemangiomas were female.[65]

In a large series of patients with PHACE(S) syndrome, Poetke and colleagues[64] reported that 12% of patients with PHACE(S) also had intracranial hemangiomas. In their study, the term "intracranial hemangiomas" described extra-axial, meningeal-based, contrast-enhancing masses. These masses were often noted in the cerebellopontine angle. They demonstrated the same MRI features found in extracranial hemangiomas; that is, isointense on T1-weighted images and

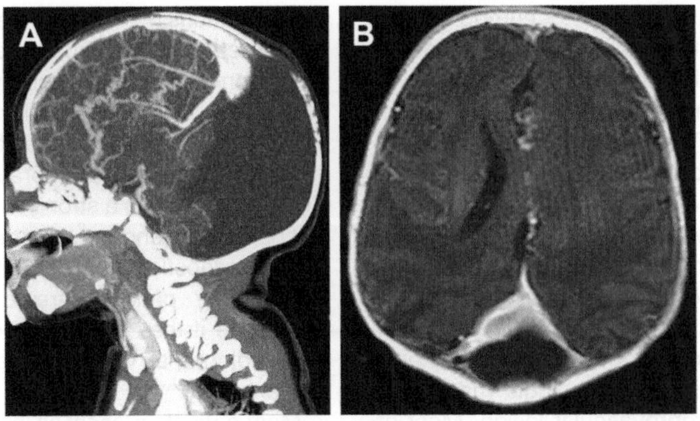

Fig. 4. Sagittal CT angiogram (*A*) and axial T1-weighted MRI (*B*) following contrast administration shows cerebral vascular malformations as well as Dandy-Walker malformation in a patient with PHACE(S).

hyperintense on T2-weighted images, suggesting that they are filled with unclotted blood. Intracranial and facial hemangiomas are often ipsilateral and behave in parallel; that is, the intracranial lesion will often demonstrate some involution with steroid therapy administered for the facial lesion.[62]

Pascual-Castroviejo[66] first demonstrated in 1978 the relationship between infantile hemangiomas and craniocervical vasculature abnormalities. He described 3 major types of abnormalities: anomalous origin or hypoplasia of major cerebral vessels, persistence of embryonic arteries, especially the trigeminal artery, and "angiomatous" malformations of intra- and extracranial blood vessels including aneurysmal dilatations and anomalous arteries mostly located at the carotid siphon and hypothalamus. The most common congenital vascular anomalies associated with PHACE(S) include an aberrant origin or course of major cerebral vessels, arterial absence or agenesis, saccular aneurysms, arterial dysplasia, and persistence of fetal anastomoses.[63] Progressive vasculopathy associated with PHACE(S) was first demonstrated by Burrows and colleagues.[63,67] In that series, progressive arterial obstruction led to ischemic stroke in 4 patients. Less commonly, patients with PHACE(S) can develop moyamoyalike progressive vasculopathy and resultant ischemic strokes. Burrows and colleagues[67] reported that of the 4 patients in their study with PHACE(S) and ischemic strokes, 3 had moyamoyalike collateral vessel proliferation. Among other studies reporting acute ischemic infarct in patients with a clear diagnosis of PHACE(S), the average age of symptom onset was 8.8 months, with ages ranging from 3 to 18 months. The most common presenting symptoms of infarct in these patients were seizures and hemiparesis.

Focal cerebral dysplasia rarely occurs in association with this syndrome. Lesions reported in patients with PHACE(S) include pachygyria, polymicrogyria, cortical thickening, heterotopic gray matter, and cerebral volume loss. The lesions also tend to occur ipsilateral to the facial hemangioma.[63,68]

Treating children with PHACE(S) is difficult because they are simultaneously at risk for ischemia as well as hemorrhage. There are no established guidelines for treatment of these patients, but there are many reports describing the use of corticosteroids and aspirin. Burrows and colleagues[67] suggest that therapies used to treat cutaneous hemangiomas may be helpful in treating the cerebrovascular disease associated with PHACE(S). In their series, 9 of 10 patients with PHACE(S) and ischemic strokes were treated with systemic corticosteroids or interferon therapies, which promote the regression of hemangiomas by modulating the cytokine pathways that regulate angiogenesis. However, one should consider that inhibition of angiogenesis in a patient with moyamoyalike vasculopathy could prevent formation of the collateral circulation necessary to maintain cerebral blood flow, potentially leading to ischemia and infarcts. Strater and colleagues[69] recommended starting aspirin therapy in patients with PHACE(S) suffering from acute ischemic infarct, as there is at least a 6% risk of recurrent stroke in infants with acute ischemic infarct beyond 6 months of age.

WYBURN-MASON SYNDROME

In 1943, Wyburn-Mason[70] studied 27 patients with retinal AVMs and found 81% also had intracranial AVMs. The syndrome he described is now known to be a congenital neurocutaneous syndrome of ipsilateral AVMs of the midbrain, vascular abnormalities affecting the visual pathway (often retinal or orbital AVMs), and facial nevi. The mean age at diagnosis is 23 years for males and 16 years for females.[71] Although there are no strict diagnostic criteria for the syndrome, the presence of all 3 classic features are generally not required for a diagnosis of Wyburn-Mason syndrome.

It is likely that Wyburn-Mason syndrome is the result of an abnormality in the primitive vascular mesoderm that is shared by the developing optic cup and anterior neural tube. Disturbance of these developing tissues before the seventh week of gestation leads to persistence of primitive vascular tissues, affecting both the eye and ipsilateral mesencephalon.[71] Disturbances that occur after the seventh week typically affect only 1 of the 2 structures.[72] However, bilateral cases of Wyburn-Mason syndrome have been reported and are more difficult to explain developmentally.[73]

Facial nevi characteristic of Wyburn-Mason syndrome include angiomas affecting the skin in the distribution of the trigeminal nerve. Dayani and colleagues[71] found that 14 of the 27 patients in their study exhibited facial nevi, whereas Theron and colleagues[74] found that 8 of 25 patients had them. These lesions may also affect deeper structures such as frontal or maxillary sinuses or the mandible. Manipulation of these lesions may lead to significant hemorrhage.

Retinal and orbital AVMs are also associated with Wyburn-Mason syndrome, but are not required for diagnosis. Approximately 30% of Wyburn-Mason patients have retinal AVMs.[71] These lesions commonly present with a progressive or acute decline in visual acuity, proptosis, papillary defects, optic atrophy, and visual field defects. Retinal AVMs are typically more stable than intracranial AVMs.[71] Patients presenting with retinal AVMs should undergo MRI and MRA imaging of the brain and orbit to detect additional AVMs. Changes in retinal AVMs have not been shown to have predictive value in the behavior of cerebral vascular malformations.[75]

The presentation of patients with intracranial AVMs is variable. They are most commonly found in the hypothalamus, thalamus, optic chiasm, and suprasellar area. Many patients are asymptomatic, but among those who experience symptoms, the most common presenting complaints are headaches, retro-orbital pain, and hemiparesis.[71] Patients may also present with developmental delay, irritability, cerebellar dysfunction, or Parinaud's syndrome. Like nonsyndromic AVMs, these lesions may present with spontaneous rupture. The treatment for patients with Wyburn-Mason syndrome is controversial. Occasionally, patients may be managed conservatively, with close observation for changes in lesions.[71] Surgical, radiosurgical, or endovascular treatment of AVMs can be performed with the same indications, risks, and benefits of AVMs not associated with the syndrome.

KLIPPEL-TRENAUNAY SYNDROME

Klippel-Trenaunay is a congenital syndrome characterized by cutaneous nevi, venous varices, and hemihypertrophy of bones and soft tissues, usually involving one of the extremities. This syndrome may also be associated with lesions characteristic of the Sturge-Weber syndrome, such as leptomeningeal vascular dysplasia; patients with such findings are said to have Klippel-Trenaunay-Weber syndrome.[76] Klippel-Trenaunay syndrome has also been associated with hydrocephalus, cerebral calcification, AVMs, hemimegalencephaly, and vascular malformations.[77,78] The syndrome is generally thought to occur sporadically, but some clinical manifestations have been found to cluster in families, suggesting a possible autosomal dominant inheritance pattern.[79] The cutaneous vascular nevi in Klippel-Trenaunay syndrome include port-wine stains, hemangiomas, or lymphangiomas.

Hemimegalencephaly, a congenital hamartomatous overgrowth of all or part of a cerebral hemisphere with changes in sulcation and pachygyria, is associated with Klippel-Trenaunay syndrome.[80] When present, hemimegalencephaly occurs on the same side as the cutaneous lesion and bony and soft tissue hypertrophy.[76,81] Hemimegalencephaly may be asymptomatic or may present with retardation or seizures.[82] Torregrosa and colleagues[76] found 18% of patients in their series had cerebral hemihypertrophy. The cause of this abnormality is unknown, but some authors have speculated that it may be attributable to mosaicism resulting in asymmetrical growth of the endo-, meso-, and ectoderm, which must occur before these 3 layers differentiate.[83,84]

There are approximately 24 reported cases of spinal AVMs associated with Klippel-Trenaunay syndrome in the literature.[85] Djindjian and colleagues[86] described 5 cases of Klippel-Trenaunay-Weber syndrome associated with intramedullary AVMs. Retromedullary arteriovenous fistulas and extradural thoracic AVMs have also been reported.[87,88] Treatment of these lesions does not differ from that for spinal vascular malformations not associated with the syndrome.

SINUS PERICRANII

Sinus pericranii is a rare and usually asymptomatic vascular condition in which there is an abnormal communication between the extracranial and intradural venous system through diploic veins in the skull. The condition was first described in 1845 by Hecker and again characterized in 1850 by Stromeyer as a "blood bag on the skull, in connection with the veins of the diploe and through these with the sinuses of the brain."[89–91] Sinus pericranii is typically diagnosed in childhood and may increase in size. Children often present at birth with a nonpulsatile soft tissue mass. A thrill can sometimes be felt with palpation of the lesion. The anomalous vessels enlarge with crying or when applying a Valsalva maneuver to create increased intracranial pressure, and diminish with compression or elevation of the head.[90] These lesions are typically located in the midline and frontally, although they can be located anywhere on the skull.[92]

The differential diagnosis of sinus pericranii is broad and includes subgaleal hematoma, pseudomeningocele, dermoid cysts, epidermoid cysts, hemangiomas, arteriovenous malformations, growing skull fracture, and skin lesions resulting in a subcutaneous soft scalp mass.[90,93,94] The work-up for these lesions typically begins with skull x-rays, head computed tomography (CT), or brain MRI looking for bony defects or associated cortical changes. Cranial ultrasound with color flow Doppler can demonstrate blood flow between the intradural venous sinuses into the extracranial lesion. Digital subtraction cerebral angiography remains the gold standard for diagnosis; however, CT angiography and magnetic resonance venogram are becoming increasingly useful aids for diagnosis and preventing the need for more invasive testing.

Most patients with sinus pericranii are asymptomatic, but they occasionally experience headaches, nausea, vertigo, local discomfort, mild cardiac failure, and signs and symptoms related to an associated vascular anomaly.[90,92] There is an association with intracranial venous anomalies, including vein of Galen hypoplasia, vein of Galen malformations, dural sinus malformations, solitary developmental venous anomalies, and intraosseous AVMs.[92,93,95–97]

Sinus pericranii can arise either as congenital lesions or acquired after trauma. The etiology of congenital sinus pericranii is unknown. Their association with developmental venous anomalies has led some to support a congenital cause from venous hypertension during the embryonic period, thereby altering early intracranial venous development.[93] The natural history of sinus pericranii is largely unknown, but prognosis is thought to be favorable as most show no change in size after puberty. Although rare, spontaneous involution of sinus pericranii has been reported in the literature.[90,98] The decision to offer surgical treatment is often based on cosmetic concerns. Although uncommon, sinus pericranii can occasionally lead to life-threatening complications from thrombosis or massive scalp hemorrhage.[90,93,94] Surgical treatment is aimed at prevention of associated complications and restoring cosmesis. Reported surgical options include craniotomy for excision of both the intradural and extracranial lesions, or local scalp incision with plugging of the boney venous channels using bone wax and bone dust.[90,98–100] Endovascular transvenous embolization for definitive treatment has been described; however, the long-term durability of this technique is unknown.[101]

VEIN OF GALEN MALFORMATION

Vein of Galen malformations are vascular anomalies of childhood that result from abnormal connections between distal branches of the choroidal and posterior cerebral arteries and the vein of Galen.[102,103] The development of these lesions occurs between weeks 6 and 11 of gestation, with a persistent embryonic prosencephalic vein of Markowski that drains into the vein of Galen.[104,105] These lesions may result in high blood flow through the fistula, occasionally resulting in an arterial steal phenomenon, ischemia, and cortical infarction.

There are 2 main classification systems used to describe vein of Galen malformations. Yasargil and colleagues[106] classified them into 4 categories in which types 1, 2, and 3 have no nidus and an artery or arteries directly connect with the vein of Galen. Type 4 malformations are true AVMs, with draining veins through the internal cerebral, basilar, or median atrial vein into the vein of Galen. Lasjaunias and colleagues[107,108] proposed another classification scheme for vein of Galen malformations, dividing them into choroidal and mural types based on location of the abnormal connection. Choroidal type malformations involve multiple fistulae, which connect with the anterior end of the median prosencephalic vein. The subependymal branches of thalamoperforators or subforniceal, pericallosal, or choroidal arteries supply choroidal type malformations. The fistula is located in the wall of the median prosencephalic vein in mural-type malformations. The posterior choroidal and collicular arteries supply mural-type malformations.

Vein of Galen malformations have an incidence rate of 1 in 25,000 deliveries and represent about 30% to 50% of all vascular malformations in children.[109–111] With the increasing use of prenatal ultrasound and MRI, in utero diagnosis is becoming more common.[102] Neonates typically present with macrocephaly, bruits, dilated orbital veins, and high-output heart failure. Infants present with symptoms attributable to hydrocephalus or seizures from focal compression on adjacent CNS structures. Older children and adults present with headaches, cognitive dysfunction, subarachnoid hemorrhage, and focal neurologic deficits.[110,112] The estimated morbidity and mortality for each hemorrhagic event in the pediatric population is 50% and 5% to 10%, respectively.[113–115] Neonatal presentation is the most common, encompassing 90% of cases, and carries a worse prognosis.[105] The presence or absence of cortical ischemia and high-output cardiac failure are the most important factors in determining prognosis.[105]

Endovascular embolization has become the treatment of choice for vein of Galen malformations.[114,116] Determining which children to treat and when to offer treatment has been controversial. Lasjaunias and colleagues[108,117] reviewed their single-institution series of patients with vein of Galen malformations treated over a 20-year period. Of the 371 patients evaluated, 233 were treated with endovascular embolization. In this series, 10.6% of patients died despite or because of treatment. Of the surviving patients, 10.4% survived with severe disability, 15.6% with moderate disability, and 74.0% were neurologically normal. Lasjaunias and colleagues developed a pediatric scoring system to better determine the timing of treatment and when treatment should be withheld in patients with vein of Galen malformations.[102,108,117] Giebprasert and colleagues[102] suggest that a small subgroup of patients will have a good outcome with conservative management and are unlikely to require surgical intervention. Their criteria for conservative management included mild or well-controlled congestive heart failure; the absence of parenchymal loss, calcifications, hydrocephalus, tonsillar herniation, or evidence of arterial steal on imaging; a high neonatal admission score; and findings suggestive of low-flow shunts (2 or fewer arterial feeding vessels, no deep veinous drainage, or no jugular bulb stenosis). Poor prognosis is suggested by severe heart failure with multiorgan failure, or a combination of brain damage, poor clinical status, calcifications on imaging, arterial steal, and an overall poor clinical status. For patients in whom treatment is considered, the timing of treatment remains controversial. Giebprasert and colleagues[102] suggest more urgent treatment if the patient exhibits deterioration of cardiac function, arterial steal, developing hydrocephalus, progressive jugular bulb stenosis, or developmental delay. For all patients, close follow-up is suggested with a brain MRI at least at birth and between 4 to 5 months of age. If the patient remains clinically and radiologically stable, then treatment is offered at 4 to 5 months of age.[102,105]

BLUE RUBBER BLEB NEVUS SYNDROME

Blue rubber blev nevus syndrome (BRBN) syndrome is a rare congenital disorder first described by Gascoyen in 1860.[118] He took note of the association between cutaneous vascular nevi and gastrointestinal bleeding. Bean[119] coined the unique term "blue rubber bleb nevus syndrome" in 1958 to describe the cutaneous vascular malformations that "have the look and feel of rubber nipples." BRBN primarily involves the skin and gastrointestinal tract. However, vascular lesions may be present in other organs, including lung, pleura, pericardium, heart, liver, spleen, peritoneum, tongue, skeletal muscle, urogenital system, eye, and nasopharynx.[120] The cutaneous lesions are malformations of venules or capillaries with a cyanotic appearance and an elevated nipplelike center. Gastrointestinal malformations typically involve the small intestines and often bleed causing iron deficiency anemia. CNS involvement of BRBN was first described in 1978 by Waybright and colleagues.[121] Patients with BRBN of the CNS typically present with seizures, developmental delay, or focal neurologic deficits. There have been 8 reported cases in the literature of BRBN with CNS involvement. These lesions are readily seen on brain MRI as multiple enhancing vascular lesions, cortical atrophy, or venous sinus malformations.[122]

MELAS

The acronym MELAS refers to a syndrome characterized by *m*itochondrial myopathy (M), *e*ncephalopathy (E), and *l*actic (L) *a*cidosis (A) with *s*trokelike (S) episodes. MELAS is one of the most frequently occurring mitochondrial encephalomyopathies. It is maternally inherited, with onset usually in the first decade of life. Strokelike episodes often occur before the age of 15 years. The clinical course is highly variable, ranging from asymptomatic to progressive muscle weakness, lactic acidosis, cognitive dysfunction, seizures, strokelike episodes, encephalopathy, and death.[123] MELAS is associated with many point mutations in mitochondrial DNA, over 80% of which occur in the dihydrouridine loop of the mitochondrial transfer RNA. There is currently no clear consensus on diagnostic criteria for MELAS. It is usually diagnosed by muscle biopsy that demonstrates ragged-red fibers, COX-negative fibers, and abnormally shaped mitochondria with paracrystalline inclusions. Diagnosis is further confirmed by demonstration of a biochemical respiratory chain defect or one of the known mutations that causes MELAS.[124] Most affected children meet early milestones normally. They may present later with headaches, recurrent vomiting, seizures, and neurologic deficits resembling ischemic strokes. Many also complain of easy fatigability, short stature, and progressive sensorineural hearing loss.[125]

The strokelike episodes associated with MELAS are recurrent cerebral events that do not conform to discreet vascular territories. These episodes may be transient and nondisabling. Pathogenesis of the strokelike episodes remains unknown, but 2 major theories have been proposed. The first attributes them to mitochondrial angiopathy, with degenerative changes in small arteries and arterioles. The second suggests that these are likely nonischemic events and attributes them to mitochondrial cytopathy characterized by increased capillary permeability, hyperperfusion, neuronal vulnerability, and hyperexcitability.[126] A specific mechanism for this has been proposed by Iizuka and colleagues[127]: mitochondrial dysfunction in a localized area may cause neuronal hyperexcitability, which then leads to depolarization of adjacent neurons and epileptic activity that spreads to the surrounding cortex. This activity causes increased capillary permeability, leading to the edematous lesions seen predominantly in the cortex on imaging during the strokelike episodes. This is supported by the finding of local cerebral hyperemia that may reflect vasodilation in response to local metabolic acidosis in the area of infarct.[128]

There is no clear treatment paradigm for MELAS, although the results of recent medical therapies have been encouraging. L-arginine is an amino acid that plays an important role in endothelial-dependent vascular relaxation. Koga and colleagues[129–132] found decreased plasma concentrations of L-arginine in patients with MELAS compared with controls in both the acute phase of strokelike episodes and the period between episodes. Patients treated with L-arginine during the acute phase of strokelike episodes had symptoms that were significantly improved. Oral administration of L-arginine decreased the frequency and severity of strokelike episodes, and improved endothelial function to that of controls at 2-year follow-up.

RADIATION-INDUCED VASCULOPATHY

Intracranial vasculopathy is occasionally seen following radiotherapy to the head and neck.[133–135] Vasculopathy following radiation is much more common in small vessels than in medium and large vessels.[136] A review of 345 patients who underwent therapeutic radiation for a primary brain tumor found that 9.6% had vascular abnormalities on neuroimaging.[137] Most reported cases presented with vasculopathy many years following radiation treatment, but presentations as early as 15 months after treatment have been described.[138] Radiation-induced vascular disorders include thrombosis, hemorrhage, aneurysm formation, arterial dissection, moyamoya syndrome, fibrinous exudates, telangiectasias, vascular fibrosis/hyalinization with luminal stenosis, and fibrinoid vascular necrosis.[139] A large review by Scott and colleagues[140] found that among 345 patients, 10 had vessel ectasia or narrowing, 12 had moyamoya disease, and 3 had hemorrhagic radiation vasculopathy.

Endothelial cells are an actively proliferating site within the brain and are, therefore, one of the most vulnerable to radiation toxicity. Huvos and colleagues[141] demonstrated that accelerated atheroma formation, rather than inflammation, is likely the pathologic process induced by radiation in large arteries. Histologic studies of vessels exposed to therapeutic radiation revealed fibrous thickening of the adventitia, intimal hyperplasia, hyaline thickening, and exuberant loose connective tissue production with relative sparing of the media.[138] Changes are most often noted in small cerebral arteries and white matter, often sparing medium- and large-sized arteries.[142,143]

Individual risk factors for radiation-induced vascular disease are not well defined but, in general, younger patients are more vulnerable.[139] Biologic data and case reports suggest that radiation involving the circle of Willis and patients who have neurofibromatosis type 1 may be at increased risk of developing moyamoyalike vascular changes.[137,140] In a study by Scott and colleagues,[140] among 15 cases of postradiation moyamoya, 8 were treated for hypothalamic-optic gliomas and 4 for craniopharyngioma. The same study also suggests that the development of moyamoya after radiation is both dose- and time-dependent.[137] This may also prove to be true of other vascular changes associated with radiation.

Guidelines for evaluation and treatment of radiation-induced vasculopathies are not clearly defined. In general, clinical deterioration not explained by tumor recurrence should prompt evaluation by MRI, MRA, or conventional angiography. Treatment varies depending on the specific type and extent of vascular abnormality, but in general, is the same as treatment for similar abnormalities not caused by radiation.

REFERENCES

1. Acciarri N, Galassi E, Giulioni M, et al. Cavernous malformations of the central nervous system in the pediatric age group. Pediatr Neurosurg 2009;45:81–104.
2. Herter T, Brandt M, Szuwart U. Cavernous hemangiomas in children. Childs Nerv Syst 1988;4:123–7.
3. Mazza C, Scienza R, Beltramello A, et al. Cerebral cavernous malformations (cavernomas) in the pediatric age-group. Childs Nerv Syst 1991;7:139–46.
4. Rigamonti D, Hadley MN, Drayer BP, et al. Cerebral cavernous malformations. Incidence and familial occurrence. N Engl J Med 1988;319:343–7.
5. Clatterbuck RE, Eberhart CG, Crain BJ, et al. Ultrastructural and immunocytochemical evidence that an incompetent blood-brain barrier is related to the pathophysiology of cavernous malformations. J Neurol Neurosurg Psychiatry 2001;71:188–92.
6. Russell DS, Rubenstein LJ. Russell & Rubenstein's pathology of tumors of the nervous system. Baltimore (MD): Williams & Wilkins; 1989.
7. Bicknell JM. Familial cavernous angioma of the brain stem dominantly inherited in Hispanics. Neurosurgery 1989;24:102–5.
8. Hayman LA, Evans RA, Ferrell RE, et al. Familial cavernous angiomas: natural history and genetic study over a 5-year period. Am J Med Genet 1982;11:147–60.
9. Labauge P, Laberge S, Brunereau L, et al. Hereditary cerebral cavernous angiomas: clinical and genetic features in 57 French families. Societe Francaise de Neurochirurgie. Lancet 1998;352:1892–7.
10. Mason I, Aase JM, Orrison WW, et al. Familial cavernous angiomas of the brain in an Hispanic family. Neurology 1988;38:324–6.
11. Mottolese C, Hermier M, Stan H, et al. Central nervous system cavernomas in the pediatric age group. Neurosurg Rev 2001;24:55–73.
12. Pozzati E, Acciarri N, Tognetti F, et al. Growth, subsequent bleeding, and de novo appearance of cerebral cavernous angiomas. Neurosurgery 1996;38:662–70.
13. Zabramski JM, Wascher TM, Spetzler RF, et al. The natural history of familial cavernous malformations: results of an ongoing study. J Neurosurg 1994;80:422–32.
14. Pozzati E, Giuliani G, Nuzzo G, et al. The growth of cerebral cavernous angiomas. Neurosurgery 1989;25:92–7.
15. Kattapong VJ, Hart BL, Davis LE. Familial cerebral cavernous angiomas: clinical and radiologic studies. Neurology 1995;45:492–7.
16. Notelet L, Chapon F, Khoury S, et al. Familial cavernous malformations in a large French kindred: mapping of the gene to the CCM1 locus on chromosome 7q. J Neurol Neurosurg Psychiatry 1997;63:40–5.
17. Labauge P, Brunereau L, Laberge S, et al. Prospective follow-up of 33 asymptomatic patients with familial cerebral cavernous malformations. Neurology 2001;57:1825–8.
18. Barker FG 2nd, Amin-Hanjani S, Butler WE, et al. Temporal clustering of hemorrhages from untreated cavernous malformations of the central nervous system. Neurosurgery 2001;49:15–25.
19. Lena G, Ternier J, Paz-Paredes A, et al. [Central nervous system cavernomas in children]. Neurochirurgie 2007;53:223–37 [in French].
20. Maraire JN, Awad IA. Intracranial cavernous malformations: lesion behavior and management strategies. Neurosurgery 1995;37:591–605.
21. Cohen-Gadol AA, Jacob JT, Edwards DA, et al. Coexistence of intracranial and spinal cavernous malformations: a study of prevalence and natural history. J Neurosurg 2006;104:376–81.
22. Duhem R, Vinchon M, Leblond P, et al. Cavernous malformations after cerebral irradiation during childhood: report of nine cases. Childs Nerv Syst 2005;21:922–5.
23. Narayan P, Barrow DL. Intramedullary spinal cavernous malformation following spinal irradiation. Case report and review of the literature. J Neurosurg 2003;98:68–72.
24. Porter RW, Detwiler PW, Spetzler RF, et al. Cavernous malformations of the brainstem: experience with 100 patients. J Neurosurg 1999;90:50–8.
25. Wurm G, Schnizer M, Fellner FA. Cerebral cavernous malformations associated with venous anomalies: surgical considerations. Neurosurgery 2005;57:42–58.
26. Brouillard P, Vikkula M. Genetic causes of vascular malformations. Hum Mol Genet 2007;16(Spec No 2):R140–9.
27. Dubovsky J, Zabramski JM, Kurth J, et al. A gene responsible for cavernous malformations of the brain maps to chromosome 7q. Hum Mol Genet 1995;4:453–8.
28. Hanjani SA. The genetics of cerebrovascular malformations. J Stroke Cerebrovasc Dis 2002;11:279–87.
29. Bergametti F, Denier C, Labauge P, et al. Mutations within the programmed cell death 10 gene cause cerebral cavernous malformations. Am J Hum Genet 2005;76:42–51.
30. Craig HD, Gunel M, Cepeda O, et al. Multilocus linkage identifies two new loci for a Mendelian form of stroke, cerebral cavernous malformation, at 7p15-13 and 3q25.2-27. Hum Mol Genet 1998;7:1851–8.
31. Liquori CL, Berg MJ, Siegel AM, et al. Mutations in a gene encoding a novel protein containing

a phosphotyrosine-binding domain cause type 2 cerebral cavernous malformations. Am J Hum Genet 2003;73:1459–64.
32. Liquori CL, Berg MJ, Squitieri F, et al. Low frequency of PDCD10 mutations in a panel of CCM3 probands: potential for a fourth CCM locus. Hum Mutat 2006;27:118.
33. Zawistowski JS, Serebriiskii IG, Lee MF, et al. KRIT1 association with the integrin-binding protein ICAP-1: a new direction in the elucidation of cerebral cavernous malformations (CCM1) pathogenesis. Hum Mol Genet 2002;11:389–96.
34. Zhang J, Clatterbuck RE, Rigamonti D, et al. Interaction between krit1 and icap1alpha infers perturbation of integrin beta1-mediated angiogenesis in the pathogenesis of cerebral cavernous malformation. Hum Mol Genet 2001;10:2953–60.
35. Chen L, Tanriover G, Yano H, et al. Apoptotic functions of PDCD10/CCM3, the gene mutated in cerebral cavernous malformation 3. Stroke 2009;40: 1474–81.
36. Penco S, Ratti R, Bianchi E, et al. Molecular screening test in familial forms of cerebral cavernous malformation: the impact of the Multiplex Ligation-dependent Probe Amplification approach. J Neurosurg 2009;110:929–34.
37. Lee JW, Kim DS, Shim KW, et al. Management of intracranial cavernous malformation in pediatric patients. Childs Nerv Syst 2008;24:321–7.
38. Xia C, Zhang R, Mao Y, et al. Pediatric cavernous malformation in the central nervous system: report of 66 cases. Pediatr Neurosurg 2009;45:105–13.
39. Guttmacher AE, Marchuk DA, White RI Jr. Hereditary hemorrhagic telangiectasia. N Engl J Med 1995;333:918–24.
40. Porteous ME, Burn J, Proctor SJ. Hereditary haemorrhagic telangiectasia: a clinical analysis. J Med Genet 1992;29:527–30.
41. Bayrak-Toydemir P, Mao R, Lewin S, et al. Hereditary hemorrhagic telangiectasia: an overview of diagnosis and management in the molecular era for clinicians. Genet Med 2004;6:175–91.
42. Sharathkumar AA, Shapiro A. Hereditary haemorrhagic telangiectasia. Haemophilia 2008;14:1269–80.
43. Aassar OS, Friedman CM, White RI Jr. The natural history of epistaxis in hereditary hemorrhagic telangiectasia. Laryngoscope 1991;101:977–80.
44. Vase P, Grove O. Gastrointestinal lesions in hereditary hemorrhagic telangiectasia. Gastroenterology 1986;91:1079–83.
45. Plauchu H, de Chadarevian JP, Bideau A, et al. Age-related clinical profile of hereditary hemorrhagic telangiectasia in an epidemiologically recruited population. Am J Med Genet 1989;32: 291–7.
46. Maher CO, Piepgras DG, Brown RD Jr, et al. Cerebrovascular manifestations in 321 cases of hereditary hemorrhagic telangiectasia. Stroke 2001;32:877–82.
47. Shovlin CL, Guttmacher AE, Buscarini E, et al. Diagnostic criteria for hereditary hemorrhagic telangiectasia (Rendu-Osler-Weber syndrome). Am J Med Genet 2000;91:66–7.
48. Fulbright RK, Chaloupka JC, Putman CM, et al. MR of hereditary hemorrhagic telangiectasia: prevalence and spectrum of cerebrovascular malformations. AJNR Am J Neuroradiol 1998;19:477–84.
49. Willemse RB, Mager JJ, Westermann CJ, et al. Bleeding risk of cerebrovascular malformations in hereditary hemorrhagic telangiectasia. J Neurosurg 2000;92:779–84.
50. Mont'Alverne F, Musacchio M, Tolentino V, et al. Giant spinal perimedullary fistula in hereditary haemorrhagic telangiectasia: diagnosis, endovascular treatment and review of the literature. Neuroradiology 2003;45:830–6.
51. Brown RD Jr, Wiebers DO, Forbes G, et al. The natural history of unruptured intracranial arteriovenous malformations. J Neurosurg 1988;68:352–7.
52. Jane JA, Kassell NF, Torner JC, et al. The natural history of aneurysms and arteriovenous malformations. J Neurosurg 1985;62:321–3.
53. Ondra SL, Troupp H, George ED, et al. The natural history of symptomatic arteriovenous malformations of the brain: a 24-year follow-up assessment. J Neurosurg 1990;73:387–91.
54. Spetzler RF, Hargraves RW, McCormick PW, et al. Relationship of perfusion pressure and size to risk of hemorrhage from arteriovenous malformations. J Neurosurg 1992;76:918–23.
55. Aesch B, Lioret E, de Toffol B, et al. Multiple cerebral angiomas and Rendu-Osler-Weber disease: case report. Neurosurgery 1991;29:599–602.
56. Kadoya C, Momota Y, Ikegami Y, et al. Central nervous system arteriovenous malformations with hereditary hemorrhagic telangiectasia: report of a family with three cases. Surg Neurol 1994;42: 234–9.
57. Willinsky RA, Lasjaunias P, Terbrugge K, et al. Multiple cerebral arteriovenous malformations (AVMs). Review of our experience from 203 patients with cerebral vascular lesions. Neuroradiology 1990;32:207–10.
58. Roman G, Fisher M, Perl DP, et al. Neurological manifestations of hereditary hemorrhagic telangiectasia (Rendu-Osler-Weber disease): report of 2 cases and review of the literature. Ann Neurol 1978;4:130–44.
59. Boillot O, Bianco F, Viale JP, et al. Liver transplantation resolves the hyperdynamic circulation in hereditary hemorrhagic telangiectasia with hepatic involvement. Gastroenterology 1999;116:187–92.
60. Frieden IJ, Reese V, Cohen D. PHACE syndrome. The association of posterior fossa brain

malformations, hemangiomas, arterial anomalies, coarctation of the aorta and cardiac defects, and eye abnormalities. Arch Dermatol 1996;132:307–11.
61. Metry DW, Dowd CF, Barkovich AJ, et al. The many faces of PHACE syndrome. J Pediatr 2001;139: 117–23.
62. Judd CD, Chapman PR, Koch B, et al. Intracranial infantile hemangiomas associated with PHACE syndrome. AJNR Am J Neuroradiol 2007;28:25–9.
63. Heyer GL, Millar WS, Ghatan S, et al. The neurologic aspects of PHACE: case report and review of the literature. Pediatr Neurol 2006;35:419–24.
64. Poetke M, Frommeld T, Berlien HP. PHACE syndrome: new views on diagnostic criteria. Eur J Pediatr Surg 2002;12:366–74.
65. Hirsch JF, Pierre-Kahn A, Renier D, et al. The Dandy-Walker malformation. A review of 40 cases. J Neurosurg 1984;61:515–22.
66. Pascual-Castroviejo I. Vascular and nonvascular intracranial malformation associated with external capillary hemangiomas. Neuroradiology 1978;16: 82–4.
67. Burrows PE, Robertson RL, Mulliken JB, et al. Cerebral vasculopathy and neurologic sequelae in infants with cervicofacial hemangioma: report of eight patients. Radiology 1998;207:601–7.
68. Grosso S, De Cosmo L, Bonifazi E, et al. Facial hemangioma and malformation of the cortical development: a broadening of the PHACE spectrum or a new entity? Am J Med Genet A 2004; 124:192–5.
69. Strater R, Becker S, von Eckardstein A, et al. Prospective assessment of risk factors for recurrent stroke during childhood—a 5-year follow-up study. Lancet 2002;360:1540–5.
70. Wyburn-Mason R. Arteriovenous aneurysm of midbrain and retina, facial naevi and mental changes. Brain 1943;66:163–203.
71. Dayani PN, Sadun AA. A case report of Wyburn-Mason syndrome and review of the literature. Neuroradiology 2007;49:445–56.
72. Ponce FA, Han PP, Spetzler RF, et al. Associated arteriovenous malformation of the orbit and brain: a case of Wyburn-Mason syndrome without retinal involvement. Case report. J Neurosurg 2001;95: 346–9.
73. Kim J, Kim OH, Suh JH, et al. Wyburn-Mason syndrome: an unusual presentation of bilateral orbital and unilateral brain arteriovenous malformations. Pediatr Radiol 1998;28:161.
74. Theron J, Newton TH, Hoyt WF. Unilateral retinocephalic vascular malformations. Neuroradiology 1974;7:185–96.
75. Augsburger JJ, Goldberg RE, Shields JA, et al. Changing appearance of retinal arteriovenous malformation. Albrecht Von Graefes Arch Klin Exp Ophthalmol 1980;215:65–70.
76. Torregrosa A, Marti-Bonmati L, Higueras V, et al. Klippel-Trenaunay syndrome: frequency of cerebral and cerebellar hemihypertrophy on MRI. Neuroradiology 2000;42:420–3.
77. Cristaldi A, Vigevano F, Antoniazzi G, et al. Hemimegalencephaly, hemihypertrophy and vascular lesions. Eur J Pediatr 1995;154:134–7.
78. Williams DW 3rd, Elster AD. Cranial CT and MR in the Klippel-Trenaunay-Weber syndrome. AJNR Am J Neuroradiol 1992;13:291–4.
79. Aelvoet GE, Jorens PG, Roelen LM. Genetic aspects of the Klippel-Trenaunay syndrome. Br J Dermatol 1992;126:603–7.
80. Wolpert SM, Cohen A, Libenson MH. Hemimegalencephaly: a longitudinal MR study. AJNR Am J Neuroradiol 1994;15:1479–82.
81. Anlar B, Yalaz K, Erzen C. Klippel-Trenaunay-Weber syndrome: a case with cerebral and cerebellar hemihypertrophy. Neuroradiology 1988;30: 360.
82. Chen PC, Shu WC. Klippel-Trenaunay-Weber syndrome with hemimegalencephaly: report of one case. Zhonghua Min Guo Xiao Er Ke Yi Xue Hui Za Zhi 1996;37:138–41.
83. Dean JC, Cole GF, Appleton RE, et al. Cranial hemihypertrophy and neurodevelopmental prognosis. J Med Genet 1990;27:160–4.
84. Stephan MJ, Hall BD, Smith DW, et al. Macrocephaly in association with unusual cutaneous angiomatosis. J Pediatr 1975;87:353–9.
85. Rohany M, Shaibani A, Arafat O, et al. Spinal arteriovenous malformations associated with Klippel-Trenaunay-Weber syndrome: a literature search and report of two cases. AJNR Am J Neuroradiol 2007;28:584–9.
86. Djindjian M, Djindjian R, Hurth M, et al. Spinal cord arteriovenous malformations and the Klippel-Trenaunay-Weber syndrome. Surg Neurol 1977;8: 229–37.
87. Alexander MJ, Grossi PM, Spetzler RF, et al. Extradural thoracic arteriovenous malformation in a patient with Klippel-Trenaunay-Weber syndrome: case report. Neurosurgery 2002;51:1275–9.
88. Benhaiem-Sigaux N, Zerah M, Gherardi R, et al. A retromedullary arteriovenous fistula associated with the Klippel-Trenaunay-Weber syndrome. A clinicopathologic study. Acta Neuropathol 1985; 66:318–24.
89. Bollar A, Allut AG, Prieto A, et al. Sinus pericranii: radiological and etiopathological considerations. Case report. J Neurosurg 1992;77:469–72.
90. Rozen WM, Joseph S, Lo PA. Spontaneous involution of two sinus pericranii—a unique case and review of the literature. J Clin Neurosci 2008;15: 833–5.
91. Stromeyer. About sinus pericranii (translating of original 1850 text). Surg Neurol 1993;40:3–4.

92. Gandolfo C, Krings T, Alvarez H, et al. Sinus pericranii: diagnostic and therapeutic considerations in 15 patients. Neuroradiology 2007;49:505–14.
93. Nomura S, Kato S, Ishihara H, et al. Association of intra- and extradural developmental venous anomalies, so-called venous angioma and sinus pericranii. Childs Nerv Syst 2006;22:428–31.
94. Vinas FC, Valenzuela S, Zuleta A. Literature review: sinus pericranii. Neurol Res 1994;16:471–4.
95. Beers GJ, Carter AP, Ordia JI, et al. Sinus pericranii with dural venous lakes. AJNR Am J Neuroradiol 1984;5:629–31.
96. Nakasu Y, Nakasu S, Minouchi K, et al. Multiple sinus pericranii with systemic angiomas: case report. Surg Neurol 1993;39:41–5.
97. Sakai K, Namba K, Meguro T, et al. Sinus pericranii associated with a cerebellar venous angioma—case report. Neurol Med Chir (Tokyo) 1997;37:464–7.
98. Higuchi M, Fujimoto Y, Ikeda H, et al. Sinus pericranii: neuroradiologic findings and clinical management. Pediatr Neurosurg 1997;27:325–8.
99. Kaido T, Kim YK, Ueda K. Diagnostic and therapeutic considerations for sinus pericranii. J Clin Neurosci 2006;13:788–92.
100. Lo PA, Besser M, Lam AH. Sinus pericranii: a clinical and radiological review of an unusual condition. J Clin Neurosci 1997;4:247–52.
101. Brook AL, Gold MM, Farinhas JM, et al. Endovascular transvenous embolization of sinus pericranii. Case report. J Neurosurg Pediatr 2009;3:220–4.
102. Geibprasert S, Krings T, Armstrong D, et al. Predicting factors for the follow-up outcome and management decisions in vein of Galen aneurismal malformations. Childs Nerv Syst 2009 [Epub ahead of print].
103. Papanagiotou P, Rohrer T, Grunwald IQ, et al. Vein of Galen aneurysmal malformation treated with Onyx. Arch Neurol 2009;66:906–7.
104. Lasjaunias P, Alvarez H, Rodesch G, et al. Aneurysmal malformation of the vein of Galen, followup of 120 children treated between 1984 and 1994. Intervent Neuroradiol 1996;2:15–26.
105. Muquit S, Shah M, Bassi S. Vein of Galen malformation presenting in adulthood. Br J Neurosurg 2008;22:692–4.
106. Yasargil MG. Microneurosurgery, vol. IIIB. Stuttgart (Germany): Georg Thieme Verlag; 1988. 323–57.
107. Berenstein A, Lasjaunias P. Arteriovenous fistulas of the brain. Surgical neuroangiography: endovascular treatment of cerebral lesions. Berlin: Springer-Verlag; 1993. 267–317.
108. Lasjaunias PL, Chng SM, Sachet M, et al. The management of vein of Galen aneurysmal malformations. Neurosurgery 2006;59:S184–94.
109. Lasjaunias P, Hui F, Zerah M, et al. Cerebral arteriovenous malformations in children. Management of 179 consecutive cases and review of the literature. Childs Nerv Syst 1995;11:66–79.
110. Shinkar RM, Clarke P. Images in paediatrics. Vein of Galen aneurysmal malformation presenting as prominent scalp veins. Arch Dis Child 2008;93:1006.
111. Smith ER, Butler WE, Ogilvy CS. Surgical approaches to vascular anomalies of the child's brain. Curr Opin Neurol 2002;15:165–71.
112. Gold AP, Ransohoff JR, Carter S. Vein of Galen malformation. Acta Neurol Scand 1964;40(Suppl 11):5.
113. Gerosa MA, Cappellotto P, Licata C, et al. Cerebral arteriovenous malformations in children (56 cases). Childs Brain 1981;8:356–71.
114. Jankowitz BT, Vora N, Jovin T, et al. Treatment of pediatric intracranial vascular malformations using Onyx-18. J Neurosurg Pediatr 2008;2:171–6.
115. Wilkins RH. Natural history of intracranial vascular malformations: a review. Neurosurgery 1985;16:421–30.
116. van der Schaaf I, Fransen H. Endovascular treatment of vein of Galen aneurysmal malformation. JBR-BTR 2009;92:25–8.
117. Lasjaunias P, Berenstein A, terBrugge KG. Surgical neuroangiography: clinical and interventional aspects in children. 2nd edition. Berlin: Springer-Verlag; 2006.
118. Gascoyen M. Case of naevus involving the parotid gland, and causing death from suffocation: naevi of the viscera. Trans Pathol Soc Lond 1860;11:267.
119. Bean WB. Vascular spiders and related lesions of the skin. Springfield (MA): Thomas; 1958.
120. Moodley M, Ramdial P. Blue rubber bleb nevus syndrome: case report and review of the literature. Pediatrics 1993;92:160–2.
121. Waybright EA, Selhorst JB, Rosenblum WI, et al. Blue rubber bleb nevus syndrome with CNS involvement and thrombosis of a vein of Galen malformation. Ann Neurol 1978;3:464–7.
122. Park CO, Park J, Chung KY. Blue rubber bleb nevus syndrome with central nervous system involvement. J Dermatol 2006;33:649–51.
123. Scaglia F, Northrop JL. The mitochondrial myopathy encephalopathy, lactic acidosis with stroke-like episodes (MELAS) syndrome: a review of treatment options. CNS Drugs 2006;20:443–64.
124. Finsterer J. [MELAS syndrome as a differential diagnosis of ischemic stroke]. Fortschr Neurol Psychiatr 2009;77:25–31 [in German].
125. Longo N, Schrijver I, Vogel H, et al. Progressive cerebral vascular degeneration with mitochondrial encephalopathy. Am J Med Genet A 2008;146:361–7.
126. Ohama E, Ohara S, Ikuta F, et al. Mitochondrial angiopathy in cerebral blood vessels of mitochondrial encephalomyopathy. Acta Neuropathol 1987;74:226–33.

127. Iizuka T, Sakai F. Pathogenesis of stroke-like episodes in MELAS: analysis of neurovascular cellular mechanisms. Curr Neurovasc Res 2005;2: 29–45.
128. Gropen TI, Prohovnik I, Tatemichi TK, et al. Cerebral hyperemia in MELAS. Stroke 1994;25:1873–6.
129. Koga Y, Akita Y, Junko N, et al. Endothelial dysfunction in MELAS improved by L-arginine supplementation. Neurology 2006;66:1766–9.
130. Koga Y, Akita Y, Nishioka J, et al. MELAS and L-arginine therapy. Mitochondrion 2007;7:133–9.
131. Koga Y, Akita Y, Nishioka J, et al. L-arginine improves the symptoms of strokelike episodes in MELAS. Neurology 2005;64:710–2.
132. Koga Y, Ishibashi M, Ueki I, et al. Effects of L-arginine on the acute phase of strokes in three patients with MELAS. Neurology 2002;58:827–8.
133. Bowen J, Paulsen CA. Stroke after pituitary irradiation. Stroke 1992;23:908–11.
134. Grenier Y, Tomita T, Marymont MH, et al. Late post-irradiation occlusive vasculopathy in childhood medulloblastoma. Report of two cases. J Neurosurg 1998;89:460–4.
135. Painter MJ, Chutorian AM, Hilal SK. Cerebrovasculopathy following irradiation in childhood. Neurology 1975;25:189–94.
136. Omura M, Aida N, Sekido K, et al. Large intracranial vessel occlusive vasculopathy after radiation therapy in children: clinical features and usefulness of magnetic resonance imaging. Int J Radiat Oncol Biol Phys 1997;38:241–9.
137. Ullrich NJ, Robertson R, Kinnamon DD, et al. Moyamoya following cranial irradiation for primary brain tumors in children. Neurology 2007;68:932–8.
138. Maher CO, Raffel C. Early vasculopathy following radiation in a child with medulloblastoma. Pediatr Neurosurg 2000;32:255–8.
139. Perry A, Schmidt RE. Cancer therapy-associated CNS neuropathology: an update and review of the literature. Acta Neuropathol 2006;111:197–212.
140. Scott RM, Smith JL, Robertson RL, et al. Long-term outcome in children with moyamoya syndrome after cranial revascularization by pial synangiosis. J Neurosurg 2004;100:142–9.
141. Huvos AG, Leaming RH, Moore OS. Clinicopathologic study of the resected carotid artery. Analysis of sixty-four cases. Am J Surg 1973;126:570–4.
142. Laitt RD, Chambers EJ, Goddard PR, et al. Magnetic resonance imaging and magnetic resonance angiography in long term survivors of acute lymphoblastic leukemia treated with cranial irradiation. Cancer 1995;76:1846–52.
143. Paakko E, Talvensaari K, Pyhtinen J, et al. Late cranial MRI after cranial irradiation in survivors of childhood cancer. Neuroradiology 1994;36:652–5.

Diagnosis and Management of Arteriovenous Malformations in Children

Toba N. Niazi, MD[a], Paul Klimo Jr, MD, MPH, Maj, USAF[b,*], Richard C.E. Anderson, MD[c], Corey Raffel, MD, PhD[d,e]

KEYWORDS

- Arteriovenous malformation • Pediatric
- Children • Treatment • Outcomes • Surgery
- Radiosurgery • Embolization

Cerebral arteriovenous malformations (AVMs) are congenital lesions thought to arise because of failure of embryogenesis during the differentiation of vascular channels into mature arteries, capillaries, and veins, which results in direct arteriovenous shunts without intervening capillary beds.[1] Three major types of AVMs have been identified: (1) the more common high-flow variant with a compact nidus and few arterial feeders and draining veins; (2) the rarer diffuse variant with low-flow and multiple en-passage arterial feeders and draining veins[2,3]; and (3) the recently described linear, vein-based configuration with multiple arterial feeders draining into a single, usually superficial, vein.[4] Cerebral AVMs most often become symptomatic in the second to fourth decades of life, presenting with hemorrhage, seizures, or progressive neurologic deficits. Despite the congenital nature of the disease, cerebral AVMs are less commonly discovered in children than in adults, with children composing only 3% to 19% of AVM patients.[5,6]

Intracranial hemorrhage is the most frequent clinical presentation of AVMs in children and adults, and 80% to 85% of pediatric patients suffer a hemorrhagic event as the initial presenting symptom compared with their adult counterparts who present with hemorrhage in 50% to 65% of cases.[5–9] Hemorrhagic events from an AVM in children have been associated with a 25% mortality rate, whereas the mortality rate from hemorrhage in adults is 6% to 10%.[10,11] One explanation for this discrepancy is the propensity of posterior fossa (**Fig. 1**) and deep-seated AVMs (eg, in the basal ganglia) to hemorrhage in children. The annual rate of rebleeding in the pediatric population may be higher than that seen in the adult population (2%–4% in children vs 1%–3% in adults), although not all investigators are in agreement with this assertion.[8] If this risk of hemorrhage or rehemorrhage is stratified (projected) over a 50-year horizon to account for a child's longer life expectancy, the probability of rehemorrhage is in the order of 65%. The high cumulative risk of

[a] Department of Neurosurgery, Primary Children's Medical Center, University of Utah, 100 North Mario Capecchi Drive, Salt Lake City, UT, USA
[b] 88th Medical Group, SGOS/SGCXN, 4881 Sugar Maple Drive, Wright-Patterson Air Force Base, OH 45433, USA
[c] Department of Neurosurgery, Columbia University College of Physicians and Surgeons, 710 West 168th Street, Room 213, New York, NY 10032, USA
[d] Section of Pediatric Neurosurgery, Nationwide Children's Hospital, Columbus, OH, USA
[e] Department of Neurological Surgery, The Ohio State University College of Medicine, 700 Children's Drive, Columbus, OH 43205, USA
* Corresponding author.
E-mail address: atomkpnk@yahoo.com

Neurosurg Clin N Am 21 (2010) 443–456
doi:10.1016/j.nec.2010.03.012
1042-3680/10/$ – see front matter. Published by Elsevier Inc.

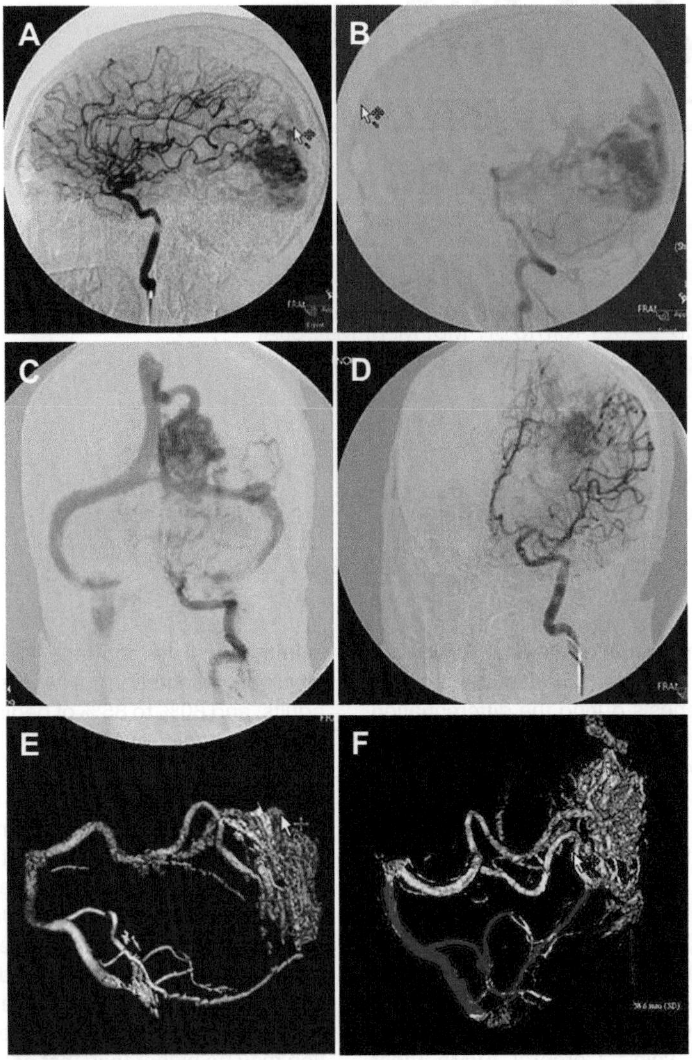

Fig. 1. (*A–F*) Large left occipital lobe AVM supplied predominantly by dilated left parietal, occipital, and calcarine arteries off the posterior cerebral artery. There is also supply from distal branches of the left middle cerebral artery and angular and temporo-occipital arteries.

hemorrhage during the long potential life span of the pediatric patient with an AVM underscores the importance of treating even asymptomatic AVMs in children. The natural history, pathology, diagnosis, and treatment of cerebral AVMs are discussed in this article.

INCIDENCE AND NATURAL HISTORY

Matson[12] evaluated 34 pediatric patients and declared AVM "the most frequent abnormality of intracranial circulation in childhood." Excluding hemorrhages of prematurity and early infancy, AVM is the most common cause of spontaneous intraparenchymal hemorrhage in children. Hence, a spontaneous intraparenchymal hemorrhage in a child should be considered an AVM until proven otherwise. Because most children diagnosed with AVMs undergo initial treatment emergently, the natural history of AVMs in the pediatric population is not well understood. As stated previously, children more likely present with hemorrhage than do adults, who tend to display presumed ischemic symptoms of headache, dementia, seizures, and progressive neurologic dysfunction.[11,13] Fewer than 15% of pediatric patients with AVM present with a chronic seizure disturbance, whereas epilepsy, which is presumed to develop from hypoxia caused by steal phenomenon associated with the adjacent AVM, occurs as a presenting symptom in 20% to 67% of adult patients with AVMs.[14]

As with presenting symptoms, there seem to be differences between young and old patients with AVM with regards to location and mortality rates. There is a higher incidence of AVMs located in the posterior fossa in children, whereas in adults AVMs are more likely to be supratentorial.[15] A higher percentage of AVMs are located in the basal ganglia and thalamus in children, and such lesions are more prone to bleeding.[1,8,16] The hemorrhagic effects of AVMs are less tolerable in the posterior fossa, and the outcome can be catastrophic. Fults and Kelly[15] reported mortality in 4 of 6 patients with infratentorial AVMs. Celli and colleagues[10] showed that intracerebral hemorrhages in children demonstrate a more violent pattern, as shown by a higher frequency of intraparenchymal and intraventricular hemorrhage. Humphreys and colleagues[6] suggested that this phenomenon is related to the "progressive biologic activity of the malformation in children." However, no evidence suggests that the vessels in a pediatric AVM are more fragile than those in an adult AVM.

Many investigators have tried to elucidate factors predictive of hemorrhage or rehemorrhage of AVMs. The size of the malformation has been extensively investigated. Some investigators have found that smaller AVMs have a greater propensity to hemorrhage.[17] Waltimo[18] demonstrated that the smaller the malformation, the more likely it is to bleed. Spetzler and colleagues[19] also noted an inverse relationship between the size of the AVM and the hemorrhage and explained this phenomenon by the differences in arterial feeding pressure between large and small AVMs. However, according to numerous reports larger AVMs are more at risk to rupture.[20–22]

As previously stated, some studies suggest that children have a higher incidence of hemorrhage than adults, but there are also data to the contrary.[20,21] Fullerton and colleagues[23] found the annual risk to be 2.0% for children and 2.2% for adults. Previous history of hemorrhage, especially within the first 5 years, and deep-seated or infratentorial AVMs have been shown consistently in the literature to be risk factors.[20–22,24–27] Other factors that may play a role include exclusive deep venous drainage,[17,21,25] female sex,[28] associated aneurysms (pedicle or intranidal),[25,29,30] and diffuse AVM morphology.[26]

PATHOLOGY

AVMs may form anywhere in the embryonic brain but most originate above the tentorium, where their roots extend over the hemispheric surfaces and dig deep into the cortex. There is a structural defect in the formation of the arteriolar capillary network that is normally present between arteries and veins within the substance of the brain. The exact mechanism by which these malformations form is unknown; however, it is hypothesized that most malformations occur during the third week of embryogenesis, before the embryo reaches 40 mm in length. Mullan and colleagues[31] postulated that the origin of the cerebral AVM relates to the sequential formation and absorption of surface veins, which occur during the 40- to 80-mm embryonal stage. The shunting that ensues if there is an absence of capillary communication between the arterial and venous channels elevates intraluminal venous pressure and produces ectasia and muscularization so that hybrid vessels with both venous and arterial characteristics are formed. In children, these lesions are often hidden within the subcortical tissues and supplied by a straightened dilated artery, which may be the only superficial hallmark of the lesion. In contrast, adult lesions consist of a tangled, tortuous mass of vessels covered by opacified and thickened arachnoid on the surface of the brain. Surrounding these lesions is evidence of prior hemorrhage proved by hemosiderin staining and atrophy of the surrounding parenchyma because of ischemia caused by steal phenomenon. Over time, the lesion is molded by pressure differentials and enlarges insidiously, only becoming symptomatic after childhood. These postnatal and delayed factors contribute to the development of and the symptoms attributed to these lesions.

The reason why an AVM becomes hemorrhagic in childhood in some affected individuals has yet to be elucidated. Shin and colleagues[32] surmised that these lesions are nonstatic in nature and are involved in active angiogenesis and remodeling, especially in younger patients. The theory that growth factors are more potent in the pediatric population and contribute to pediatric AVMs has been investigated. Sonstein and colleagues[33] examined the role of growth factors, specifically vascular endothelial growth factor (VEGF), as a mediator of angiogenesis in AVM development and noted a positive correlation. They noted an increase in VEGF in pediatric patients who had previously undergone complete obliteration of their AVMs with microsurgical resection and had a recurrence of lesions.

DIAGNOSIS

Most AVMs in pediatric patients do not come to clinical attention unless they hemorrhage. The high mortality rate of hemorrhagic events associated with an AVM underscores the importance of accurate diagnosis. Advances in imaging modalities have greatly contributed to the ease in diagnosis of intracerebral hemorrhages caused by AVMs. Computed tomography (CT) is often the initial study performed, and it shows the presence of an intracranial hemorrhage and any calcification. Contrast enhancement can be used to help elucidate the presence of large draining veins and varices. CT angiography can further detail the vascular nature of the hemorrhage and provide a rough estimate of the location, size, and drainage of an AVM, particularly if further imaging has to be delayed for emergent surgical decompression.

Magnetic resonance imaging (MRI) of the brain with and without gadolinium enhancement and with magnetic resonance angiography (MRA) sequences is often obtained for patients with AVMs for several reasons: (1) the high resolution of MRI helps with the localization of the lesion; (2) comparison of contrast, noncontrast, and gradient echo sequences helps to rule out other hemorrhagic lesions, such as tumors and cavernous malformations; (3) MRA sequences can help delineate the vascular anatomy of the lesion; and (4) volumetric sequences can be obtained to allow frameless stereotactic guidance intraoperatively if desired.

Conventional 4-vessel cerebral angiography remains the gold standard (**Figs. 2–5**) for the diagnosis of AVMs. Using subtraction and magnification techniques, angiography clearly defines the characteristics of the lesion—size; location; feeding vessels; draining veins; location of the nidus; presence of associated vascular lesions, such as pedicle or intranidal aneurysms; and anomalies of the venous side, such as ectasia, varices, and stenosis. Angiography also allows evaluation of the dynamic blood flow through and around AVMs. Ninety percent of AVMs are located in the supratentorial compartment, and most of them are fed by the middle cerebral artery (see **Fig. 2**).[13] Although there are typically many arterial feeders that contribute to the AVM, the major venous drainage in children is most frequently through a solitary large cortical vein or a single vein draining into the deep venous system. Aneurysms associated with AVMs, which can occur in many locations including feeding arteries, the nidus, and veins, tend to occur more commonly in adults than in children. During an 8-year period at Columbia University, for example, AVM-associated aneurysms were observed in 41% of adult AVMs but only in 26% of pediatric AVMs. Intranidal aneurysms have also been reported to be more frequent in adults (9%) than in children (<2%).[34,35]

Occasionally, vascular malformations are angiographically occult. Most occult malformations are cavernous; however, angiographically occult AVMs are often found in the region of the middle cerebral artery, with small hemorrhages, and these small malformations may be responsible for intracerebral hemorrhage of unknown cause.[32] Caution

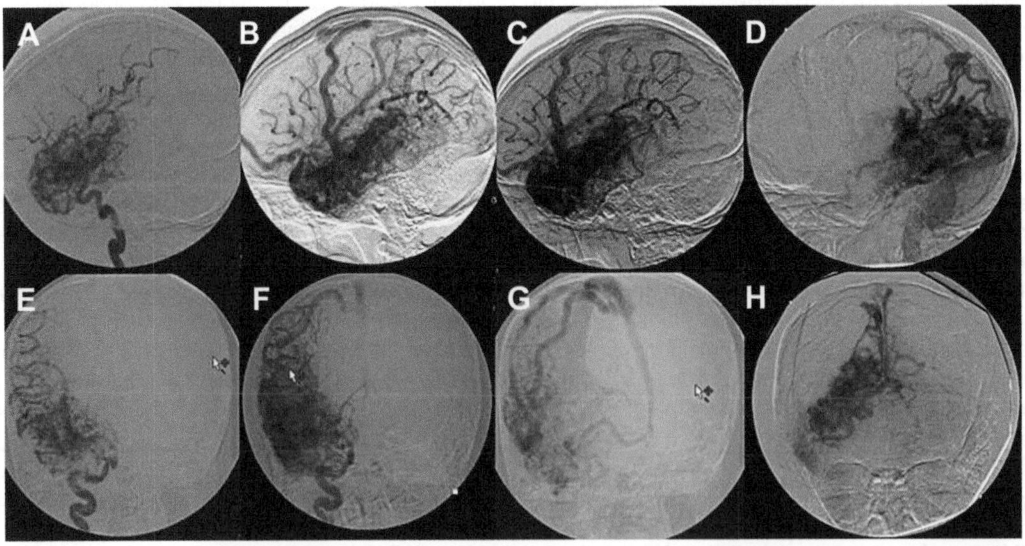

Fig. 2. (*A–H*) Right cerebral hemisphere AVM measuring 5 × 4 × 11 cm supplied by the right middle cerebral artery, right posterior cerebral artery, and distal right anterior cerebral artery vasculature. This AVM also has extracranial cerebral artery supply. This lesion was treated with a combination of stereotactic radiosurgery and embolization.

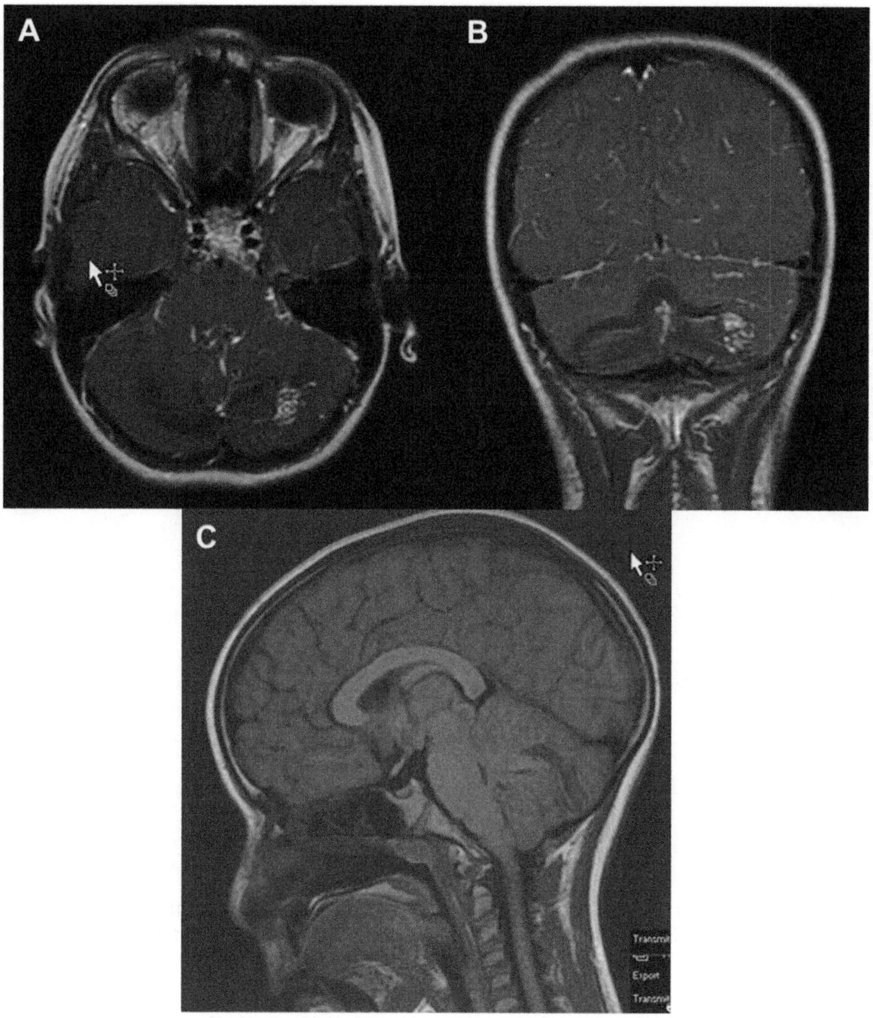

Fig. 3. (*A–C*) Left cerebellar hemisphere AVM measuring 1.5 cm with surrounding edema and hemorrhage. This lesion was amenable to surgical excision.

must be taken in children and young adults who present with an acute spontaneous intraparenchymal hematoma with a negative imaging workup (CT angiography, MRA, conventional angiography). The hematoma can compress and obscure the AVM; therefore, delayed imaging as the clot dissolves and retracts is mandatory. Jordan and colleagues[36] provided an excellent example of this. They reported the case of a 4-year-old boy who presented with a spontaneous intracerebral hemorrhage, in whom a subsequent MRI/MRA done within 24 hours did not reveal the source of the hemorrhage. Follow-up CT and MRI done at 2 weeks, 2 months, and 7 months were all negative. A year after the initial presentation he developed a recurrent hemorrhage; a digital subtraction angiogram revealed an AVM, which was successfully removed. This example also illustrates the need for conventional angiography on initial presentation because small AVMs often cannot be seen on traditional MRI/MRA sequences.

TREATMENT

General Considerations

Treatment of AVMs focuses on the complete obliteration or resection of the vascular lesion to prevent future recurrence of hemorrhage and to preserve and restore neurologic function. Success of the treatment depends on the location and size of the AVM, its hemodynamic properties, the clinical condition of the patient, and the treatment modality selected. The armamentarium available for AVM management has grown with technological advances and now includes microsurgical

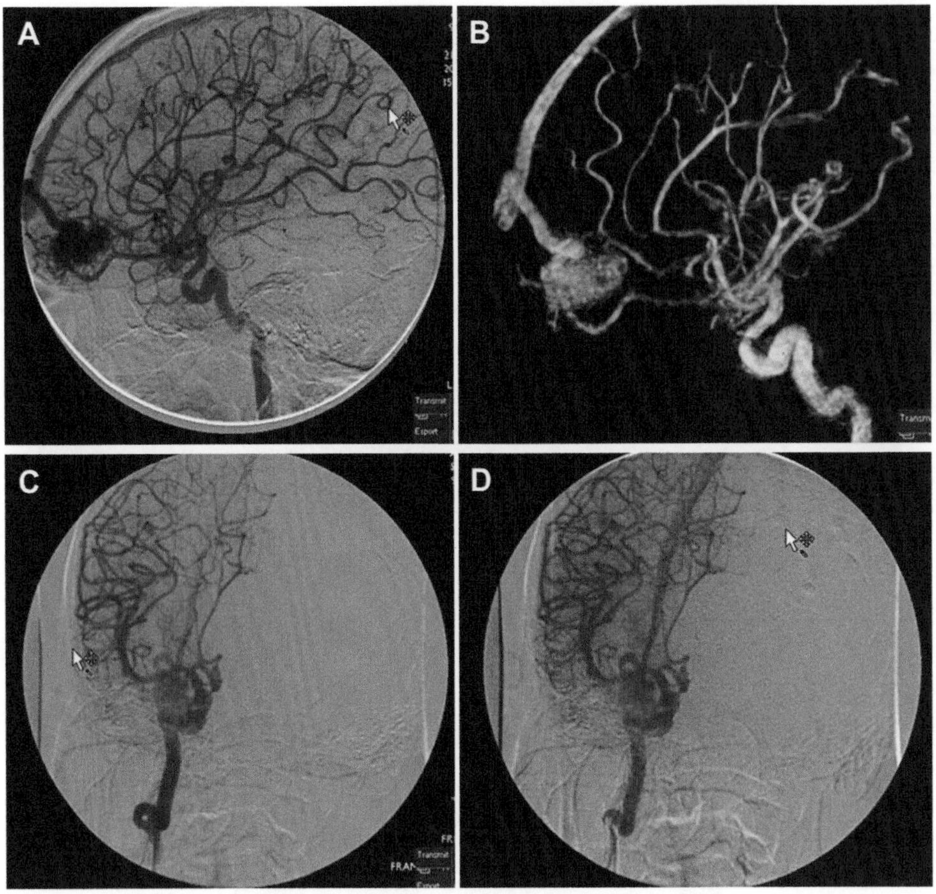

Fig. 4. (*A–D*) Right inferior frontal AVM supplied via the orbitofrontal and frontopolar arteries with superficial drainage. There is an early draining vein that is detected from the distal branch of the left calcarine artery.

resection, endovascular embolization, radiosurgery, and any combination of these modalities.

Although earlier series emphasized the role of conservative management of pediatric AVMs,[37,38] this philosophy has largely been abandoned except in those AVMs where treatment is deemed excessively morbid or ineffective. Early studies suggested that more aggressive management was only necessary in certain clinical situations. For instance, So[38] recommended surgical intervention for those children presenting with hemorrhage alone, whereas Kelly and

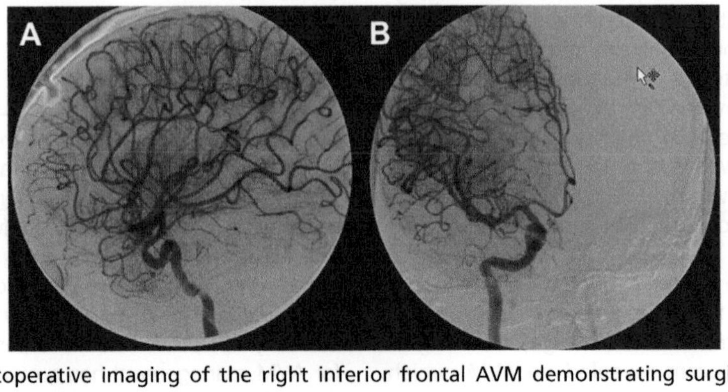

Fig. 5. (*A, B*) Postoperative imaging of the right inferior frontal AVM demonstrating surgical extirpation of the AVM.

colleagues[39] recommended that surgical intervention only be considered for infants with massive lesions, children with large hematomas and associated mass effect, and patients with refractory seizures. However, Gerosa and colleagues[37] correctly indicated that pediatric AVMs necessitated surgery regardless of the presence or absence of hemorrhage because of the poor results they noted with conservative management in their series of patients. Although microsurgical resection will be the primary treatment in most patients, a multidisciplinary approach involving the surgeon, endovascular neurosurgeon or interventional neuroradiologist, and radiation oncologist is an excellent strategy to determine the optimal treatment on a patient-by-patient basis.

Surgical Resection

The optimal management of intracranial AVMs in children remains controversial. Surgery offers the potential benefit of immediate cure and allows the surgeon to remove a hematoma. However, there are several factors that need to be considered to determine the best treatment for the child. The age and size of the patient should be considered. In infants, who have a low total blood volume, rapid blood loss may quickly result in loss of a large fraction of the blood volume, making AVM resection potentially a high-risk procedure. In these patients, surgical intervention should be delayed until the child is older, with a greater circulating blood volume, or another method of treatment should be considered. The location of the AVM is also an important factor when considering surgery. In an AVM in a highly eloquent area, such as the basal ganglia, brainstem, or motor or visual cortex, the location may entirely rule out surgery or may raise the risk of postoperative deficits to unacceptably high levels for the patient and family.

Microsurgical resection may be considered the treatment of choice in those AVMs that fall into Spetzler-Martin (SM) grades I to III because of the high rate of obliteration of the lesion that can be achieved and the low rates of associated morbidity and mortality.[5,8,37,40] In a series of 40 patients, Hoh and colleagues[8] demonstrated that the 20 patients who underwent surgical excision achieved complete radiologic obliteration of their AVM. Six of the 20 patients underwent preoperative embolization, and all had AVMs that were SM grades I to III, except 1 patient, whose AVM was SM grade IV. Schaller and Schramm[41] reported a 98.4% cure rate in their series of 62 patients with AVM, including children and adults with SM grade I to III AVMs. Kiris and colleagues[1] presented a series of 20 pediatric patients with surgically treated SM grade I to III AVMs with an 89% cure rate, and 90% of the patients had excellent clinical outcomes. The excellent outcomes in these and other studies taken in conjunction with the disadvantages of radiosurgery (see Radiosurgery section) make surgery an attractive primary treatment modality for patients with AVMs of SM grades I to III, especially if there is a history of hemorrhage. The role of surgery in higher-grade AVMs (SM grades IV and V) has not been assessed in the pediatric population. Most data are based on the adult age group, and no consensus has been reached on the optimal management of these lesions. Ferch and Morgan[42] examined 46 patients with SM grade IV or V lesions, compared the morbidity and mortality of operatively and non-operatively high-grade lesions, and identified surgical risk factors for increased morbidity in this population. Twenty-nine patients underwent surgery, and 17 were conservatively managed. An average follow-up period of 33 months demonstrated a decline in neurologic function in 27% of conservatively managed cases because of intracranial hemorrhage, progressive neurologic deficits, and seizures. The surgical group of patients was divided into those with a deep perforating arterial supply and/or meningeal recruitment and those without a deep component. In those patients with a deep component, there was a combined morbidity and mortality of 44%, and in those who lacked a deep component, there was a combined morbidity and mortality of 10%. This result was statistically significant, and the investigators concluded that there was a high rate of operative morbidity in patients harboring SM grade IV and V lesions. However, given the inherent poor natural history of these lesions, some patients, such as those lacking a deep perforating arterial supply, may benefit more from surgery. Patients harboring high-grade lesions with deep arterial supply are probably better treated with a multimodal therapy using radiosurgery and embolization.

Surgical Pearls

Although individual surgeons may have unique strategies to achieve a complete resection of an AVM, there are key steps that most surgeons would consider critical in obtaining a successful, angiographically proven outcome. This section discusses some of these common steps and those that are more controversial.

A careful analysis of the preoperative imaging studies, especially the angiogram, is crucial. Features that should be carefully examined are the location and size of the nidus, the number and location of feeding arteries (particularly deep feeders), and the number and location of draining veins. Although preoperative embolization is not done routinely in all institutions, many would believe that it is a good option if the procedure can be done safely (eg, the younger the patient, the more technically challenging the case) and if it provides a significant benefit to the surgeon. For example, it would be a good option for those AVMs that have a single major arterial feeder or feeders that are difficult to access surgically. If the AVM is large, multistaged embolization may be required (often 2 or 3 stages). Surgical resection is typically planned for the day after the last embolization. If it is a small AVM, surgery is done after a single embolization.

Intraoperatively, clear instructions must be given to the anesthesiologist to keep the systolic blood pressure at normal or 10% to 20% below normal for age. A generous craniotomy should be performed with or without frameless stereotaxy. The resection should proceed by staying strictly in the gliotic brain adjacent to the AVM, cauterizing the numerous arterial feeders, and advancing in a circumferential fashion. Feeding arteries are often found underneath draining veins. It is critical to stay outside the nidus because it is difficult to control bleeding from it. The primary draining vein should be the last structure to be cauterized and cut, and this procedure is followed by removal of the AVM en bloc.

Many surgeons obtain an angiogram either intraoperatively if the quality of the images is satisfactory or in an angiography suite with the patient still intubated and sedated. If the angiogram reveals residual nidus or a persistently early draining vein, then resection is continued until the angiogram is deemed negative.

Embolization

Technological advances and improvements in catheter technique, design, and embolization devices have increased the use of endovascular treatment in the adjunctive treatment of pediatric AVMs. Endovascular treatment has become the standard of care in other pediatric vascular entities such as vein of Galen malformations. It is important to recognize, however, that embolization by itself is unlikely to be a permanent solution to pediatric AVMs. Wisoff and Berenstein[43] demonstrated that they were rarely able to obtain a cure with embolization alone but that staged embolizations were of great use in the treatment of large AVMs. A decrease in the symptoms caused by the AVM was often seen after embolization; however, over time recruitment of new vasculature would occur without a more definitive treatment. Wisoff and Berenstein[43] also demonstrated that although there was clinical improvement, hemorrhage risk did not decrease after embolization alone. Frizzel and Fisher[44] reviewed a series of 1246 patients who underwent only embolization of their AVMs and found that only 5% of the patients had complete obliteration of their AVM. Further adjunctive measures had to be undertaken to eradicate the AVM. Wikholm and colleagues[45] substantiated this finding with their series of 192 patients who had SM grade III to IV lesions that were not amenable to surgical resection and instead were treated with embolization only. Of the 192 patients in their series, only 13% had complete obliteration of their lesions.

However, as an adjunctive treatment to surgery and/or radiosurgery, this modality has proven to be of great benefit. Bristol and colleagues[46] reported their series of 83 children who underwent treatment of their AVMs using multimodal therapies including surgical resection, embolization, and radiosurgery. More than 50% of the patients in this series underwent adjunctive treatment with embolization or radiosurgery, and embolization was the preferred treatment modality.

Some children may not need preoperative embolization for low–SM grade lesions or will not be able to get this adjunctive therapy if they require emergent surgical intervention. Small AVMs tend to have tortuous vessels and small branches that are difficult to cannulate and embolize. As briefly discussed in the previous section, in those children with SM grade II to V lesions, embolization plays an important role to help decrease the bulk of the lesion to allow for definitive surgical extirpation without excessive blood loss. This technique may be a favored over radiosurgical adjuvant treatment in larger lesions because of the increased risk of radiation edema that is noted in patients with AVM volumes greater than 3 mL.[47] In neonates, there is the added pressure of attempting to cannulate small vessels for access, and this can pose an added risk to the patients if multiple treatment sessions are necessary. Rarely, a general surgeon is necessary in these cases to provide direct access via a cutdown technique exposing the vessel followed by primary repair of the vessel. The periprocedural morbidity and mortality rate of endovascular treatment is typically very low but may be as high as 11.8%.[48] Kim and colleagues[48] reported a series of 153 patients in which 1 patient died and 17 patients suffered unexpected neurologic deficits immediately after embolization, 5 of whom recovered during the follow-up period.

Neuroembolic substances also exhibit toxicity at certain dosages, and these dosages are less in children because of the circulating blood volume and the size of the patient involved. Endovascular options will continue to evolve and improve and should be incorporated into the treatment paradigm for adjunctive treatment in the pediatric population on an individualized case-by-case basis.

Radiosurgery

Since its advent in 1951,[49] stereotactic radiosurgery has evolved significantly and is now being used to treat a host of neurosurgical diseases. Radiosurgery has long been an adjunctive modality in the treatment of deep-seated or large adult cerebral AVMs. Because of the concerns of exposing the developing brain to ionizing radiation, only recently has information about radiosurgery of pediatric AVMs become available. Stereotactic radiosurgery was first used for the treatment of pediatric AVMs in the late 1980s in an effort to treat this population with minimally invasive means. Radiosurgery was used in an effort to avoid surgical intervention in children with deep-seated lesions or lesions in eloquent areas of the cortex.[50] The goal was to obtain a complete angiographic obliteration without inducing new neurologic deficits.

During the last 2 decades, 20 retrospective studies (**Table 1**) have been performed to look at the efficacy and safety of stereotactic radiosurgery in the pediatric population.[8,50–68] In children, the obliteration rate varies between 27% 3 years after radiosurgery and 95% 5 years after radiosurgery.[69,70] Levy and colleagues[56] described a series of 53 children who underwent at least 36 months of imaging follow-up after radiosurgery and assessed the obliteration rates in these children. They stratified their obliteration results in terms of AVM volume (group 1, ≤3 mL; group 2, >3 mL to ≤10 mL; group 3, >10 mL), and the median marginal dose that each child received was 20 Gy. They had excellent obliteration rates; 80% of patients in group 1 and 65% of patients in group 2 achieved obliteration. The only patient in group 3 did not achieve complete obliteration. This is not surprising given the large volume of AVM defined as group 3. Of the 53 patients, 49 (93%) returned to their neurologic baseline and functional activity levels after radiosurgery. Complications in the series were infrequent and included 1 patient with brainstem edema and persistent ataxia 4 months after treatment and 1 patient with transient pulmonary edema. Four patients experienced hemorrhagic events after radiosurgical treatment at 30, 40, 84, and 96 months after radiosurgery. Three of these 4 patients had residual neurologic impairment after the intracranial hemorrhage, and 1 patient died because of intracranial hemorrhage 40 months after radiosurgical treatment. Overall, the investigators concluded that radiosurgery was safe and efficacious for selected children with AVMs as was evidenced by successful obliteration and low morbidity and mortality rates.

Pollock and colleagues[70] found that the major variable associated with obliteration of pediatric AVMs was the AVM score, which consists of the patient's age, volume of AVM, and location of AVM. A higher rate of complete obliteration was noted in those patients with a smaller volume of AVM and a higher marginal dose.[56] There was also a positive correlation between time to obliteration and younger age. However, during the interval between treatment and complete obliteration there continues to be a risk of hemorrhage, which continues to place these patients at risk of neurologic compromise.

The long-term effects of ionizing radiation from radiosurgery on the developing nervous system have not yet been fully evaluated because of the paucity of data. Reyns and colleagues[63] reported a 5% permanent neurologic deficit rate in a series of 100 pediatric patients with AVM who underwent stereotactic surgery with a mean dose of 15 to 25 Gy and a follow-up of greater than 36 months. Radiation-induced changes are seen on MRI in as many as 32% of pediatric patients treated with stereotactic radiosurgery; however, only a fraction of these go on to experience permanent neurologic deficits.[52] Friedman and colleagues[71] reported that a 12-Gy volume was a predictor of future permanent neurologic complication. Delayed cyst formation has also been observed in this population and is also associated with a higher maximal treatment dose, a larger AVM volume, and the lobar location of the AVM.[72] Evaluation of the incidence of intracranial malignancy after radiosurgery in childhood has yet to be fully assessed. To date, 4 cases of radiosurgery-associated malignancy have been reported in the literature; however, the full effect of this treatment modality on the pediatric population is not known.[73] No standard median dose has been consistently used, with doses ranging from 14 to 30 Gy. Furthermore, different machines, including the Gamma Knife and the linear accelerator, have been used, making evaluation of this treatment modality difficult. All studies to date have been retrospective, nonrandomized studies in which selection bias is undoubtedly present.

Table 1
Studies evaluating the safety and efficacy of stereotactic radiosurgery for treatment of AVMs in children

Author, year	Number of Patients (n)	Modality	Age Range (y)	Dose Range (Gy)	Follow-up (%)	Obliteration (%)	Complications/Deficits		
							Transient	Permanent	Death
Altschuler et al,[50] 1989	18	GK	2–18	17.5–25	83 (15/18)	20 (3/18)	1	0	0
Loeffler et al,[57] 1990	8	LINAC	6–20	16.5–20	100 (8/8)	63 (5/8)	0	0	0
Yamamoto et al,[67] 1992	9	GK	9–16	15–30	100 (9/9)	67 (6/9)	0	0	0
Tanaka et al,[66] 1996	23	GK	2–15	20.5	91 (21/23)	95 (20/23)	0	0	0
Gertszen et al,[77] 1996	15	GK	2–17	15–25	100 (15/15)	40 (6/15)	0	0	0
Nicolato et al,[78] 1997	7	GK	5–16	23.6–25.8	85 (6/7)	33 (2/7)	1	0	0
Levy et al,[56] 2000	53	GK	2–17	15–25	100 (53/53)	74 (39/53)	0	4	2
Hoh et al,[8] 2000	15	PB	1–18	8–26	60 (9/15)	47 (7/15)	0	1	1
Amendola et al,[51] 2000	31	GK	7–19	20–25	100 (31/31)	71 (22/31)	0	0	0
Smyth et al,[65] 2002	31	GK	3–17	3.4–17.5	100 (31/31)	35 (11/31)	0	2	0
Shin et al,[64] 2002	100	GK	4–19	17–28	82 (82/100)	87 (71/82)	2	3	1
Nataf et al,[59] 2003	57	LINAC	7–15	18–28	86 (49/57)	61 (30/57)	0	0	1
Maity et al,[58] 2004	17	LINAC	5–18	16–18	100 (17/17)	53 (9/17)	1	3	0
Nicolato et al,[60] 2005	63	GK	5–16	16–26	74 (47/63)	79 (31/63)	1	1	0
Fuss et al,[54] 2005	7	IMRS	7–18	17.5–20	86 (6/7)	33 (2/7)	0	0	0
Cohen-Gadol and Pollock,[53] 2006	38	GK	7–18	16–25	100 (38/38)	66 (23/38)	1	0	0
Zabel-du Bois et al,[68] 2006	22	LINAC	4–16	15–20	100 (22/22)	64 (14/22)	0	0	0
Nicolato et al,[62] 2006	62	GK	5–20	14–26.4	100 (62/62)	85 (53/62)	1	1	0
Reyns et al,[63] 2007	100	LINAC	2–16	15–25	100 (100/100)	70 (70/100)	1	8	1
Buis et al,[52] 2008	22	LINAC	6–20	15–21	100 (22/22)	68 (15/22)	0	1	1

Abbreviations: GK, Gamma Knife; IMRS, intensity-modulated radiosurgery; LINAC, linear accelerator; PB, proton beam.

FOLLOW-UP

There is an increasingly recognized phenomenon of late AVM recurrence, even after angiographic cure.[3,40,46,74–76] Klimo and colleagues[3] recently reviewed the literature and identified 29 published cases of recurrent AVMs, of which 20 (69%) were that of children. They also found that diffuse-type AVMs were more likely to develop a recurrence. The longest reported interval between total surgical removal and recurrence is 19 years.[76] Maher and Scott[4] recently reported the Children's Hospital Boston experience, in which 4 patients had recurrence—2 occurring 1 year after surgery, 1 at 3 years, and another at 11 years. This growing literature presents a challenge to the treating physician: How long should the child be monitored and with what imaging modality? Maher and Scott[4] noted that they performed a follow-up angiogram at 1 year and MRI studies annually for at least 5 years. At Columbia University, if the immediate postoperative angiogram is negative, another delayed angiogram is typically performed 5 years later or when the child reaches adulthood.

SUMMARY

The optimal management for pediatric AVMs remains controversial. Children with intracranial AVMs represent a special challenge in that they harbor unacceptable lifelong risks of hemorrhage and potential neurologic deficits. Treatment of these lesions has evolved during the last century with advances in the medical, surgical, and technological fronts. Treatment of pediatric AVMs should be undertaken in a multidisciplinary fashion, and patients should be evaluated on a case-by-case basis to determine the best treatment regimen to preserve neurologic function and eradicate the AVM with the lowest risk of mortality. Microsurgical resection remains the gold standard for the treatment of accessible pediatric AVMs, especially in cases with intracranial hemorrhage. Only in the last two decades have embolization and radiosurgery been used in this population. Although embolization alone does not provide complete obliteration of AVMs, this modality provides a useful adjunct to microsurgery and can greatly assist the surgeon, prevent significant blood loss, and decrease the volume of AVM to be resected. Radiosurgery provides an alternative treatment approach in those patients with large AVMs, deep-seated or eloquently located AVMs, or recurrent AVMs. The long-term effects of this treatment modality have yet to be elucidated. In children, long-term follow-up with repeated diagnostic imaging is important despite complete obliteration of the lesion to rule out the small possibility of AVM recurrence.

REFERENCES

1. Kiris T, Sencer A, Sahinbas M, et al. Surgical results in pediatric Spetzler-Martin grades I-III intracranial arteriovenous malformations. Childs Nerv Syst 2005;21(1):69–74 [discussion: 75–6].
2. Chin LS, Raffel C, Gonzalez-Gomez I, et al. Diffuse arteriovenous malformations: a clinical, radiological, and pathological description. Neurosurgery 1992; 31(5):863–8 [discussion: 868–9].
3. Klimo P Jr, Rao G, Brockmeyer D. Pediatric arteriovenous malformations: a 15-year experience with an emphasis on residual and recurrent lesions. Childs Nerv Syst 2007;23(1):31–7.
4. Maher CO, Scott RM. Linear vein-based arteriovenous malformations in children. J Neurosurg Pediatr 2009;4(1):12–6.
5. Di Rocco C, Tamburrini G, Rollo M. Cerebral arteriovenous malformations in children. Acta Neurochir (Wien) 2000;142(2):145–56 [discussion: 156–8].
6. Humphreys RP, Hendrick EB, Hoffman HJ. Arteriovenous malformations of the brainstem in childhood. Childs Brain 1984;11(1):1–11.
7. Millar C, Bissonnette B, Humphreys RP. Cerebral arteriovenous malformations in children. Can J Anaesth 1994;41(4):321–31.
8. Hoh BL, Ogilvy CS, Butler WE, et al. Multimodality treatment of nongalenic arteriovenous malformations in pediatric patients. Neurosurgery 2000; 47(2):346–57 [discussion: 357–8].
9. Mori K, Murata T, Hashimoto N, et al. Clinical analysis of arteriovenous malformations in children. Childs Brain 1980;6(1):13–25.
10. Celli P, Ferrante L, Palma L, et al. Cerebral arteriovenous malformations in children. Clinical features and outcome of treatment in children and in adults. Surg Neurol 1984;22(1):43–9.
11. Kondziolka D, Humphreys RP, Hoffman HJ, et al. Arteriovenous malformations of the brain in children: a forty year experience. Can J Neurol Sci 1992; 19(1):40–5.
12. Matson DD. Neurosurgery of infancy and childhood. Springfield (IL): CC Thomas; 1969.
13. Perret G, Nishioka H. Report on the cooperative study of intracranial aneurysms and subarachnoid hemorrhage. Section VI. Arteriovenous malformations. An analysis of 545 cases of cranio-cerebral arteriovenous malformations and fistulae reported to the cooperative study. J Neurosurg 1966;25(4): 467–90.
14. Leblanc R, Feindel W, Ethier R. Epilepsy from cerebral arteriovenous malformations. Can J Neurol Sci 1983;10(2):91–5.

15. Fults D, Kelly DL Jr. Natural history of arteriovenous malformations of the brain: a clinical study. Neurosurgery 1984;15(5):658–62.
16. Humphreys RP, Hoffman HJ, Drake JM, et al. Choices in the 1990s for the management of pediatric cerebral arteriovenous malformations. Pediatr Neurosurg 1996;25:277–85.
17. Langer DJ, Lasner TM, Hurst RW, et al. Hypertension, small size, and deep venous drainage are associated with risk of hemorrhagic presentation of cerebral arteriovenous malformations. Neurosurgery 1998;42(3):481–6 [discussion: 487–9].
18. Waltimo O. The relationship of size, density and localization of intracranial arteriovenous malformations to the type of initial symptom. J Neurol Sci 1973;19(1):13–9.
19. Spetzler RF, Hargraves RW, McCormick PW, et al. Relationship of perfusion pressure and size to risk of hemorrhage from arteriovenous malformations. J Neurosurg 1992;76(6):918–23.
20. Hernesniemi JA, Dashti R, Juvela S, et al. Natural history of brain arteriovenous malformations: a long-term follow-up study of risk of hemorrhage in 238 patients. Neurosurgery 2008;63(5):823–9 [discussion: 829–31].
21. Stapf C, Mast H, Sciacca RR, et al. Predictors of hemorrhage in patients with untreated brain arteriovenous malformation. Neurology 2006;66(9): 1350–5.
22. Stefani MA, Porter PJ, terBrugge KG, et al. Large and deep brain arteriovenous malformations are associated with risk of future hemorrhage. Stroke 2002;33(5):1220–4.
23. Fullerton HJ, Achrol AS, Johnston SC, et al. Long-term hemorrhage risk in children versus adults with brain arteriovenous malformations. Stroke 2005; 36(10):2099–104.
24. Arnaout OM, Gross BA, Eddleman CS, et al. Posterior fossa arteriovenous malformations. Neurosurg Focus 2009;26(5):E12.
25. Khaw AV, Mohr JP, Sciacca RR, et al. Association of infratentorial brain arteriovenous malformations with hemorrhage at initial presentation. Stroke 2004; 35(3):660–3.
26. Pollock BE, Flickinger JC, Lunsford LD, et al. Factors that predict the bleeding risk of cerebral arteriovenous malformations. Stroke 1996;27(1):1–6.
27. da Costa L, Wallace MC, Ter Brugge KG, et al. The natural history and predictive features of hemorrhage from brain arteriovenous malformations. Stroke 2009;40(1):100–5.
28. Yamada S, Takagi Y, Nozaki K, et al. Risk factors for subsequent hemorrhage in patients with cerebral arteriovenous malformations. J Neurosurg 2007; 107(5):965–72.
29. Meisel HJ, Mansmann U, Alvarez H, et al. Cerebral arteriovenous malformations and associated aneurysms: analysis of 305 cases from a series of 662 patients. Neurosurgery 2000;46(4):793–800 [discussion: 800–2].
30. Redekop G, TerBrugge K, Montanera W, et al. Arterial aneurysms associated with cerebral arteriovenous malformations: classification, incidence, and risk of hemorrhage. J Neurosurg 1998;89(4): 539–46.
31. Mullan S, Mojtahedi S, Johnson DL, et al. Embryological basis of some aspects of cerebral vascular fistulas and malformations. J Neurosurg 1996; 85(1):1–8.
32. Shin M, Maruyama K, Kurita H, et al. Analysis of nidus obliteration rates after Gamma Knife surgery for arteriovenous malformations based on long-term follow-up data: the University of Tokyo experience. J Neurosurg 2004;101(1):18–24.
33. Sonstein WJ, Kader A, Michelsen WJ, et al. Expression of vascular endothelial growth factor in pediatric and adult cerebral arteriovenous malformations: an immunocytochemical study. J Neurosurg 1996; 85(5):838–45.
34. Graf CJ, Perret GE, Torner JC. Bleeding from cerebral arteriovenous malformations as part of their natural history. J Neurosurg 1983;58(3):331–7.
35. Ostergaard JR. Association of intracranial aneurysm and arteriovenous malformation in childhood. Neurosurgery 1984;14(3):358–62.
36. Jordan LC, Jallo GI, Gailloud P. Recurrent intracerebral hemorrhage from a cerebral arteriovenous malformation undetected by repeated noninvasive neuroimaging in a 4-year-old boy. Case report. J Neurosurg Pediatr 2008;1(4):316–9.
37. Gerosa MA, Cappellotto P, Licata C, et al. Cerebral arteriovenous malformations in children (56 cases). Childs Brain 1981;8(5):356–71.
38. So SC. Cerebral arteriovenous malformations in children. Childs Brain 1978;4(4):242–50.
39. Kelly J, Alvarez RD, Roland PY. Arteriovenous malformation presenting as a complex pelvic mass with ureteral obstruction. A case report. J Reprod Med 1998;43(10):916–8.
40. Hladky JP, Lejeune JP, Blond S, et al. Cerebral arteriovenous malformations in children: report on 62 cases. Childs Nerv Syst 1994;10(5):328–33.
41. Schaller C, Schramm J. Microsurgical results for small arteriovenous malformations accessible for radiosurgical or embolization treatment. Neurosurgery 1997;40(4):664–72 [discussion: 672–4].
42. Ferch RD, Morgan MK. High-grade arteriovenous malformations and their management. J Clin Neurosci 2002;9(1):37–40.
43. Wisoff JH, Berenstein A. Interventional neuroradiology. In: Edwards MSB, Hoffman HJ, editors. Cerebral vascular disease in children and adolescents. Baltimore (MD): Williams and Wilkins; 1989. p. 139–57.

44. Frizzel RT, Fisher WS 3rd. Cure, morbidity, and mortality associated with embolization of brain arteriovenous malformations: a review of 1246 patients in 32 series over a 35-year period. Neurosurgery 1995;37(6):1031–9 [discussion: 1039–40].
45. Wikholm G, Lundqvist C, Svendsen P. Embolization of cerebral arteriovenous malformations: part I–technique, morphology, and complications. Neurosurgery 1996;39(3):448–57 [discussion: 457–9].
46. Bristol RE, Albuquerque FC, Spetzler RF, et al. Surgical management of arteriovenous malformations in children. J Neurosurg 2006;105(Suppl 2): 88–93.
47. Kiran NA, Kale SS, Vaishya S, et al. Gamma Knife surgery for intracranial arteriovenous malformations in children: a retrospective study in 103 patients. J Neurosurg 2007;107(Suppl 6):479–84.
48. Kim LJ, Albuquerque FC, Spetzler RF, et al. Postembolization neurological deficits in cerebral arteriovenous malformations: stratification by arteriovenous malformation grade. Neurosurgery 2006;59(1):53–9 [discussion: 53–9].
49. Leksell L. Sterotaxic radiosurgery in trigeminal neuralgia. Acta Chir Scand 1971;137(4):311–4.
50. Altschuler EM, Lunsford LD, Coffey RJ, et al. Gamma Knife radiosurgery for intracranial arteriovenous malformations in childhood and adolescence. Pediatr Neurosci 1989;15(2):53–61.
51. Amendola BE, Wolf A, Coy SR, et al. Radiosurgery for intracranial arteriovenous malformations in children. J Radiosurg 2000;3:159–64.
52. Buis DR, Dirven CM, Lagerwaard FJ, et al. Radiosurgery of brain arteriovenous malformations in children. J Neurol 2008;255(4):551–60.
53. Cohen-Gadol AA, Pollock BE. Radiosurgery for arteriovenous malformations in children. J Neurosurg 2006;104(Suppl 6):388–91.
54. Fuss M, Salter BJ, Caron JL, et al. Intensity-modulated radiosurgery for childhood arteriovenous malformations. Acta Neurochir (Wien) 2005;147(11): 1141–9 [discussion: 1149–50].
55. Gerszten PC, Adelson PD, Kondziolka D, et al. Seizure outcome in children treated for arteriovenous malformations using Gamma Knife radiosurgery. Pediatr Neurosurg 1996;24(3):139–44.
56. Levy EI, Niranjan A, Thompson TP, et al. Radiosurgery for childhood intracranial arteriovenous malformations. Neurosurgery 2000;47(4):834–41 [discussion: 841–2].
57. Loeffler JS, Rossitch E Jr, Siddon R, et al. Role of stereotactic radiosurgery with a linear accelerator in treatment of intracranial arteriovenous malformations and tumors in children. Pediatrics 1990;85(5): 774–82.
58. Maity A, Shu HK, Tan JE, et al. Treatment of pediatric intracranial arteriovenous malformations with linear-accelerator-based stereotactic radiosurgery: the University of Pennsylvania experience. Pediatr Neurosurg 2004;40(5):207–14.
59. Nataf F, Schlienger M, Lefkopoulos D, et al. Radiosurgery of cerebral arteriovenous malformations in children: a series of 57 cases. Int J Radiat Oncol Biol Phys 2003;57(1):184–95.
60. Nicolato A, Foroni R, Seghedoni A, et al. Leksell Gamma Knife radiosurgery for cerebral arteriovenous malformations in pediatric patients. Childs Nerv Syst 2005;21(4):301–7 [discussion: 308].
61. Nicolato A, Lupidi F, Sandri MF, et al. Gamma Knife radiosurgery for cerebral arteriovenous malformations in children/adolescents and adults. Part I: differences in epidemiologic, morphologic, and clinical characteristics, permanent complications, and bleeding in the latency period. Int J Radiat Oncol Biol Phys 2006;64(3):904–13.
62. Nicolato A, Lupidi F, Sandri MF, et al. Gamma Knife radiosurgery for cerebral arteriovenous malformations in children/adolescents and adults. Part II: differences in obliteration rates, treatment-obliteration intervals, and prognostic factors. Int J Radiat Oncol Biol Phys 2006;64(3):914–21.
63. Reyns N, Blond S, Gauvrit JY, et al. Role of radiosurgery in the management of cerebral arteriovenous malformations in the pediatric age group: data from a 100-patient series. Neurosurgery 2007; 60(2):268–76 [discussion: 276].
64. Shin M, Kawamoto S, Kurita H, et al. Retrospective analysis of a 10-year experience of stereotactic radio surgery for arteriovenous malformations in children and adolescents. J Neurosurg 2002;97(4): 779–84.
65. Smyth MD, Sneed PK, Ciricillo SF, et al. Stereotactic radiosurgery for pediatric intracranial arteriovenous malformations: the University of California at San Francisco experience. J Neurosurg 2002; 97(1):48–55.
66. Tanaka T, Kobayashi T, Kida Y, et al. Comparison between adult and pediatric arteriovenous malformations treated by Gamma Knife radiosurgery. Stereotact Funct Neurosurg 1996;66(Suppl 1):288–95.
67. Yamamoto M, Jimbo M, Ide M, et al. Long-term follow-up of radiosurgically treated arteriovenous malformations in children: report of nine cases. Surg Neurol 1992;38(2):95–100.
68. Zabel-du Bois A, Milker-Zabel S, Huber P, et al. Pediatric cerebral arteriovenous malforma tions: the role of stereotactic linac-based radiosurgery. Int J Radiat Oncol Biol Phys 2006;65(4): 1206–11.
69. Pollock BE, Kondziolka D, Flickinger JC, et al. Magnetic resonance imaging: an accurate method to evaluate arteriovenous malformations after stereotactic radiosurgery. J Neurosurg 1996;85(6): 1044–9.

70. Pollock BE, Flickinger JC, Lunsford LD, et al. Factors associated with successful arteriovenous malformation radiosurgery. Neurosurgery 1998;42(6):1239–44 [discussion: 1244–7].
71. Friedman WA, Bova FJ, Bollampally S, et al. Analysis of factors predictive of success or complications in arteriovenous malformation radiosurgery. Neurosurgery 2003;52(2):296–307 [discussion: 307–8].
72. Izawa M, Hayashi M, Chernov M, et al. Long-term complications after Gamma Knife surgery for arteriovenous malformations. J Neurosurg 2005; 102(Suppl):34–7.
73. McIver JI, Pollock BE. Radiation-induced tumor after stereotactic radiosurgery and whole brain radiotherapy: case report and literature review. J Neurooncol 2004;66(3):301–5.
74. Ali MJ, Bendok BR, Rosenblatt S, et al. Recurrence of pediatric cerebral arteriovenous malformations after angiographically documented resection. Pediatr Neurosurg 2003;39(1):32–8.
75. Andaluz N, Myseros JS, Sathi S, et al. Recurrence of cerebral arteriovenous malformations in children: report of two cases and review of the literature. Surg Neurol 2004;62(4):324–30 [discussion: 330–1].
76. Higuchi M, Bitoh S, Hasegawa H, et al. [Marked growth of arteriovenous malformations 19 years after resection: a case report]. No Shinkei Geka 1991;19: 75–8 [in Japanese].
77. Gerszten PC, Adelson PD, Kondziolka D, et al. Seizure outcome in children treated for arteriovenous malformations using gamma knife radiosurgery. Pediatr Neurosurg 1996;24(3):139–44.
78. Nicolato A, Gerosa M, Ferraresi P, et al. Stereotactic radiosurgery for the treatment of arteriovenous malformations in childhood. J Neurosurg Sci 1997; 41(4):359–71.

Stereotactic Radiosurgery for Pediatric Arteriovenous Malformations

Andrew B. Foy, MD[a], Nicholas Wetjen, MD[a], Bruce E. Pollock, MD[a,b,*]

KEYWORDS

- Radiosurgery • Arteriovenous malformation
- Pediatric neurosurgery

Children with intracranial arteriovenous malformations (AVMs) have a high lifetime risk of hemorrhage, and appropriate treatment of these lesions in children is critical. It is estimated that 12% to 18% of all open resections for intracranial AVMs are performed on children.[1–4] Children are more likely than adults to present with hemorrhage, which often leads to significant morbidity, and mortality rates as high as 25% have been reported.[5] The annual hemorrhage rate from intracranial AVMs has been estimated to be between 2% and 4%, and some have suggested that the yearly risk of hemorrhage from AVMs may be higher in the pediatric population.[6–8] The options for treatment of intracranial AVMs in the pediatric population include open microsurgical resection of the nidus, embolization of feeding vessels, stereotactic radiosurgery (SRS), or a combination of these treatments. The role of SRS in the treatment of children with AVMs is the topic of this review.

INDICATIONS AND PATIENT CHARACTERISTICS

While firmly established as a treatment of AVMs in adults, concerns regarding the potential toxicity of radiation to the developing nervous system delayed the widespread use of SRS for children with intracranial AVMs.[9] Modern series of children treated with radiosurgery for AVMs, though, have shown this treatment modality to be effective and safe. While microsurgical resection is generally considered the treatment of choice for AVMs that can be resected safely, SRS is more often recommended for AVMs in critical cortical areas and deep brain locations such as the thalamus, basal ganglia, and brainstem.[10] An additional consideration for pediatric patients is that SRS may be better tolerated than surgical resection when significant intraoperative blood loss is anticipated. An important difference when comparing outcomes of microsurgical resection and SRS for AVMs is that patients remain at risk for hemorrhage following SRS until the AVM has gone on to complete obliteration. Also, while the early morbidity following SRS in children has been documented in several studies to be relatively low, the life expectancy of pediatric patients with AVMs is many decades and the long-term risk of SRS is not yet fully defined.

Over the last decade, several modern retrospective reviews have been published on the use of SRS in pediatric patients harboring AVMs.

Funding/Conflict of Interest: None.

[a] Department of Neurologic Surgery, Mayo Clinic and Foundation, 200 First Street SW, Rochester, MN 55905, USA

[b] Department of Radiation Oncology, Mayo Clinic and Foundation, 200 First Street SW, Rochester, MN 55905, USA

* Corresponding author. Department of Neurologic Surgery, Mayo Clinic and Foundation, 200 First Street SW, Rochester, MN 55905.

E-mail address: wetjen.nicholas@mayo.edu

Neurosurg Clin N Am 21 (2010) 457–461
doi:10.1016/j.nec.2010.03.002
1042-3680/10/$ – see front matter

These reports suggest that pediatric patients are more likely than adults to present with hemorrhage. Not surprisingly, the number of patients undergoing SRS who have had a prior hemorrhage ranges from 53% to 79% of patients.[11–19] The average age of children undergoing SRS is remarkably similar over several series from different institutions, ranging from 11 to 15 years old.[11–19] The available series have not shown a significant difference in the male to female ratio of children treated with SRS.

RADIOSURGICAL TECHNIQUE

The technique for SRS varies from center to center depending on the method of radiation delivery and local practice. At the Mayo Clinic, the procedure is performed under general anesthesia for all patients younger than 13 years, with older children undergoing either general anesthesia or monitored anesthesia care based on the child's maturity level and the preference of the patient's parents. A stereotactic headframe is placed on the patient and a stereotactic magnetic resonance imaging (MRI) scan with gadolinium administration is performed for dose planning. In the majority of patients, biplanar stereotactic angiography is also used, and both imaging modalities are imported into the computer workstation. At the authors' institution, radiosurgery is performed using the Leksell Gamma Knife (Elekta Instruments, Inc, Norcross, GA, USA). The authors recently reported on 38 children undergoing Gamma Knife AVM radiosurgery. Of these, 32 were treated in a single session and 6 were treated with staged-volume radiosurgery.[11,20] The median margin dose in this series was 20 Gy (range, 16–25 Gy). The mean marginal dose in the available large studies of SRS for childhood AVMs ranges from 16.7 to 23.8 Gy.[11–19] In a study by Smyth and colleagues,[19] a multivariate analysis of factors associated with AVM obliteration following SRS for childhood AVMs showed a tenfold increase in obliteration rates in patients who had a treatment margin dose of 18 Gy or more. Although some centers have used pre-radiosurgical embolization as a method to reduce the AVM size in preparation for SRS, recent studies have questioned the usefulness of embolization as a meaningful adjunct to SRS.[21] Because the utility of this technique is not established, the authors do not recommend embolization before radiosurgery for their patients.

OUTCOMES AND PREDICTORS OF SUCCESS

The goal of AVM radiosurgery is nidus obliteration and reduction in annual hemorrhage rate. Recent studies have documented a total AVM obliteration rate between 61% and 86% with average follow-up between 26 and 71 months.[11–18] Smyth and colleagues[19] reported a lower obliteration rate than comparable studies. This group reported an obliteration rate of 35% with a mean follow-up of 62 months. Of note is that this center used a lower mean marginal dose (16.7 Gy) than most other reports (18.5–23 Gy), and on multivariate analysis showed a much higher rate of obliteration when the mean marginal dose prescribed was 18 Gy or higher. The lower obliteration rate likely reflects the lower mean marginal dose prescribed. While most pediatric patients with AVMs present with hemorrhage and the ultimate goal of treatment is to reduce the risk of intracranial hemorrhage, radiosurgery also seems to have a positive effect on seizure outcome for children presenting with AVM-associated seizure disorders. Although there are fewer studies regarding the seizure outcome following SRS for childhood AVMs, most series suggest a 50% to 90% improvement in seizure burden after SRS.[12,13,22]

The volume of the AVMs treated with radiosurgery has been variable across institutions reporting significant experience treating childhood AVMs. Studies have reported an average treated volume between 1.7 cm^3 and 5.37 cm^3.[11–19] Many studies have documented a statistically significant decrease in obliteration rate for larger volume AVMs. Levy and colleagues[12] reported a series of 53 children treated with SRS for AVMs with at least 36 months of follow-up. On multivariate analysis the only factor associated with obliteration rate in their series was AVM volume. Shin and colleagues,[18] in a series of 100 patients, found that age younger than 12 years, smaller AVM volume and diameter, and Spetzler-Martin grade of III or less were associated with improved obliteration rate. Nicolato and colleagues[15] observed that younger age and lower Spetzler-Martin grade correlated with improved obliteration rate, and that Spetzler-Martin grade and noneloquent location correlated with improved time to obliteration after treatment with SRS. In one recent series, Pan and colleagues[16] reported a significantly higher average volume treated (11.7 cm^3) than for previous studies, but this group was still able to achieve a relatively high obliteration rate for large AVMs (64%).

In the series from their own center, the authors observed a 68% obliteration rate with a median follow-up of 42 months.[11] None of the patients suffered a new neurologic deficit after treatment despite the majority of patients having Spetzler-Martin grade III or higher AVMs. The authors also showed that the radiosurgery-based AVM score[23,24] was useful in predicting outcomes in children treated with SRS. Age is one of the key measures in the radiosurgery-based AVM score (along with AVM volume and location). The authors found that children with a radiosurgery-based AVM score less than 1 had an 88% chance of excellent outcome compared with a 52% chance in children who had a score greater than 1. Other centers tested the radiosurgery-based AVM system and found that it effectively predicted outcomes after radiosurgery for pediatric AVMs.[25]

HEMORRHAGE RISK AND MORBIDITY

Whereas direct surgical resection of an AVM nidus immediately removes the hemorrhage risk in children harboring AVMs, radiosurgery has a much longer interval between treatment and obliteration of the AVM nidus. This factor is of particular concern, as hemorrhage is the most common presenting symptom in children and the vast majority of children treated with SRS in the literature presented with intracranial hemorrhage. The post-radiosurgery hemorrhage rate in large modern series is between 1.3% and 8.2%.[11–19] The annual bleeding rate following radiosurgery is between 0.56% and 4.3%. In the study by Smyth and colleagues[19] an overall 8% bleeding rate was found, with a rate of 4.3% per year over the first 3 years following treatment. Shin and colleagues[18] found that posterior fossa AVMs were at a significantly greater risk of posttreatment hemorrhage. Rare deaths have been reported following SRS due to hemorrhage.[17,18] Permanent neurologic morbidity following SRS is low in reported series. In the authors' own series, one patient presented with an intraventricular hemorrhage following treatment but had no permanent neurologic morbidity. No patient had new permanent neurologic morbidity after treatment. Other series have put the risk of neurologic morbidity between 0% and 6%.[12,13,16,17,19] One method to reduce the incidence of post-radiosurgical hemorrhage is to delay SRS for at least 6 months after a patient's most recent bleeding event. By waiting this interval, the period of highest risk of AVM rebleeding has passed and the annual risk of hemorrhage is again approximately 2% to 4%.

It should also be mentioned that children who undergo successful SRS or microsurgery for intracranial AVM should be followed closely, as recurrence of these lesions has been documented in the pediatric population.[3–5,26–29] Many have hypothesized that AVM vessels in childhood have a more immature phenotype than adult AVM vessels. It is possible that immature, angiographically undetectable AVM vessels may persist after treatment and lead to delayed regrowth of an AVM nidus.[28] Furthermore, recanalization of previously obliterated AVM vessels may account for regrowth in the pediatric population.[27] It is advised that children with documented AVM obliteration continue to be followed into adulthood to rule out regrowth of these lesions. Lastly, one must consider the risk of radiation-induced tumors in this population with an extended life expectancy. Whereas the risk of second tumor formation is between 2% and 3% following fractionated radiation therapy, the risk of radiation-induced tumors after radiosurgery has been estimated to be approximately 1 in 1000 or less. Rowe and colleagues[28] from the National Center for Stereotactic Radiosurgery in Sheffield compared the incidence of new central nervous system malignancies in their patient population with the national incidence in the United Kingdom. Based on more than 30,000 patient-years of follow-up, they did not find an increased incidence in their radiosurgical patients compared with the age- and sex-adjusted national cohort. The primary weakness of this study is the relative short mean follow-up interval (6.1 years) after radiosurgery relative to the life expectancy of patients having radiosurgery for benign conditions. Neurocognitive deficits after small-volume, single-session radiosurgery have not been reported.

MAYO CLINIC EXPERIENCE

In 2006 the authors published their experience on pediatric AVM radiosurgery for 38 patients managed between 1990 and 2001.[11] To date, the authors have now performed AVM radiosurgery for a total of 60 AVM patients 18 years or younger. Excluded from further analysis are 3 patients managed early in the series with had partial AVM treatment and 9 patients without any (n = 2) or less than 12 months of clinical and radiologic follow-up (n = 7). The median age of the remaining 48 patients (20 boys, 28 girls) was 15 years (range, 3–18 years). Twenty-seven patients (57%) had a previous hemorrhage, whereas 10 patients (21%) had headaches, 7 patients (15%) had seizures, and 4 patients (8%) had their AVM discovered incidentally. The AVM locations included the cerebral hemispheres (n = 32), thalamus (n = 11), brainstem (n = 2), basal ganglia (n = 2), and cerebellum (n = 1).

Single-session radiosurgery was performed for 43 patients and 5 patients underwent staged-volume procedures. A median of 6 isocenters of radiation (range, 1–25) were used to cover a median AVM volume of 3.5 cm^3 (range, 0.2–32.5 cm^3). The median AVM margin dose was 18 Gy (range, 15–25 Gy) and the median maximum radiation dose was 36 Gy (range, 22–50 Gy). The median modified radiosurgery-based AVM score was 0.93 (range, 0.26–3.47).[30] Twelve patients (25%) underwent repeat radiosurgery at a median of 52 months (range, 41–73 months) after their initial radiosurgical procedure. The median follow-up after radiosurgery was 73.5 months (range, 12–151 months).

Nidus obliteration was confirmed in 25 patients (52%) after their initial radiosurgery by angiography (n = 16) or MRI (n = 9). Five additional patients had AVM obliteration after repeat radiosurgery, for a total obliteration rate of 63%. Three patients (6%) had radiation-related deficits after initial (n = 1) or repeat radiosurgery (n = 2). One patient had diplopia from a third nerve paresis after initial radiosurgery of a midbrain AVM, one patient developed hand numbness after repeat radiosurgery of a thalamic AVM, and one patient developed an intentional tremor after repeat radiosurgery of a thalamic AVM. No patient had AVM bleeding following radiosurgery. No patient has had a documented neurocognitive decline or radiation-induced tumor after radiosurgery. Patients with a modified AVM score of less than 1 more frequently had nidus obliteration without new deficits (23/30, 77%) compared with patients with a modified AVM score greater than 1 (6/18, 33%) ($P = .005$, Fisher Exact test).

COMPARISON WITH ADULT OUTCOMES FOLLOWING SRS

The number of studies on AVM radiosurgery in children is far fewer than the published experience of adult AVM radiosurgery. However, it is unclear whether these data can be directly applied to the pediatric population. Many believe that AVM vessels in children have less mature morphology, and that children with AVMs may have a more nebulous natural history. The fact that AVMs treated in childhood have the capacity in rare instances to reoccur has been touted as evidence of the dynamic character of these lesions in childhood.[26,31] Obliteration rates in pediatric patients may be better when compared with adult patients. A study by Tanaka and colleagues[32] reported outcomes for 26 pediatric and 76 adult patients following SRS for intracranial AVMs. Both groups of patients had similar characteristics with regard to AVM grade, treated volume, and radiation dose. Complete obliteration was noted in 45% of adults and 72% of children 1 year after treatment; this rose to 85% for adults and 95% for children 2 years after treatment. Complications were only seen in the adult population (radiation necrosis and bleeding); however, the population of pediatric patients was smaller.

More recently, Nicolato and colleagues[15] reported similar findings in a cohort of 62 children and 193 adult patients. Overall obliteration rates were found to be similar in adults and children (87.6% and 85.5%, respectively); however, the pediatric cohort had a statistically significant decrease in the time to obliteration following treatment and a higher actuarial obliteration rate 36 months after treatment. Although the radiobiological basis of this difference is not clear, it is hypothesized that the endothelium of childhood AVMs has a more robust reaction to radiation. Nicolato and colleagues[14] also showed in a similar study that children had a similar hemorrhage risk during the latency period between treatment and nidus obliteration and that children had a slightly smaller rate of permanent neurologic morbidity following SRS for AVMs, although this difference was not statistically significant. It should be noted, however, that there were statistically significant differences between the cohort of adults and the cohort of children. The pediatric cohort had a significantly greater number of deep-seated AVMs treated with SRS, and children presented with hemorrhage at a much higher rate.[14] Pan and colleagues[16] also recently reviewed their experience with 105 pediatric patients and 458 adult patients treated with SRS for intracranial AVMs. Their results stand in some contrast to the previous reports. Pan and colleagues found that obliteration rates were lower in children for medium-sized (3–10 cm^3) AVMs compared with those of the adult cohort (57.5% compared with 77.9%).

SUMMARY

Stereotactic radiosurgery is a safe and effective option for properly selected pediatric AVM patients. SRS is of particular benefit for children with critically located or deep lesions for which surgical resection would pose a tremendous risk to the patient. The time to AVM obliteration appears to be shorter in children when compared with adult AVM patients.

REFERENCES

1. Celli P, Ferrante L, Palma L, et al. Cerebral arteriovenous malformations in children. Clinical features and outcome of treatment in children and in adults. Surg Neurol 1984;22:43.
2. D'Aliberti G, Talamonti G, Versari PP, et al. Comparison of pediatric and adult cerebral arteriovenous malformations. J Neurosurg Sci 1997;41:331.
3. Humphreys RP, Hoffman HJ, Drake JM, et al. Choices in the 1990s for the management of

pediatric cerebral arteriovenous malformations. Pediatr Neurosurg 1996;25:277.
4. Kahl W, Kessel G, Schwarz M, et al. Arterio-venous malformations in childhood: clinical presentation, results after operative treatment and long-term follow-up. Neurosurg Rev 1989;12:165.
5. Kondziolka D, Humphreys RP, Hoffman HJ, et al. Arteriovenous malformations of the brain in children: a forty year experience. Can J Neurol Sci 1992;19:40.
6. Menovsky T, van Overbeeke JJ. Cerebral arteriovenous malformations in childhood: state of the art with special reference to treatment. Eur J Pediatr 1997;156:741.
7. Ondra SL, Troupp H, George ED, et al. The natural history of symptomatic arteriovenous malformations of the brain: a 24-year follow-up assessment. J Neurosurg 1990;73:387.
8. Smith ER, Butler WE, Ogilvy CS. Surgical approaches to vascular anomalies of the child's brain. Curr Opin Neurol 2002;15:165.
9. Altschuler EM, Lunsford LD, Coffey RJ, et al. Gamma knife radiosurgery for intracranial arteriovenous malformations in childhood and adolescence. Pediatr Neurosci 1989;15:53.
10. Pollock BE, Gorman DA, Brown PD. Radiosurgery for arteriovenous malformations of the basal ganglia, thalamus, and brainstem. J Neurosurg 2004;100:210.
11. Cohen-Gadol AA, Pollock BE. Radiosurgery for arteriovenous malformations in children. J Neurosurg 2006;104(Suppl 6):388.
12. Levy EI, Niranjan A, Thompson TP, et al. Radiosurgery for childhood intracranial arteriovenous malformations. Neurosurgery 2000;47:834.
13. Nataf F, Schlienger M, Lefkopoulos D, et al. Radiosurgery of cerebral arteriovenous malformations in children: a series of 57 cases. Int J Radiat Oncol Biol Phys 2003;57:184.
14. Nicolato A, Lupidi F, Sandri MF, et al. Gamma knife radiosurgery for cerebral arteriovenous malformations in children/adolescents and adults. Part I: differences in epidemiologic, morphologic, and clinical characteristics, permanent complications, and bleeding in the latency period. Int J Radiat Oncol Biol Phys 2006;64:904.
15. Nicolato A, Lupidi F, Sandri MF, et al. Gamma knife radiosurgery for cerebral arteriovenous malformations in children/adolescents and adults. Part II: differences in obliteration rates, treatment-obliteration intervals, and prognostic factors. Int J Radiat Oncol Biol Phys 2006;64:914.
16. Pan DH, Kuo YH, Guo WY, et al. Gamma knife surgery for cerebral arteriovenous malformations in children: a 13-year experience. J Neurosurg Pediatr 2008;1:296.
17. Reyns N, Blond S, Gauvrit JY, et al. Role of radiosurgery in the management of cerebral arteriovenous malformations in the pediatric age group: data from a 100-patient series. Neurosurgery 2007;60:268.
18. Shin M, Kawamoto S, Kurita H, et al. Retrospective analysis of a 10-year experience of stereotactic radio surgery for arteriovenous malformations in children and adolescents. J Neurosurg 2002;97:779.
19. Smyth MD, Sneed PK, Ciricillo SF, et al. Stereotactic radiosurgery for pediatric intracranial arteriovenous malformations: the University of California at San Francisco experience. J Neurosurg 2002;97:48.
20. Pollock BE, Kline RW, Stafford SL, et al. The rationale and technique of staged-volume arteriovenous malformation radiosurgery. Int J Radiat Oncol Biol Phys 2000;48:817.
21. Andrade-Souza YM, Ramani M, Scora D, et al. Embolization before radiosurgery reduces the obliteration rate of arteriovenous malformations. Neurosurgery 2007;60:443.
22. Gerszten PC, Adelson PD, Kondziolka D, et al. Seizure outcome in children treated for arteriovenous malformations using gamma knife radiosurgery. Pediatr Neurosurg 1996;24:139.
23. Andrade-Souza YM, Zadeh G, Ramani M, et al. Testing the radiosurgery-based arteriovenous malformation score and the modified Spetzler-Martin grading system to predict radiosurgical outcome. J Neurosurg 2005;103:642.
24. Pollock BE, Flickinger JC. A proposed radiosurgery-based grading system for arteriovenous malformations. J Neurosurg 2002;96:79.
25. Zabel-du Bois A, Milker-Zabel S, Huber P, et al. Pediatric cerebral arteriovenous malformations: the role of stereotactic linac-based radiosurgery. Int J Radiat Oncol Biol Phys 2006;65:1206.
26. Kader A, Goodrich JT, Sonstein WJ, et al. Recurrent cerebral arteriovenous malformations after negative postoperative angiograms. J Neurosurg 1996;85:14.
27. Lindqvist M, Karlsson B, Guo WY, et al. Angiographic long-term follow-up data for arteriovenous malformations previously proven to be obliterated after gamma knife radiosurgery. Neurosurgery 2000;46:803.
28. Rowe J, Grainger A, Walton L, et al. Risk of malignancy after gamma knife stereotactic radiosurgery. Neurosurgery 2007;60:60.
29. Rodriguez-Arias C, Martinez R, Rey G, et al. Recurrence in a different location of a cerebral arteriovenous malformation in a child after radiosurgery. Childs Nerv Syst 2000;16:363.
30. Pollock BE, Flickinger JC. Modification of the radiosurgery-based arteriovenous malformation grading system. Neurosurgery 2008;63:239.
31. Schmit BP, Burrows PE, Kuban K, et al. Acquired cerebral arteriovenous malformation in a child with moyamoya disease. Case report. J Neurosurg 1996;84:677.
32. Tanaka T, Kobayashi T, Kida Y, et al. [The comparison between adult and pediatric AVMs treated by gamma knife radiosurgery]. No Shinkei Geka 1995; 23(9):773 [in Japanese].

Classification and Endovascular Management of Pediatric Cerebral Vascular Malformations

Timo Krings, MD, PhD, FRCP(C)[a,b,c,*], Sasikhan Geibprasert, MD[d,e], Karel terBrugge, MD, FRCP(C)[a]

KEYWORDS

- Endovascular management
- Pediatric cerebral vascular malformations
- Classification

Before treating pediatric vascular malformation, 2 basic principles have to be taken into account that may seem trivial but still have an effect on management strategies. The first principle is that the understanding of a disease should precede its treatment. In vascular malformations, little is known about their cause, pathophysiology, or natural history, and the numerous different classification schemes that should aid in the understanding of arteriovenous (AV) shunts testify to this lack of knowledge. In addition, advances in diagnostic tools for pretreatment risk assessment as well as continuously improved treatment modalities are likely to further change the way these vascular malformations are managed. The second basic principle is that children are not small adults; vascular malformations in the pediatric population differ significantly from the adult population. Therefore, classification schemes used for and derived from the experience in treating adults are not likely to be compatible with the treatment protocols in children. As a particular example, the adult-based classification of AV shunting lesions that is related to the expected surgical outcome of AV malformations is particularly inappropriate in children, in whom (1) cerebral eloquence is difficult to assess because of the remodeling potential, particularly in the first few years of life, (2) most lesions are fistulas or multifocal, (3) the drainage usually affects the entire venous system, and (4) the potential for recovery is different. In addition, the anatomic and physiologic characteristics of the neonatal and infant brain (including hydrovenous peculiarities and immaturity of myelination) create a specific group of nonhemorrhagic symptoms and therapeutic challenges that are not encountered in adults.

[a] Division of Neuroradiology, Department of Medical Imaging, Toronto Western Hospital, University of Toronto, 399 Bathurst Street, 3MCL – 429, Toronto, ON M5T 2S8, Canada
[b] Department of Neuroradiology, University Hospital Aachen, Pauwelsstraße 30, Aachen 52074, Germany
[c] Service de Neuroradiologie Diagnostique et Therapeutique, CHU Le-Kremlin-Bicetre, 78, rue du Général Leclerc, Cedex, Paris 94275, France
[d] Department of Diagnostic Imaging, The Hospital for Sick Children, University of Toronto, 555 University Avenue, Toronto, ON M5G 1X8, Canada
[e] Department of Radiology, Ramathibodi Hospital, Mahidol University, 270 Rama VI Road, Ratchatewi, Bangkok 10400, Thailand
* Corresponding author. Division of Neuroradiology, Department of Medical Imaging, Toronto Western Hospital, University of Toronto, 399 Bathurst Street, 3MCL – 429, Toronto, ON M5T 2S8, Canada.
E-mail address: timo.krings@uhn.on.ca

Neurosurg Clin N Am 21 (2010) 463–482
doi:10.1016/j.nec.2010.03.010
1042-3680/10/$ – see front matter

This article discusses different approaches to classifying pediatric vascular malformations and describes the endovascular management options. The difficulty in classifying pediatric cerebral vascular malformations is reflected by the large variety of different approaches that have been used for these rare diseases. These classifications may be based on symptoms, pathomechanisms, patient's age, or morphologic features. Each of these classifications may have specific advantages, but the fact that no uniform classification has yet been decided on testifies to their specific drawbacks.

PATHOMECHANICAL CLASSIFICATION

A clinical and pathomechanical classification can lead to the following subcategories: certain high-flow shunts (ie, fistulous pial AV malformations) can lead to macrocrania, hydrocephalus, and psychomotor developmental retardation as a result of hydrovenous disorders, and cardiac insufficiency caused by cardiac overload. Venous congestion that can be caused by a high input (fistulous lesions) or a reduced outflow (secondary stenosis of the outflow pattern) may lead to cognitive decline or epilepsy. Even if signs of venous congestion are not present, a long pial course of the draining vein may indicate that venous drainage restriction is present in a large area, increasing the risk of venous congestion and subsequent epilepsy.[1] Conversely, a short vein that drains almost directly into a dural sinus is unlikely to interfere with the normal pial drainage. If epilepsy was present in a patient with this kind of angioarchitecture, the magnetic resonance imaging (MRI) should be scrutinized for signs of perinidal gliosis or hemosiderosis as the cause of the patient's symptoms. Mass effect is a rare pathomechanism that may result from large venous ectasias or the nidus proper compressing critical structures and may lead to epilepsy, neurologic deficits, and even hydrocephalus.[2] Arterial steal has been associated with clinical findings such as migraine and focal neurologic symptoms that most often are transitory in nature.[3] With the advent of new imaging modalities such as functional MRI and perfusion-weighted MRI it has now become possible to visualize whether or not the symptoms of a patient can be attributed to a true steal. Hemorrhage in AV shunting lesions may be caused by angioarchitectural risk factors such as venous outlet stenoses or intranidal aneurysms (**Table 1**).[4,5] One advantage of this classification is that it may be used to guide therapies, because it relates the pathomechanism to the clinical findings. Therefore, in patients with high-flow shunts and problems that indicate venous congestion or in patients with arterial steal, treatment should be aimed to reduce the AV shunting volume, which can be achieved by endovascular techniques. In patients with epilepsy from perifocal gliosis, or in patients presenting with mass effect, endovascular treatment may be less indicated. Surgical resection or decompression with possible preoperative embolization are likely to be more beneficial in these cases.

AGE-RELATED CLASSIFICATION

A classification of pediatric vascular malformations according to the patient's age is helpful in predicting what type of vascular malformations will be encountered, but does not explain why the predominance of specific vascular malformations in specific age-groups exists. However, the major advantage of this classification is the ability to predict symptoms that are specific for each pediatric age-group.[6]

In the fetal age, prenatal MRI or ultrasound may detect high-flow fistulous lesions, vein of Galen AV malformations (VGAMs) or dural sinus malformations (DSMs). Systemic manifestations such as macrocrania with or without encephalomalacia (melting brain syndrome) and cardiac manifestations may be clinically present and point toward a bad prognosis. Similar to the fetal period, in the neonatal period, VGAMs, DSMs, and pial AV shunts are the predominant lesions; however, albeit rarer, cavernomas and arterial aneurysms have also been observed in this age-group. Systemic pathomechanisms as described earlier and hydrovenous pathomechanisms (hydrocephalus, maturation delay) are found more often in this period. Neurologic manifestations (seizures, focal deficits) point toward a hemorrhagic infarct or venous congestion. During infancy, VGAMs, pial AV shunts (more often fistulous than glomerular), DSMs, aneurysms, and cavernomas may be present. In shunting lesions, hydrodynamic disorders are the predominant pathomechanisms: the cerebrospinal fluid (CSF) reabsorption in this age-group is solely dependent on the venous (transparenchymal) drainage because the arachnoid granulations are not yet fully functional. Therefore, an increased pressure within the venous system (caused by an AV shunt) leads to retention of CSF within the ventricles with a concomitant increase in ventricular size and transependymal pressure gradient until a new equilibrium is found. Macrocrania, cognitive delay, hydrocephalus, and cerebellar tonsillar prolapse are the clinical manifestations at this stage. After

Table 1
Pathomechanical classification of AVMs

Clinical Findings	Angiographic Sign	Additional Imaging Diagnostics	Primary Pathomechanism	Treatment Rational
Neurologic deficits	Perinidal high flow and associated extranidal (remote) hypoperfusion	Perfusion-weighted MRI: extranidal hypoperfusion, Functional MRI (detection of eloquent tissues)	Steal	Reduce shunt
Neurologic deficits	Venous ectasias/pouches close to eloquent brain	MRI: compression, focal edema?, Functional MRI: detection of eloquent tissues	Mass effect	Remove mass effect
Headaches	Occipital high-flow AVM	Perfusion-weighted MRI: extranidal occipital hypoperfusion	Steal	Reduce shunt
Headaches	Large draining veins	MRI: hydrocephalus with draining veins close to the aqueduct or interventricular foramen	Mass effect	Decrease size of draining vein
Headaches	Pseudophlebitic aspect in venous phase, prolonged venous phase	MRI: edema	Venous congestion	Reduce shunt
Epilepsy	Long-standing high-flow shunts, pseudophlebitic aspect in venous phase	CT: calcifications	Venous congestion	Reduce shunt
Epilepsy	Unspecific	MRI: perinidal gliosis	Gliosis	Surgically removal
Epilepsy	Long pial course of draining vein	Unspecific	Venous restriction	Reduce shunt
Cardiac insufficiency	High-flow shunts	MRI/CT: large venous pouches	Right → left shunt	Reduce shunt
Psychomotor developmental retardation	High-flow shunts, pseudophlebitic aspect in venous phase, reduced outflow	MRI: melting brain? CT: calcifications	Venous congestion in not fully matured brain	Reduce shunt
Dementia	Pseudophlebitic aspect in venous phase	MRI: edema	Venous congestion	Reduce shunt

Abbreviation: CT, computed tomography.

2 years of age, the classic AV malformations, cavernomas, aneurysms, and dural AV shunts may be encountered. Hydrodynamic pathomechanisms become less important, whereas symptoms related to the AV shunt and its secondary effects (secondary intranidal aneurysms and venous stenoses leading to hemorrhage, arterial steal, long-standing venous congestion with epilepsy, and focal neurologic deficits) are more often observed (**Table 2**).[7]

MORPHOLOGIC CLASSIFICATION

The most widely used classification of vascular malformation is based on angioarchitectural and histomorphologic features. This purely descriptional classification leads to the well-known differentiation in dural and pial AV shunting lesions, the cavernomas, capillary telangiectasias, and developmental venous anomalies (DVAs).[8]

To differentiate these classic types, in a first step, shunting lesions have to be discerned from nonshunting lesions, the latter being cavernomas, capillary telangiectasias, and DVAs. In a second step, within the shunting lesions, those that are supplied by arteries that would normally supply the brain or the choroid plexus (pial and choroidal brain AV malformations [AVMs]) have to be differentiated from those shunts that are supplied by arteries that normally supply the dura and meninges (ie, the classic dural AV fistulae). The nonshunting lesions, on the other hand, exhibit typical neuroimaging and histologic features that in most instances allow for a further subclassification into the cavernomas, which are composed of thin-walled, dilated capillary spaces with no intervening brain tissue and blood products in varying stages of evolution, and the capillary telangiectasias, which consist of localized collections of abnormal thin-walled vascular channels interposed between normal brain parenchyma. The DVAs are nonpathologic normal variations of the venous pattern of draining the normal brain tissue distributed along transmedullary venous anastomoses (**Fig. 1**).

This angio- and histoarchitectural classification is easy to implement routinely; it is able to predict the prognosis of the vascular malformation within an affected individual and is therefore of importance for the neuroradiologist and the treating physician. However, it does not help to further our knowledge or understanding of these diseases because no information about cause or the nature of the disease can be obtained from this classification. In this purely morphologic approach, secondary changes induced by the vascular malformation itself on the adjacent vasculature may be difficult to differentiate from the malformation proper. If the pathogenesis or cause are not completely understood, therapeutic approaches may therefore be difficult to tailor to an individual malformation. In addition, although rare, certain vascular malformations do not fit into any of the proposed categories, which may result in

Table 2
Age-related classification of pediatric vascular malformations; in each age-group specific clinical presentations and disease entities are found

Age	Clinical Presentation	Type of Vascular Malformation
In utero	Congestive cardiac failure (pulse>200 beats/min, ventricular extrasystoles, tricuspid insufficiency), macrocrania, ventriculomegaly, brain loss (melting brain)	Pial high-flow AVFs, VGAMs, DSMs
Neonate	Congestive cardiac failure, multiorgan failure, coagulopathies), intracranial hemorrhage (hematomas, venous infarct, SAH), convulsions	VGAMs, pial high-flow AVFs, DSMs
Infant	Hydrovenous disorders: macrocrania, hydrocephalus, convulsions, retardation, intracranial hemorrhage (hematoma, venous infarct, SAH)	VGAMs, pial AVMs (fistulous > nidal), aneurysms, cavernomas
Child	Intracranial hemorrhage (hematoma, venous infarct, SAH), progressive neurocognitive and neurologic deficits, convulsions, headaches	Pial AVMs (nidal > fistulous), aneurysms, cavernomas, dural AV shunts

Abbreviations: AVF, arteriovenous fistula; SAH, subarachnoid hemorrhage.

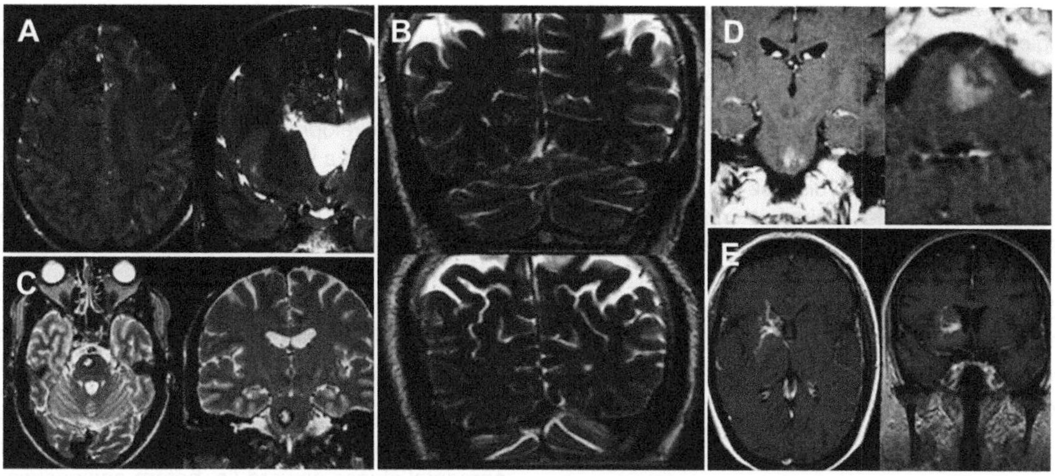

Fig. 1. Morphologic classification: these images show the classic differentiation into pial and dural AV shunting lesions (with pathologic flow voids either within the parenchyma (*A*) or within the subarachnoid space (*B*), respectively), the cavernomas with their classic mulberry shape (*C*), the capillary telangiectasias with the fluffy contrast enhancement (*D*), typically encountered in the pons), and the DVAs with their caput medusa of a dilated transmedullary vein (*E*).

a therapeutic dilemma. Moreover, cases of transitional vascular malformations point toward a spectrum of overlapping vascular disease entities rather than clear-cut categories.

We therefore propose a classification of pediatric vascular malformations that is based on the cause of the vascular malformation to account for the shortcomings mentioned earlier. Although this classification will not alter therapeutic strategies for the time being, it may enhance our knowledge about the disease beyond its pure morphologic aspect.

ETIOLOGIC CLASSIFICATION

This classification is based on the recent understanding of angio- and vasculogenesis (on the arterial and venous side) and the influence of environmental and genetic factors. To explain the concepts of this classification, we propose 3 approaches to pediatric vascular malformations: the timing, the target, and the nature of the triggering event.

The Triggering Event

The concept of the triggering event is built on the assumption that most pediatric vascular malformations can be considered as congenital malformations (ie, malformations or structural weaknesses of the vessel that have been triggered or are present before birth and that make the vessel more prone to developing, once a second hit (or second trigger) occurs, the morphologic and/or clinical vascular lesion). This concept implies that the malformations are initially quiescent and may reveal themselves only later in life, which implies a differentiation into primary (or causative) triggers and secondary (or revealing) triggers. The stages of vascular malformations based on this assumption are therefore the prepathologic stage, during which no disease exits; however, a window of exposure opens that makes the cell temporarily vulnerable for an appropriate triggering event (eg, inflammatory, infectious, radiation-induced, toxic, metabolic, or traumatic). During the genetic stage, this appropriate (or causative) trigger for the vascular target and the time produces a primary lesion (that may result in a germinal or somatic mutation or a permanent dysfunction of the vessel). If it is neither repaired nor leads to cell death, the primary local defect (although for the time being quiescent) is transmitted to later generation cells and has a clonal remote effect. At this phase, the disease is not yet morphologically apparent, but is present as a permanent structural weakness. This stage can therefore be denominated as a biologic or premorphologic stage. Later in life (in most instances postnatal), during a new window of exposure with a secondary (or revealing) trigger, a secondary mutation or an additional dysfunction allows for the phenotypic expression of the disease. This secondary trigger may appear during repeated vascular remodeling, may be related to shear stress, inflammation or trauma, or may constitute a second (somatic) mutation. At this stage, the disease manifests itself as a morphologic but not yet clinical entity (eg, incidental finding of an unruptured aneurysm). This stage is the morphologic or preclinical stage. Only after failure of biologic compensation mechanisms (intrinsic repair mechanisms), or during secondary angiopathic changes (extrinsic risk factors: hemodynamic disequilibrium, shear stresses), the already morphologically fragile disease will get symptomatic and enter the clinical, symptomatic stage (**Fig. 2**).[9]

Target of the Trigger

Development of blood vessels from differentiating endothelial cells (EC) is called vasculogenesis, whereas sprouting of new blood vessels from the preexisting ones is termed angiogenesis. Vascular endothelial growth factor (VEGF) and its receptor VEGFR2 are the most critical drivers of embryonic vessel formation. During vasculogenesis lateral and posterior mesodermal cells migrate toward the yolk sac. During their migration, the precursors aggregate to clusters, termed hemangioblastic aggregates. The peripheral cells of these aggregates flatten to differentiate into EC, whereas the centrally located cells differentiate to hematopoietic cells of the blood islands. Following this differentiation, EC surrounding these blood islands anastomose to form a capillary meshwork, which serves as a scaffold for the beginnings of circulation, before the heart starts beating.[10] It is only after the onset of heartbeat and of blood flow that the yolk sac capillary plexus is remodeled into arteries and veins in the now ongoing process of angiogenesis. Historically, it was believed that the EC of the primary capillary plexus constituted a homogenous group of cells and that further differentiation into arteries and veins occurred because of hemodynamic forces. However, in recent years, several signaling molecules were discovered, which labeled arterial or venous EC from early developmental stages onward, before the assembly of a vascular wall. Arterial EC selectively express ephrin-B2, neuropilin-1, and members of the Notch pathway, whereas other molecules are specifically expressed in the venous system only; some molecules (such as the neuropilin-2 receptor) are expressed in early stages by veins and, at later developmental stages, become restricted to lymphatic vessels.[10] These observations led to the hypothesis that the embryonic vascular system could be predetermined to an arterial, venous, or lymphatic fate from early developmental stages onward (ie, before angiogenesis and after vasculogenesis).[11] Arteries, veins, and lymphatic vessels are therefore different, molecularly defined targets. It can therefore be easily envisioned that triggering events are specific for either the arterial or the venous site. Diseases that strike only on the arterial site (aneurysms, dissections) can therefore be differentiated from diseases that are targeted against the capillary, venous, or lymphatic vessels.[12]

Timing of the Trigger

The endothelium and the media of blood vessels are derived from the mesoderm and the neural crest, respectively, with the exception of the mesencephalic region and the spinal levels, both of which originate from mesoderm. These neural crest or para-axial mesoderm cells are migrating groups of cells starting from the segmented

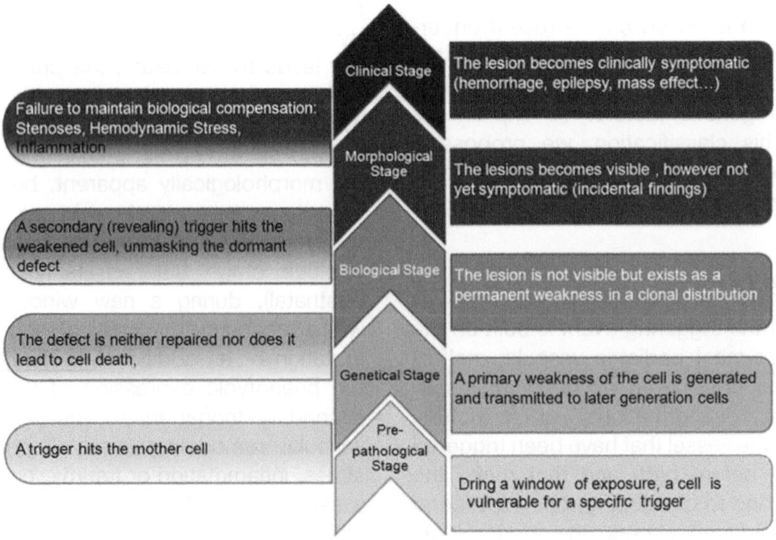

Fig. 2. The congenital nature of vascular malformations and the role of triggering events.

regions.[13] They course along predetermined paths in which daughter cells are seeded. When a defect in this migrating cell is present, the defect is transmitted to the daughter cells along its migrating path. The effect, size, area, and severity of the defect produced by the causative trigger are therefore related to the timing of the event in relation to the migration; the earlier the hit, the larger the effect on the vessels with a more widespread and severe vascular lesion. Vice versa, the later the hit, the more focal the effect and the more confined the vascular lesion. Although a germinal mutation is present in all cells, an early somatic mutation may lead to various stages of metamerically arranged defects, whereas a postnatal mutation affects only a small cluster of cells. Although congenital, some of these mutations may be revealed only later in life (such as in a failed remodeling during vascular renewal).

In the early embryonic vessel configuration (ie, during the early stages of angiogenesis and after the heart started beating) not all capillaries are integrated into the primitive circulation. In this period, the primitive circulation consists of direct transitions of arteries into veins; arterial and venous blood can flow through the same vascular channel.[10] This embryonic circulation is therefore different from the adult situation (in which blood flows through arteries into arterioles, a capillary bed, and through successively larger veins back to the heart). If this embryonic arterial-venous vessel configuration persists, large arterial-venous shunts will develop (which may be the case in certain fistulous malformations of the brain and spine). With further development of the vasculature (ie, in later embryonic and fetal stages), the area of the shunt may become more confined, again revealing the importance of the timing of the triggering event in relation to the size and effect of the vascular malformation.

Nature of the Trigger

Depending on the type of trigger, purely genetic diseases (such as hereditary hemorrhagic telangiectasia [HHT][14]) can be differentiated from purely extrinsic diseases (such as vascular traumatic lesions).[15] In between these extremes, however, triggering events with varying roles of genetic and environmental triggers can be identified.

This concept leads to the classification shown in **Table 3**, in which focal, segmental, and metameric lesions (which depend on the timing of the triggering event) are tabulated against the location of the lesion along the arteriocapillary-venous tree (as the specific target hit by the triggering event) and the nature of the trigger (ie, genetic vs nongenetic). Thus, the following classification of pediatric vascular malformations is proposed, keeping in mind that this classification has to be regarded as a spectrum of diseases and that the subclassifications presented constitute arbitrary boundaries.

MANAGEMENT STRATEGIES FOR PEDIATRIC VASCULAR MALFORMATIONS ACCORDING TO THE ETIOLOGIC CLASSIFICATION

Arterial Lesions

Focal arterial lesions

On the arterial side, aneurysms and arterial dissections are those vascular lesions that are caused by a focal effect on the arterial tree. They can be related to genetic influences (such as in arterial aneurysms associated with neurofibromatosis type 1, Ehlers-Danlos syndrome type IV, and familial immune deficiency syndrome) or to purely

Table 3
The etiologic classification of pediatric vascular malformations based on the timing, the target, and the nature of the triggering event (diseases in italics denominate a purely genetic nature of the trigger)

	Timing → Effect		
Target	**Late Hit → Focal Disease**	**Intermediate Hit → Segmental Disease**	**Early Hit → Metameric Disease**
Arterial level	Aneurysms, arterial dissections, *Ehler-Danlos syndrome IV*, *Marfan syndrome*, *NFI*	Mirror (twin) aneurysms and dissections, segmental aneurysm	PHACES
AV level	AVM, VGAM, *HHT*	Proliferative angiopathy	CAMS
Venous level	DVAs, sinus pericranii, cavernoma, *familial cavernomas*	DSM	Cerebrofacial venous metameric syndrome, *blue rubber bleb nevus*

environmental factors (such as vascular trauma). Presumably most arterial aneurysms and dissections in the pediatric age-group are related to environmental and genetic influences with intrinsic predisposing factors such as segmental vulnerability, wall matrix failure, and altered repair mechanisms on the one hand, and extrinsic triggering factors such as inflammation, (minor) trauma, and autoimmune-related causes on the other (**Fig. 3**).[16,17] Although the complete description of treatment strategies in pediatric aneurysms is beyond the scope of this article, their (dissecting, traumatic, or infectious) nature often leads to the necessity of parent vessel occlusion with the risk of subsequent stroke. Because the disease process (given its cause) is in most cases located in the vessel wall, a purely endoluminal treatment (ie, coiling of the aneurysm) is successful only in patients in whom true saccular aneurysms are present. Most aneurysms, however, are a symptom rather than the disease itself and therefore require a more thorough evaluation of their cause before treatment (**Fig. 4**).

Segmental arterial lesions

Mirror or twin aneurysms and the rarely occurring segmental aneurysms belong in this group.[18,19] Mirror aneurysms are aneurysms that occur on identical vascular segments bilaterally and may be related to vascular precursor cells that originate from a mother cell whose clones migrated to the same vessel segment within both hemispheres. These cells have been identified in quail-chicken chimera experiments and point toward a defect that occurred earlier during vasculogenesis and therefore affects a larger portion of the arterial tree (**Fig. 5**).[20] The association of cervical internal carotid artery (ICA) aneurysm with ipsilateral vertebrobasilar aneurysm is grouped in the same category. The association of a developmental error being expressed in two seemingly separate segments that are linked (from a phylogenetic and embryologic point of view) by the hypoglossal artery suggests a segmental error related to this embryonic vessel.[21] Treatment strategies in these aneurysms are similar, as discussed in the previous section; however, the treating physician

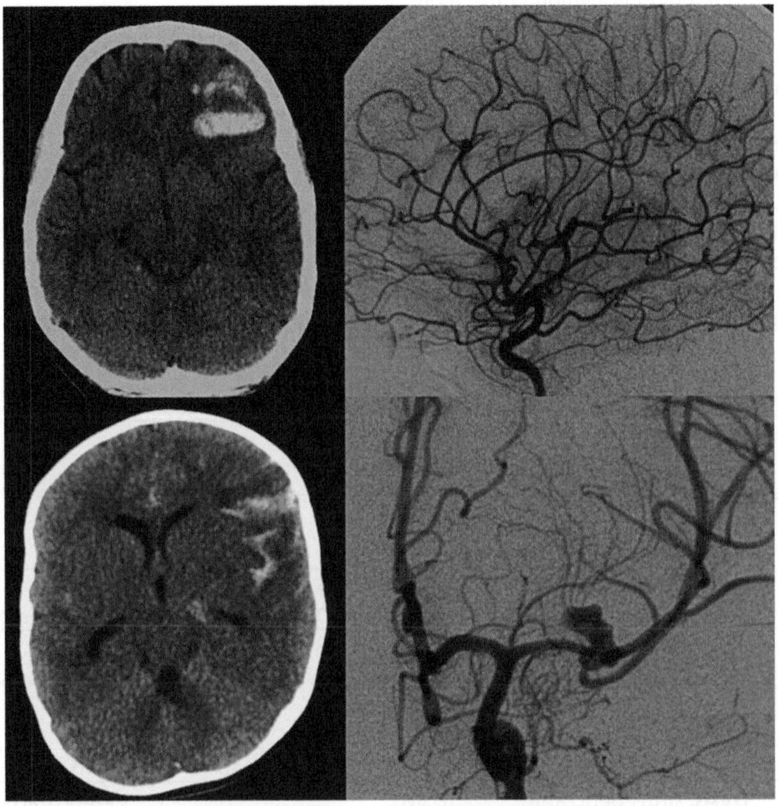

Fig. 3. Aneurysms and dissections can be regarded as focal arterial lesions. Here, 2 pediatric patients with an inflammatory aneurysm of the distal fronto-opercular branch of the middle cerebral artery (*upper row*) and a dissecting aneurysm of the left middle cerebral artery are shown.

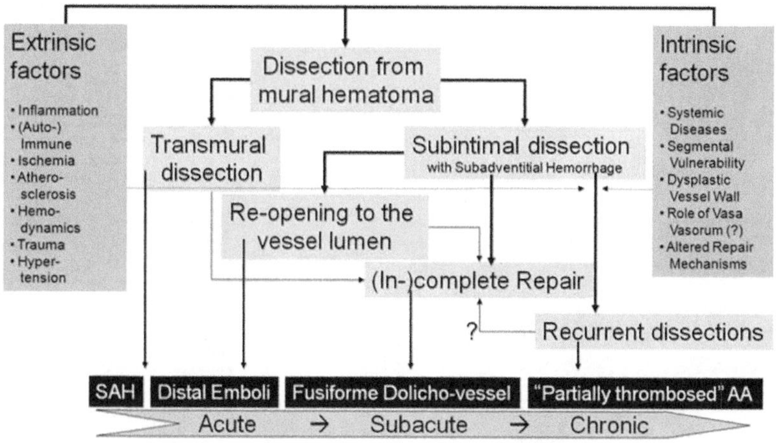

Fig. 4. It has been suggested that most pediatric aneurysms are caused by dissecting mechanisms. This graph shows the potential phenotypic expressions of dissecting diseases and their presumed cause.

has to keep in mind that the vessel wall in the affected segment may be congenitally weakened and may therefore lead to future recurrences, necessitating close imaging follow-up.

Metameric arterial lesions

When the mesodermal cells migrate to their target organs, they seed daughter cells along their predetermined paths. Once these daughter cells have migrated to their target organ, they may acquire phenotypic specificity as a result of cell-cell signaling. A defect in one of these early mesodermal cells may lead to longitudinally arranged or metameric syndromes, with multiple phenotypic expressions along the migration paths.[11] This may lead to the occurrence of seemingly unrelated (and mostly arterial) lesions, grouped according to the acronym PHACES: posterior fossa malformations, hemangiomas, arterial malformation (including the aorta and the cranial vessels with dolichosegments and stenoses), cardiac defects, eye abnormalities, and sterna raphe defects (**Fig. 6**).[22,23] Treatment of PHACES syndrome should be symptomatic and, for the hemangiomas, treatment strategies should not differ from those used for the nonsyndromal forms. With respect to the arterial anomalies, segmental dysplasias or dolichosegments do not constitute entities that should be treated and should not be misdiagnosed for AV malformations or aneurysms.

Capillary Lesions (ie, Lesions at the AV Junction)

Focal capillary lesions

A focal lesion at the AV junction may produce a shunt that can be pial, dural, or choroidal, leading to the classic AVMs,[24] choroidal AVMs

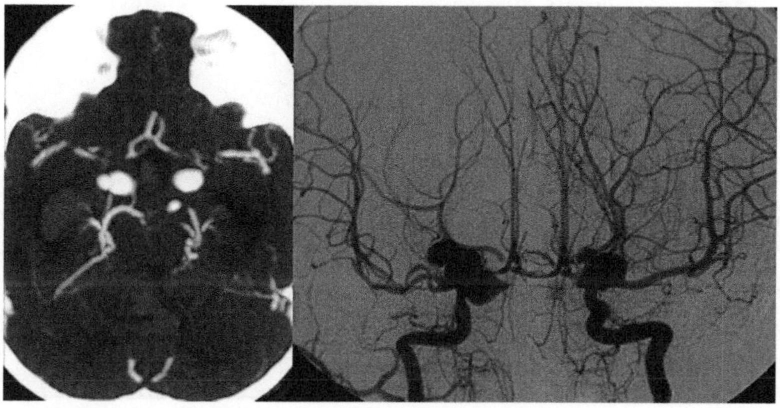

Fig. 5. Mirror (or twin) aneurysms are segmental arterial lesions because a single mother cell can give daughter cells that migrate to identical vascular segments on both cerebral hemispheres.

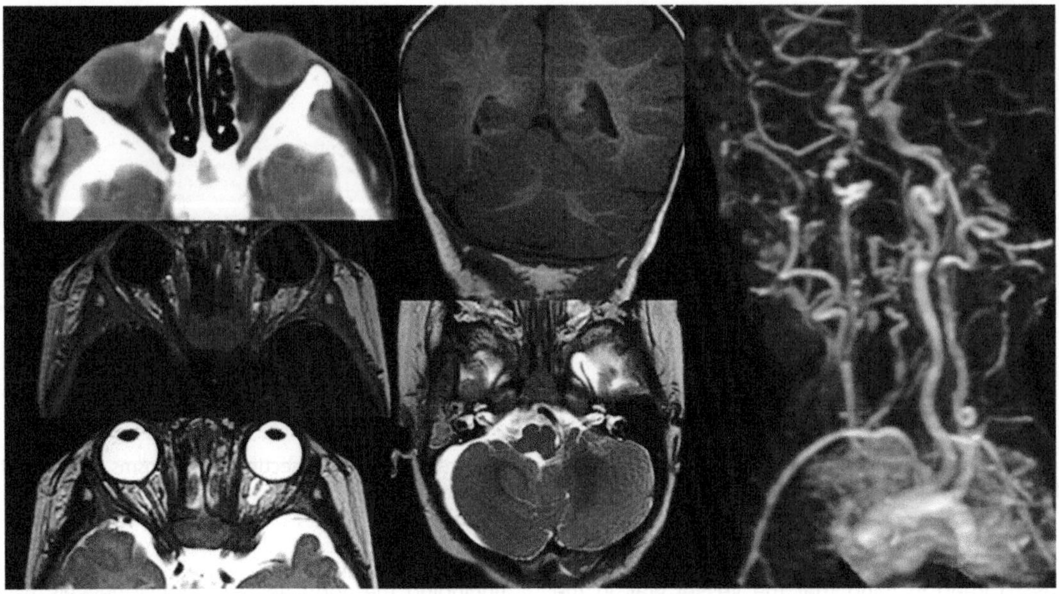

Fig. 6. Metameric arterial vascular lesion. In this 8-year-old girl, a right-sided facial hemangioma, a posterior fossa malformation, and dolichoectatic ICAs are present.

(such as the classic VGAMs),[25] or to dural AV shunts.[26] These focal AV lesions may be related to a purely genetic disease (such as HHT[27]) and encompass a spectrum of diseases: from shunting lesions with a large volume (ie, a large opening of the artery into the vein, which is, given the considerations on the timing of the event mentioned earlier, most likely related to an early causative trigger) to microshunts, and from extended shunting zones (holohemispheric AVMs) to localized nidi (**Fig. 7**).[28] Treatment strategies in these lesions are complex and related to the individual clinical presentation and AVM angioarchitecture. At least 3 different groups of patients have to be distinguished: asymptomatic patients, nonhemorrhagic symptomatic patients, and patients who became symptomatic as a result of an intracranial hemorrhage. However, in all 3 groups a careful analysis of the angioarchitecture is necessary (1) to predict further hemorrhagic and nonhemorrhagic deficits, (2) to evaluate whether the specific symptoms of an individual patient can be related to the AVM, and (3) to define the point of rupture. This analysis of the angioarchitecture not only enables

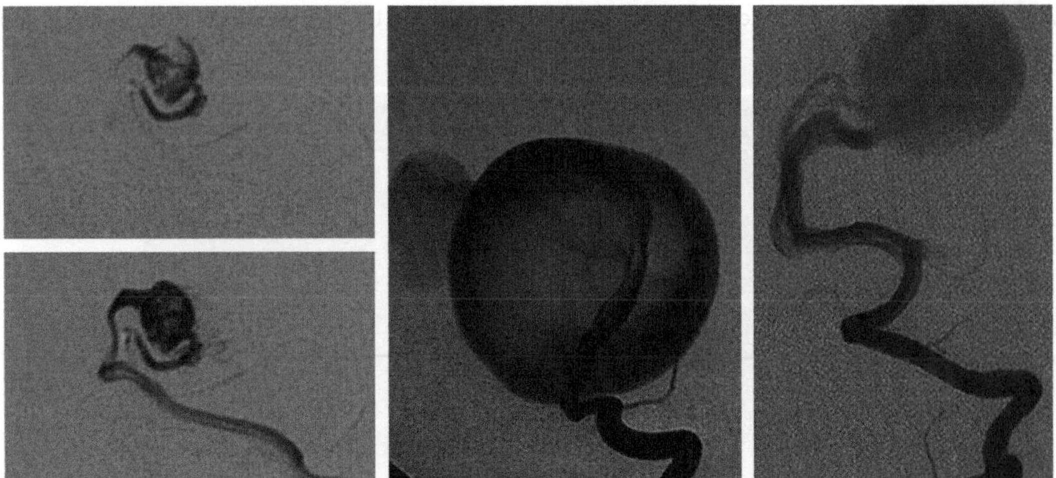

Fig. 7. Focal AV (or capillary lesions) are present in the nidal AV malformations (*right panel*) but also in the fistulous AV malformations (*middle panel*) or in the VGAMs as a special form of pediatric choroidal AV malformation.

classification according to the pathomechanical classification as pointed out in **Table 1** but also relates to future hemorrhagic risks by evaluating focal weak points. These angioarchitectural weak points are (1) intranidal aneurysms and venous ectasias[29] and (2) venous stenosis.[4]

The first investigators to state that specific angioarchitecture present in brain AV malformations make them more prone for future hemorrhage were Brown and colleagues[30] in 1988, who found that the annual risk of future hemorrhage was 3% in brain AVMs alone, and 7% per year in brain AVMs (B-AVMs) with associated pre- and intranidal aneurysms. Meisel and colleagues[29] found that among 662 patients with B-AVMs there were 305 patients with associated aneurysms and there was a significant increase in rebleed episodes in B-AVMs harboring intranidal aneurysms ($P<.002$). In the Toronto series of 759 B-AVMs, associated aneurysms were statistically significantly ($P = .015$) associated with future bleeding (**Fig. 8**).[31] It may be difficult to discern intranidal arterial aneurysms from intranidal venous ectasias, which is why these 2 angioarchitectural specificities are grouped as 1 entity in most series. Venous stenoses, on the other hand, are a separate angiographic weak point and are often seen in ruptured AVMs. The nature of the venous stenosis is not completely understood; high-flow vessel wall changes, failure in remodeling, or an increased vessel wall response to the shear stress induced by the arterialization have been proposed as potential causes. A stenotic venous outlet leads to an imbalance of pressure in various compartments of the AVM, which may induce subsequent rupture of the AVM. The compartment that is drained by the stenotic vessel should be scrutinized for contrast stagnation and, if endovascular therapy is contemplated, extreme caution has to be undertaken not to push liquid embolic agent toward the already stenosed vein, as this may lead to catastrophic results. In addition to these 2 angioarchitectural risk factors, other factors may lead to an increased risk of hemorrhage; these are deep venous drainage only, older age, and male gender.[32]

Analysis of the angioarchitecture has to be performed before contemplating therapy for an AVM; specifically, the following points have to be addressed: the nature and number of the feeding arteries, the presence or absence of flow-related aneurysms; the number of separate compartments of the malformation; any arterial or venous ectasias

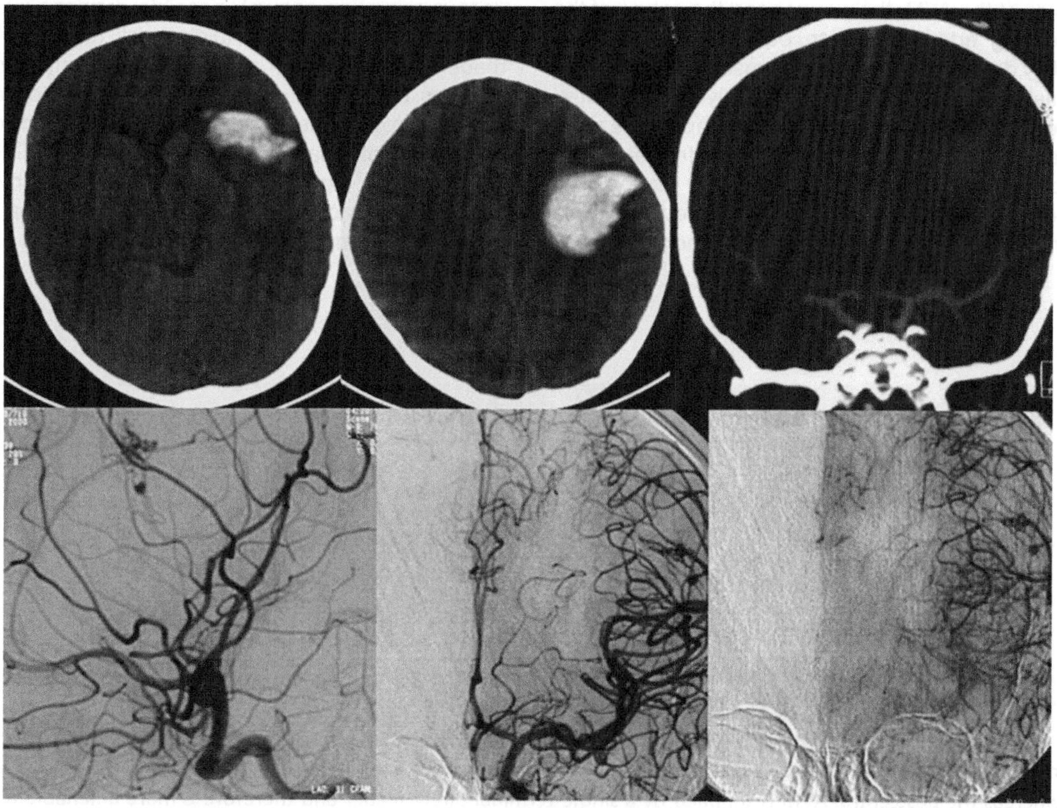

Fig. 8. In patients with AVMs, associated aneurysms should be considered as the source of bleeding.

Table 4
Features important for a treatment-based classification of B-AVMs using endovascular techniques

Artery	Flow-related aneurysms Number of feeder Type of feeder (direct vs en passage)
Nidus	Number of compartments Intranidal aneurysms Fistulous versus nidal
Veins	Stenoses Number of draining veins per compartment

near to or within the malformation; and the nature of the venous drainage (**Table 4**). On the arterial side, flow-related aneurysms (discussed in greater detail later) are typically present on branching points of the major feeding arteries. They classically resolve following treatment of the AVM and are caused by vascular remodeling following increased shear stress.[33] Although not a contraindication for endovascular treatment they present a danger to the neurointerventionalist, because flow-directed catheters are prone to enter the aneurysm rather than the distal vessels. Concerning the arterial side of the AVM, the number and the nature of the feeding arteries need to be assessed because they determine whether endovascular approaches make sense. A large number of only slightly dilated feeders make an endovascular therapy more challenging than those with a single large feeder.[34] Two basic types of feeding arteries may be encountered. Direct arterial feeders end in the AVM, while indirect arterial feeders supply the normal cortex and also supply the AVM en passage via small vessels that arise from the normal artery (**Fig. 9**).

Whereas direct feeders are safe targets for an endovascular therapy, en passage feeders may carry the risk of inadvertent arterial glue migration to distal healthy vessels. In this regard, the security margin of the catheter position has to be briefly discussed. Liquid embolic agents may cause reflux at the end of the injection. Depending on the agent, the microcatheter, the injection technique, and the skills of the operator, this reflux may be as far as 1 cm proximal to the tip of the catheter. A safe deposition of liquid embolic agent is therefore possible only if the catheter tip is distal enough to be beyond any vessel that supplies normal brain tissue. In AVMs with en passage feeders, this may not be possible, especially if the catheter is only hooked into the feeding artery and jumps backward because of the jet effect when liquid embolic agent is injected.

Moving from the artery to the angioarchitecture of the nidus, intranidal arterial aneurysms and venous varices that indicate weak points need to be recognized as well as the number of compartments and their nature (nidal vs fistulous) (**Fig. 10**). On the venous side of the AVM, the number of draining veins per compartment (the more the better for endovascular treatment if venous migration occurs), possible drainage into the deep venous system (higher risk for hemorrhage, more difficult surgical treatment), and stenosis that restrict venous outflow have to be identified to fully determine the risk of a specific AVM. This information can be obtained only by conventional digital subtraction angiography, which in our practice must still precede any treatment decision in AVMs.

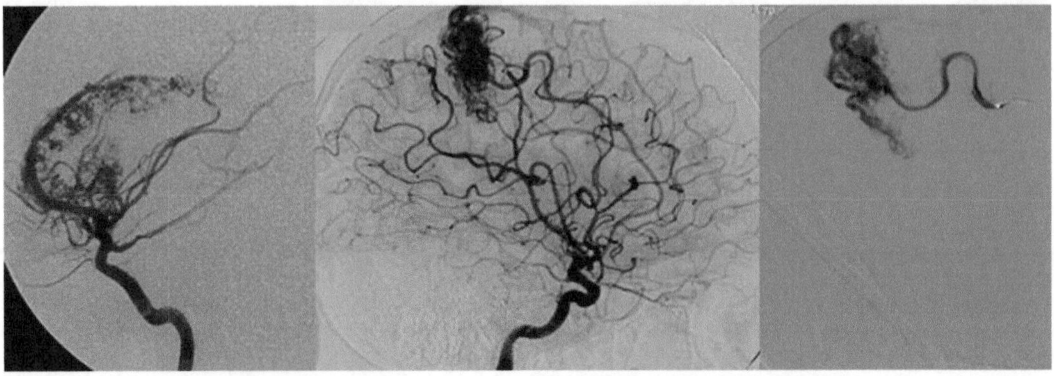

Fig. 9. Indirect versus direct feeder in 2 AVMs: the pericallosal AVM is supplied by a multitude of indirect feeders, whereas the postcentral AVM is supplied by a single-terminal direct feeder and therefore is more amenable for embolization.

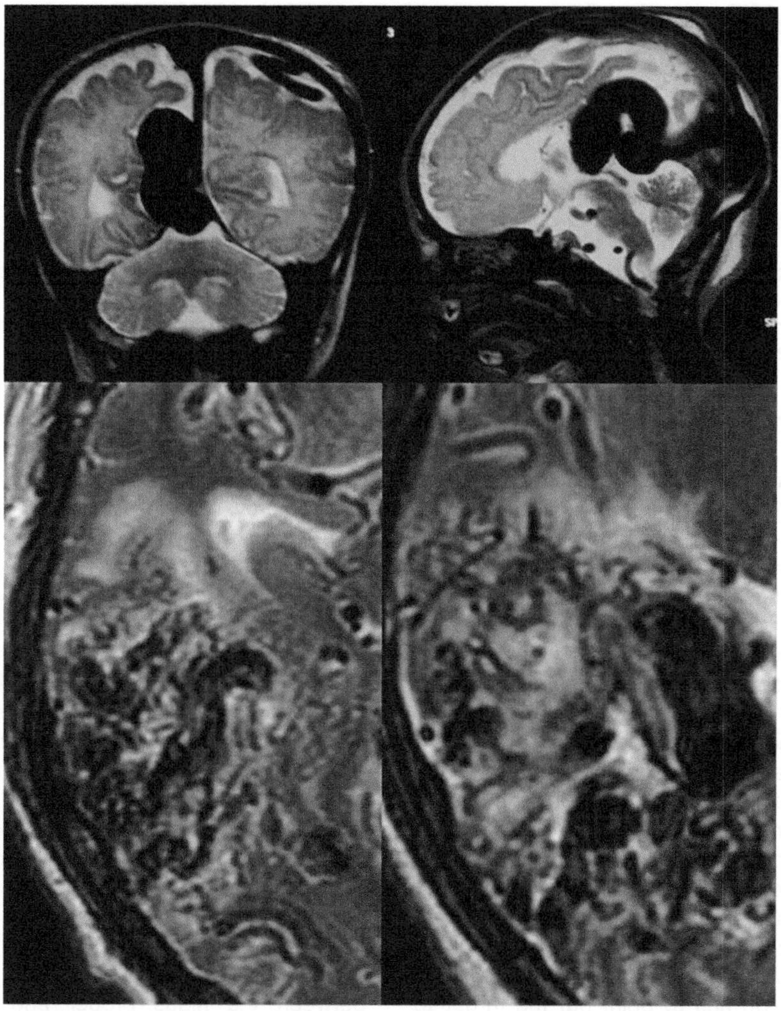

Fig. 10. Whether a nidal or a fistulous transition between arteries and veins is present can in most instances be seen from the MRI alone. This factor has major implications on the pathophysiology and on the choice of treatment modalities.

A complete cure of a pial brain AVM by endovascular means is possible in approximately 20% of all AVMs irrespective of their angioarchitecture.[35–37] Those AVMs that are favorable to a complete cure are the small, single-feeder, single-compartment AVMs that have a direct feeding artery. Because these AVMs are also good candidates for radiosurgery and open neurosurgery, a tailored team approach is preferable for each specific AVM in each individual patient, respecting their wishes and taking into consideration the clinical presentation. In most instances, endovascular therapies are used to diminish the size of an AVM before radiotherapy or surgery, to secure focal weak points in the acute and subacute stage of ruptured AVMs (**Fig. 11**) and in unruptured AVMs in which radiosurgery is contemplated, or to exclude those compartments of an AVM that may be difficult to reach during surgery. Once treatment for an AVM is decided upon, a pathway to its complete exclusion has to be agreed on by the treatment team, which should include radiosurgeons, vascular neurosurgeons, and neurointerventionalists. It does not make sense in our opinion to partially treat an AVM without a strategy on how to handle a possible residual of the AVM.

If endovascular therapy is chosen, we proceed with a predefined goal, which may mean performing what has been termed a partially targeted embolization. Such rationale is based on the outcome of a series of more than 600 patients with AVMs who were partially embolized and showed a significant decrease in hemorrhage episodes when compared with the conservatively treated series reported in the literature.[38] The

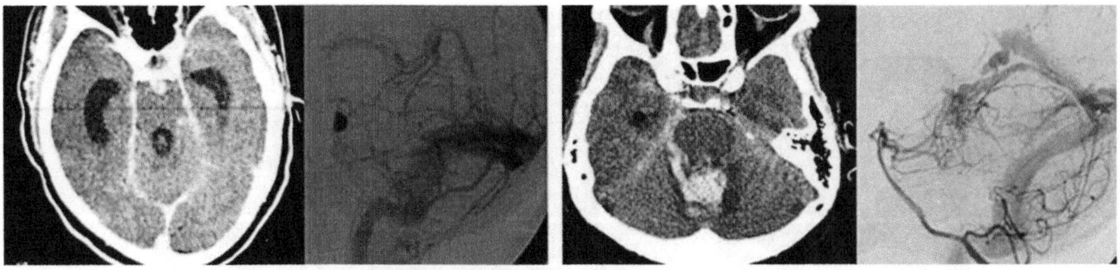

Fig. 11. In acutely ruptured AVMs, angiographic points of weakness have to be sought and can, in many instances, be secured by endovascular therapies. In these 2 examples an intranidal aneurysm with contrast stagnation as the potential source of hemorrhage and a venous stenosis with subsequent increase in intranidal pressure are visualized.

yearly hemorrhage incidence rate of patients before partial treatment was 0.062 (95% confidence interval [CI] 0.03–0.11). The observed annual rate after the start of this regime was 0.02 (95% CI 0.012–0.030).[38] Given the considerations mentioned earlier concerning focal weak points, we think that these numbers reflect the benefit of selectively embolizing specific weak compartments of an AVM, thereby providing early protection while the patient is scheduled for radiotherapy (the effects of which take more time but with higher rates of complete obliteration). In these instances the goal is to secure the AVM during the waiting period for complete occlusion. In other instances the goal may be to exclude those compartments that are difficult to reach before surgery or to diminish the size of the AVM before radiosurgery. In the latter instances, compartments in the periphery of the AVM have to be targeted, whereas in the former instances, the neurosurgeon has to point out the target to the neurointerventionalist. In combined therapies (endovascular + radiotherapy; endovascular + surgery) the relative risks of each procedure are cumulative, and embolization makes sense only if a goal is predefined before the therapy. In most instances, this goal should be reached after a maximum of 2 to 3 endovascular sessions.

For most pial AVMs, liquid embolic materials are the first choice of treatment. The therapy is performed under general monitored neuroanesthesia. We classically use a 5-F guiding catheter that is placed into the distal ICA or vertebral artery. A flow-directed microcatheter is then advanced and directed with a microguidewire or gentle contrast injections into the feeding artery and into the nidus proper using roadmap or fluoroscopy techniques. Here a wedged position of the catheter tip is sought, paying careful attention that there are no normal brain-supplying arteries distal or close to the tip of the catheter. After test injections and preparation of the catheter, the liquid embolic material is injected into the nidus, paying careful attention to avoid venous migration. Depending on the type of embolic agent and the nidus (fistulous vs nidal), the injection techniques vary. To prevent venous migration, the blood pressure may be temporarily lowered, or the jugular veins may be compressed. There is an ongoing debate into what kind of liquid embolic agent to use. Personal experience of the authors as well as published data show a higher rate of complete obliteration with the use of Onyx (40%–60%) but with a significant increased treatment associated risk for permanent morbidity and mortality (8%–12%).[39,40] Proximal occlusion of feeding arteries without penetration of the embolic material to and just beyond the site of the shunt reopens the nidus via leptomeningeal collaterals and may induce a profound neoangiogenesis, which should be avoided because subsequent endovascular therapies will not be possible. In addition, the profound neoangiogenesis makes discrimination between the nidus proper and normal brain supplying arteries nearly impossible. Therefore, in the opinion of the authors, coils and microcoils are not indicated for nidal type AVMs. These embolization materials have a place only in certain single-hole macrofistulae. Likewise, particles, especially if too large, may lead to an occlusion that is too proximal with subsequent neoangiogenesis. In addition, particles do not result in a stable occlusion in pial brain AVMs and their use at the end of a procedure is more cosmetic.

Although most AVMs have both fistulous (ie, direct transitions of arteries and veins) and glomerular (ie, shunts with an intervening network of pathologic vessels) compartments, a specific subset of purely fistulous pial AV shunts, called the pial single-hole macrofistulae, deserve special consideration. They are often present in children and should raise the suspicion of an underlying genetic disease such as HHT.[14] HHT is inherited as an autosomal-dominant trait, with varying penetrance and expressivity. Cerebral pial AV fistulas in HHT are macrofistulae with a high fistula volume and are of the single-hole type. The feeding arteries drain directly into a massively enlarged venous pouch and often there is only 1 single-feeding artery. Signs of venous congestion are typically present because of venous overload and are responsible for the patient's symptoms. Associated angiographic abnormalities include venous ectasias, venous stenoses, pial reflux, venous ischemia, calcifications, and associated arterial aneurysms. Patients are typically younger than 16 years and there is a propensity for early infancy (in our series all patients but 2 were less than 6 years old).[27] Localization of the arteriovenous fistula is either cortical supratentorial or infratentorial and deep locations are exceptional. Presenting symptoms are intracerebral hemorrhage in most patients; macrocrania, bruit, cognitive deficits, cardiac insufficiency, epilepsy, tonsillar prolapse, and hydrocephalus may also be present.

In our practice, treatment consists of superselective glue embolization to obliterate the fistulous area by pushing the glue via the artery into the venous pouch to establish a mushroom-shaped glue cast that occludes the single-hole fistula. Alternatively, coils may be used to selectively occlude the fistulous site. Because a major problem of glue embolization is the uncontrollable propagation of glue into veins with secondary venous occlusion and hemorrhage, we try to minimize this risk in these macrofistulae by using undiluted glue with tantalum powder at a position close to the venous pouch with the catheter tip pointed against the vessel wall.[27] In selected patients flow reduction with coils may be used before glue embolization (**Fig. 12**).

Segmental capillary lesions

The disease entity of proliferative angiopathy can be placed on the segmental side of the spectrum

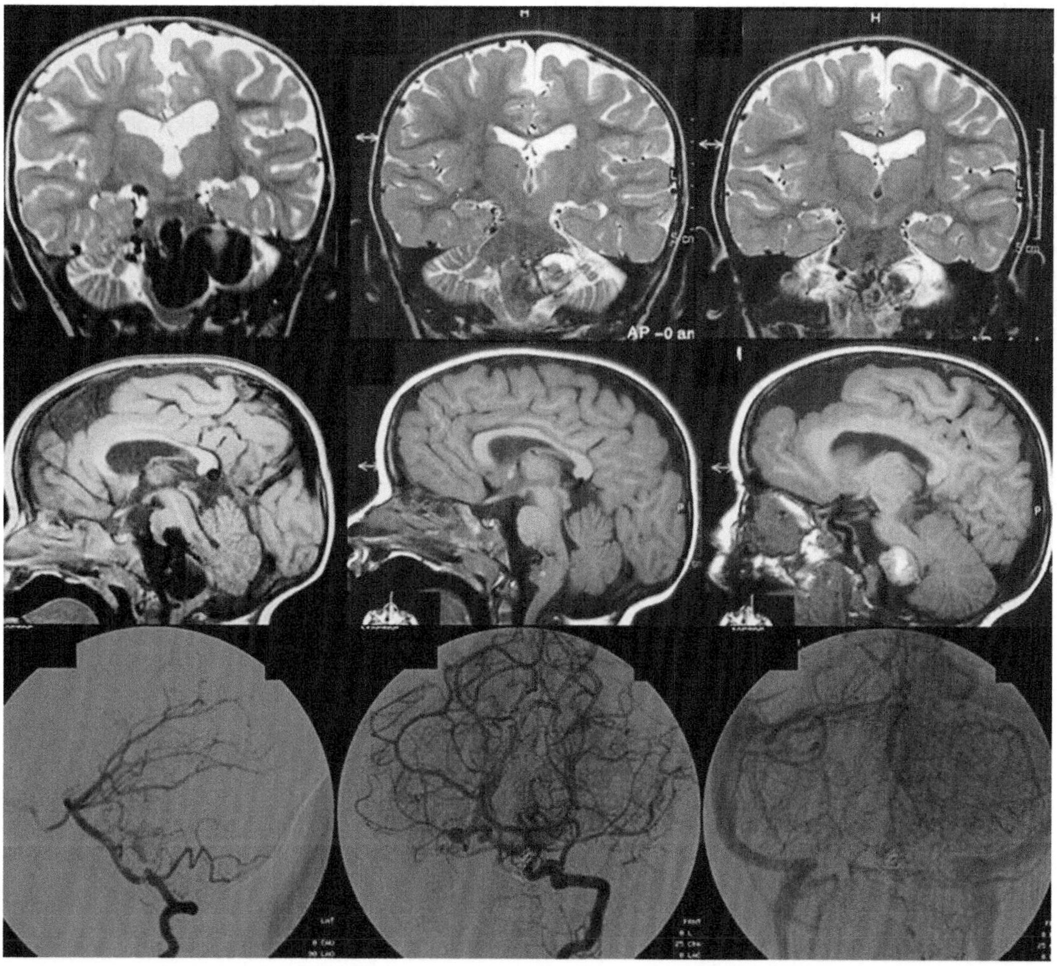

Fig. 12. Macrofistula in a child with HHT in whom as a first step, the flow was reduced by transarterial coiling of the venous pouch, followed by injection of pure glue to completely occlude the fistula.

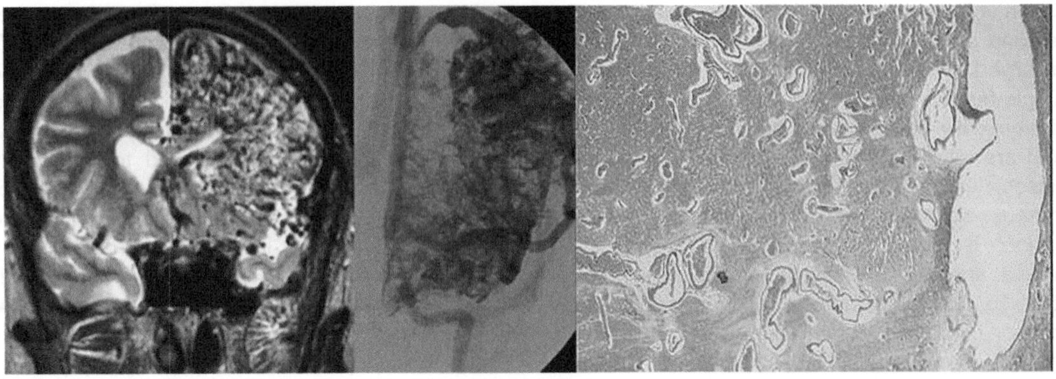

Fig. 13. Segmental AV lesions are those vascular malformations of the capillary level that have an extensive involvement of more than 1 lobe, or sometimes, the whole hemisphere. Proliferative angiopathy is the classic disease entity of this group.

of lesions at the AV junction (**Fig. 13**).[41] This vascular lesion can be regarded as separate from classic brain AVMs in angioarchitecture, natural history, clinical presentation, and, therefore, treatment. Instead of a compact or focal nidus, often multiple lobes or even a whole hemisphere are affected by a diffuse network of spaces with intermingled normal brain parenchyma. The discrepancy between the large nidus and the small shunting volume, the absence of flow-related aneurysms, the presence of diffuse angiogenesis (eg, transdural supply, progressive arterial occlusion), and the small caliber of a multitude of feeding arteries and draining veins are the angiographic hallmarks of this disease and point toward a diffuse angiogenetic activity.[42] This activity is presumably related to reduced perinidal perfusion and subsequent chronic cortical ischemia.[43] Concerning treatment strategies, surgery, radiotherapy, or nontargeted embolization of most of the malformation carry the risk of permanent neurologic deficit because of the interspersed normal neural tissue. This disease does not carry a high risk of hemorrhage; instead one of the major pathomechanisms of this disease is ischemia (which is probably multifactorial as a result of incompetent angiogenesis, steal phenomena, arterial stenosis, and capillary wall involvement). Therefore, a therapy that enhances cortical blood supply (such as calvarial burrholes) may be indicated. Similar to moyamoya-like diseases these burrholes increase the cortical blood supply by recruiting additional dural blood supply. If patients present with hemorrhage, however, endovascular treatment should be performed and aimed at fragile areas that may be identified during angiography.

Metameric capillary lesions

The association of AV malformations of the brain, the orbit (retinal and/or retrobulbar lesions), and the maxillofacial region was originally named after Bonnet-Dechaume-Blanc and Wyburn-Mason. Given the considerations mentioned earlier about

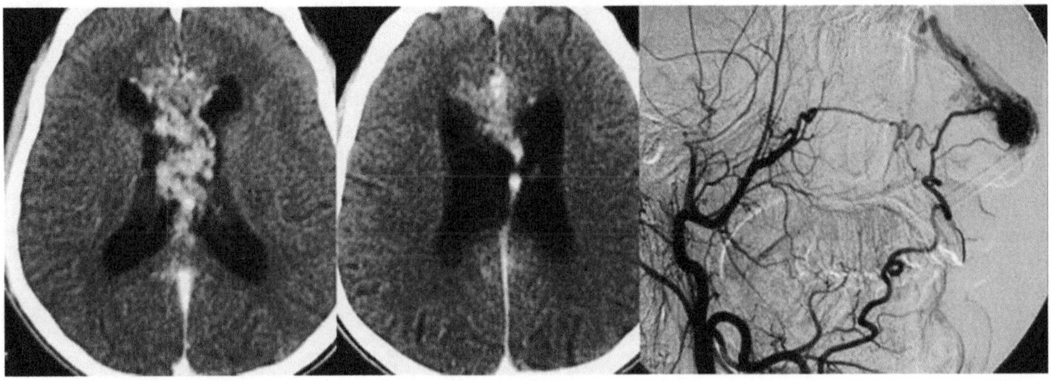

Fig. 14. The association of a corpus callosum AVM and a vascular malformation of the tip of the nose constitutes the midline prosencephalic type of a CAMS as a metameric AV vascular malformation.

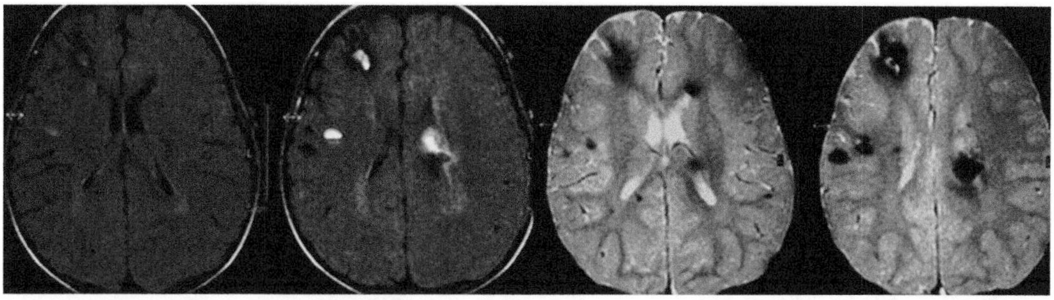

Fig. 15. Focal venous vascular lesions that are hereditary are present in some patients with multiple cavernomas.

the timing and the triggering of vascular malformations and our knowledge about the specific predetermined migration patterns of cells, it became clear that the association of different forms of AVMs follows a specific pattern that allows differentiation of different cerebrofacial AV metameric syndromes (CAMS).[11] CAMS 1 is a midline prosencephalic (olfactory) group with involvement of the hypothalamus, corpus callosum, hypophysis, and nose; CAMS 2 is a lateral prosencephalic (optic) group with involvement of the optic nerve, retina, parietotemporal-occipital lobes, thalamus, and maxilla, and CAMS 3 is a rhombencephalic (otic) group, with involvement of the cerebellum, pons, petrous bone, and mandible. The insult producing the underlying lesion develops before the migration occurs and thus before the fourth week of development. The disease spectrum may be incomplete or metachronous (**Fig. 14**).[44] Given their large size, and their potential to grow, treatment of these lesions is likely to be palliative and in our experience indicated only to focus on locally fragile areas (such as intranidal aneurysms, large shunts, compartments with venous outlet restrictions).

Venous Lesions

Focal venous lesions

In this category belong vascular malformations and variations as diverse as sinus pericranii,[45] DVAs,[46] and cavernomas.[47] Genetic forms of this category are known and present as the familial form of cavernomas, with at least 3 different gene loci identified (**Fig. 15**). These vascular malformations, although seemingly unrelated, share a defective or malformative focal development of the venous system. Transitions and combined vascular malformations exist such as a DVA draining through a sinus pericranii, a cavernoma related to a DVA, or even a true AVM draining via a DVA, underlining that this classification is a spectrum of overlapping malformations, vascular lesions, and diseases.[48] An endovascular therapy is either not possible (such as in cavernomas) or

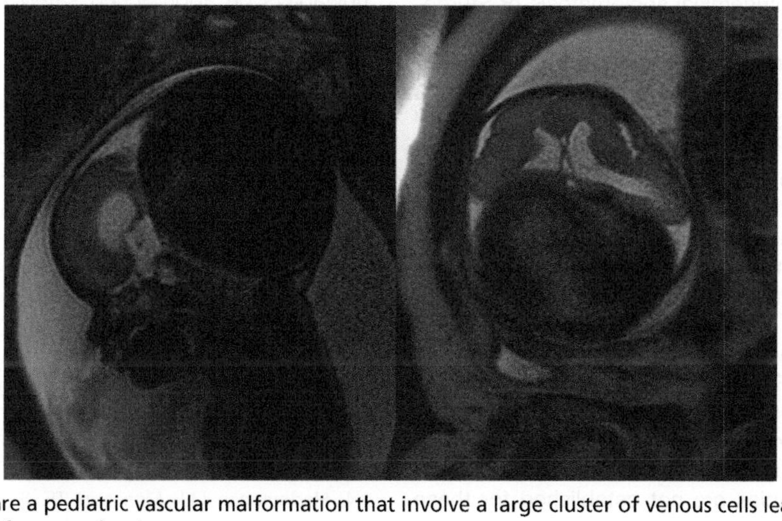

Fig. 16. DSMs are a pediatric vascular malformation that involve a large cluster of venous cells leading to extensive problems of venous development.

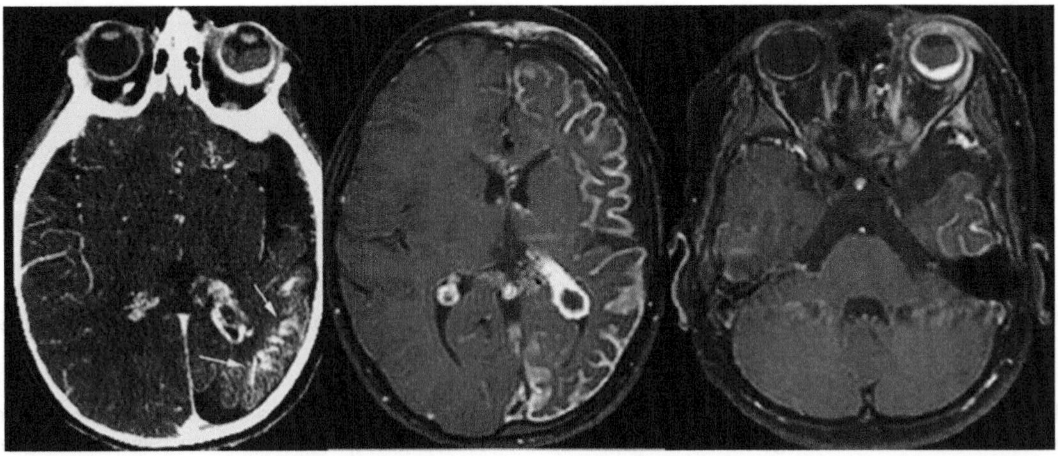

Fig. 17. Sturge-Weber syndrome can be subsumed under metameric nonhereditary venous lesions given their involvement of the face, the choroid plexus, and the cortical veins.

contraindicated (such as in most DVAs and sinus pericranii given their role in the drainage of the brain).

Segmental venous lesions

If the venous lesion affects a larger cluster of cells, more severe venous defects are encountered. The classic example is DSMs,[49] in which the development of the dural sinuses is affected (**Fig. 16**). This disease leads not only to sinus wall overgrowth and epidural confluences of venous spaces with giant lakes but also to cavernomas, sinus pericranii, DVAs, and maxillofacial malformations. The AV shunts associated with DSM add to the venous congestion of the normal brain.[50] Therefore treatment is targeted toward reduction of the shunt via a transarterial approach.

Metameric venous lesions

The encephalotrigeminal angiomatosis or Sturge-Weber syndrome is a nonfamilial disease with a skin discoloration (port wine) in the V_1 territory associated with a calcified leptomeningeal venous malformation of the ipsilateral supratentorial hemisphere, which (in relation to the CAMS mentioned earlier) may be termed cerebrofacial venous metameric syndrome.[11] Associated with the classic facial portwine stain are intracranial vascular anomalies that consist of cortical venous thrombosis with capillary venous proliferation and enlargement of the transmedullary collateral venous drainage with or without choroid plexus hypertrophy (**Fig. 17**). A genetic disease that falls into the metameric venous lesion group is the blue rubber bleb nevus syndrome, which involves multiple venous lesions (such as DVAs).[51] Endovascular therapies are not established for these diseases.

SUMMARY

The proposed classification may add to our understanding of vascular malformations because the phenotypic expression of a given vascular disease can shed light on the nature and timing of the triggering event, thereby potentially opening up treatment modalities that are directed against the triggering event rather than against the clinical manifestations or the morphologic appearance. In addition, the proposed classification may shed light on the prognosis and pathomechanisms of certain vascular malformations and may, therefore, lead to better treatment of the child afflicted with these rare and difficult diseases. For the time being, treatment in many instances is still related only to the symptoms of the disease, not to the disease process itself. However, with the methods at hand, most vascular diseases can nowadays be approached safely and with good clinical results.

REFERENCES

1. Kader A, Young WL. The effects of intracranial arteriovenous malformations on cerebral hemodynamics. Neurosurg Clin N Am 1996;7:767–81.
2. Geibprasert S, Pereira V, Krings T, et al. Hydrocephalus in unruptured brain arteriovenous malformations. Pathomechanical considerations, therapeutic implications and clinical course. J Neurosurg 2009; 110:500–7.
3. Meyer B, Schaller C, Frenkel C, et al. Physiological steal around AVMs of the brain is not equivalent to cortical ischemia. Neurol Res 1998;20(Suppl 1): S13–7.
4. Hademenos GJ, Massoud TF. Risk of intracranial arteriovenous malformation rupture due to venous

drainage impairment. A theoretical analysis. Stroke 1996;27(6):1072–83.
5. Mansmann U, Meisel J, Brock M, et al. Factors associated with intracranial hemorrhage in cases of cerebral arteriovenous malformation. Neurosurgery 2000;46(2):272–9 [discussion: 279–81].
6. Lasjaunias P, Ter Brugge K, Berenstein A. Surgical neuroangiography part 3: clinical and interventional aspects in children. 2nd edition. Berlin: Springer; 2006.
7. Lasjaunias P, Hui F, Zerah M, et al. Cerebral arteriovenous malformations in children. Management of 179 consecutive cases and review of the literature. Childs Nerv Syst 1995;11(2):66–79 [discussion: 79].
8. Bigner DD, McLendon RE, Bruner JM. Russel & Rubinstein's pathology of tumors of the nervous system. London: Arnold Publishers; 1998.
9. Lasjaunias P. A revised concept of the congenital nature of cerebral arteriovenous malformations. Intervent Neuroradiol 1997;3:275–81.
10. Eichmann A, Yuan L, Moyon D, et al. Vascular development: from precursor cells to branched arterial and venous networks. Int J Dev Biol 2005; 49:259–67.
11. Krings T, Geibprasert S, Luo CB, et al. Segmental neurovascular syndromes in children. Neuroimaging Clin N Am 2007;17(2):245–58.
12. Lasjaunias P. Segmental identity and vulnerability in cerebral arteries. Intervent Neuroradiol 2000;6: 113–24.
13. Conway EM, Collen D, Carmeliet P. Molecular mechanisms of blood vessel growth. Cardiovasc Res 2001;49(3):507–21.
14. Krings T, Ozanne A, Chng SM, et al. Neurovascular phenotypes in hereditary haemorrhagic telangiectasia patients according to age. Review of 50 consecutive patients aged 1 day-60 years. Neuroradiology 2005;47(10):711–20.
15. Krings T, Geibprasert S, Lasjaunias PL. Cerebrovascular trauma. Eur Radiol 2008;18(8):1531–45.
16. Agid R, Jonas Kimchi T, Lee SK, et al. Diagnostic characteristics and management of intracranial aneurysms in children. Neuroimaging Clin N Am 2007;17(2):153–63.
17. Lasjaunias P, Wuppalapati S, Alvarez H, et al. Intracranial aneurysms in children aged under 15 years: review of 59 consecutive children with 75 aneurysms. Childs Nerv Syst 2005;21(6):437–50.
18. Baccin CE, Krings T, Alvarez H, et al. Multiple mirror-like intracranial aneurysms. Report of a case and review of the literature. Acta Neurochir 2006; 148(10):1091–5 [discussion: 1095].
19. Krings T, Baccin CE, Alvarez H, et al. Segmental unfused basilar artery with kissing aneurysms: report of three cases and literature review. Acta Neurochir 2007;149(6):567–74 [discussion: 574].
20. Le Douarin NM, Catala M, Batini C. Embryonic neural chimeras in the study of vertebrate brain and head development. Int Rev Cytol 1997;175:241–309.
21. Holmin S, Ozanne A, Zhao WY, et al. Association of cervical internal carotid artery aneurysm with ipsilateral vertebrobasilar aneurysm in two children: a segmental entity? Childs Nerv Syst 2007;23(7):791–8.
22. Bhattacharya JJ, Luo CB, Alvarez H, et al. PHACES syndrome: a review of eight previously unreported cases with late arterial occlusions. Neuroradiology 2004;46(3):227–33.
23. Baccin CE, Krings T, Alvarez H, et al. A report of two cases with dolichosegmental intracranial arteries as a new feature of PHACES syndrome. Childs Nerv Syst 2007;23(5):559–67.
24. Fleetwood IG, Steinberg GK. Arteriovenous malformations. Lancet 2002;359(9309):863–73.
25. Alvarez H, Garcia Monaco R, Rodesch G, et al. Vein of Galen aneurysmal malformations. Neuroimaging Clin N Am 2007;17(2):189–206.
26. Geibprasert S, Pereira V, Krings T, et al. Dural arteriovenous shunts: a new classification of craniospinal epidural venous anatomical bases and clinical correlations. Stroke 2008;39(10):2783–94.
27. Krings T, Chng SM, Ozanne A, et al. Hereditary hemorrhagic telangiectasia in children: endovascular treatment of neurovascular malformations: results in 31 patients. Neuroradiology 2005; 47(12):946–54.
28. Gault J, Sarin H, Awadallah NA, et al. Pathobiology of human cerebrovascular malformations: basic mechanisms and clinical relevance. Neurosurgery 2004;55(1):1–16 [discussion: 16–7].
29. Meisel HJ, Mansmann U, Alvarez H, et al. Cerebral arteriovenous malformations and associated aneurysms: analysis of 305 cases from a series of 662 patients. Neurosurgery 2000;46(4):793–800 [discussion: 800–2].
30. Brown RD Jr, Wiebers DO, Forbes G, et al. The natural history of unruptured intracranial arteriovenous malformations. J Neurosurg 1988;68(3): 352–7.
31. Stefani MA, Porter PJ, terBrugge KG, et al. Angioarchitectural factors present in brain arteriovenous malformations associated with hemorrhagic presentation. Stroke 2002;33(4):920–4.
32. Hofmeister C, Stapf C, Hartmann A, et al. Demographic, morphological, and clinical characteristics of 1289 patients with brain arteriovenous malformation. Stroke 2000;31(6):1307–10.
33. Krings T, Geibprasert S, Pereira V, et al. Aneurysms. In: Naidich T, editor. Neuroradiology of the brain and spine. New York: Elsevier, in press.
34. Willinsky R, TerBrugge K, Montanera W, et al. Micro-arteriovenous malformations of the brain: superselective angiography in diagnosis and treatment. AJNR Am J Neuroradiol 1992;13(1):325–30.

35. Richling B, Killer M. Endovascular management of patients with cerebral arteriovenous malformations. Neurosurg Clin N Am 2000;11(1):123–45, ix.
36. Valavanis A, Yasargil MG. The endovascular treatment of brain arteriovenous malformations. Adv Tech Stand Neurosurg 1998;24:131–214.
37. Yu SC, Chan MS, Lam JM, et al. Complete obliteration of intracranial arteriovenous malformation with endovascular cyanoacrylate embolization: initial success and rate of permanent cure. AJNR Am J Neuroradiol 2004;25(7):1139–43.
38. Meisel HJ, Mansmann U, Alvarez H, et al. Effect of partial targeted N-butyl-cyano-acrylate embolization in brain AVM. Acta Neurochir 2002;144(9):879–87 [discussion: 888].
39. Katsaridis V, Papagiannaki C, Aimar E. Curative embolization of cerebral arteriovenous malformations (AVMs) with Onyx in 101 patients. Neuroradiology 2008;50(7):589–97.
40. Taylor CL, Dutton K, Rappard G, et al. Complications of preoperative embolization of cerebral arteriovenous malformations. J Neurosurg 2004;100(5):810–2.
41. Lasjaunias PL, Landrieu P, Rodesch G, et al. Cerebral proliferative angiopathy: clinical and angiographic description of an entity different from cerebral AVMs. Stroke 2008;39(3):878–85.
42. Chin LS, Raffel C, Gonzalez-Gomez I, et al. Diffuse arteriovenous malformations: a clinical, radiological, and pathological description. Neurosurgery 1992;31(5):863–8 [discussion: 868–9].
43. Ducreux D, Meder JF, Fredy D, et al. MR perfusion imaging in proliferative angiopathy. Neuroradiology 2004;46(2):105–12.
44. Wong IY, Batista LL, Alvarez H, et al. Craniofacial arteriovenous metameric syndrome (CAMS) 3–a transitional pattern between CAM 1 and 2 and spinal arteriovenous metameric syndromes. Neuroradiology 2003;45(9):611–5.
45. Gandolfo C, Krings T, Alvarez H, et al. Sinus pericranii: diagnostic and therapeutic considerations in 15 patients. Neuroradiology 2007;49(6):505–14.
46. Pereira VM, Geibprasert S, Krings T, et al. Pathomechanisms of symptomatic developmental venous anomalies. Stroke 2008;39(12):3201–15.
47. Maraire JN, Awad IA. Intracranial cavernous malformations: lesion behavior and management strategies. Neurosurgery 1995;37(4):591–605.
48. Rigamonti D, Johnson PC, Spetzler RF, et al. Cavernous malformations and capillary telangiectasia: a spectrum within a single pathological entity. Neurosurgery 1991;28(1):60–4.
49. Ozanne A, Alvarez H, Krings T, et al. [Pediatric neurovascular malformations: vein of Galen arteriovenous malformations (VGAM), pial arteriovenous malformations (pial AVM), dural sinus malformations (DSM)]. J Neuroradiol 2007;34(3):145–66 [in French].
50. Barbosa M, Mahadevan J, Wern YC, et al. Dural sinus malformations (DSM) with giant lakes in neonates and infants – review of 30 consecutive cases. Intervent Neuroradiol 2003;9:407–24.
51. Chung JI, Alvarez H, Lasjaunias P. Multifocal cerebral venous malformations and associated developmental venous anomalies in a case of blue rubber bleb nevus syndrome. Intervent Neuroradiol 2003;9:169–72.

Cavernous Malformations

Edward R. Smith, MD*, R. Michael Scott, MD

KEYWORDS

• Cavernous malformation • Epidemiology • Hemorrhage
• Natural history • Diagnosis • Surgery

DEFINITION AND HISTOLOGY

Cavernous malformations (CMs) are vascular lesions found in the central nervous system (CNS) and throughout the body. The nomenclature for these malformations can be confusing as they have been called cavernomas, cavernous angiomas, and cavernous hemangiomas. CMs have come to the attention of pediatric neurosurgeons because of their capacity to affect children through hemorrhage, seizure, focal neurologic deficits, and headache.

CMs are composed of a compact mass of sinusoidal-type vessels contiguous with one another and with no intervening normal parenchyma. These well-circumscribed unencapsulated masses are identified grossly as having a purple lobulated mulberry appearance (**Fig. 1**). Calcifications may be present grossly and microscopically. Cysts containing old hemorrhage products may be present and may help explain the controversial phenomenon of growth of these lesions, providing a substrate for neovascularization following hemorrhage. Surrounding tissue may be gliotic and stained from previous hemorrhage with green, yellow, or brown discoloration.

EPIDEMIOLOGY

CMs are relatively rare lesions, with an estimated prevalence of 0.4% to 0.5% in autopsy and magnetic resonance imaging (MRI) studies.[1–4] An incidence of 0.43 diagnoses per 100,000 people per year has been reported.[5] Symptomatic lesions manifest in all age groups. The peak incidence of presentation is usually in the third to fourth decade without a gender preponderance.[4,6] Affected children seem to be clustered in 2 age groups: infants and toddlers less than 3 years of age and children in early puberty aged 12 to 16 years.[7,8]

Most cases are sporadic (50%–80%), that is, there is no family history of CMs.[1,4] A single CM is found in 75% of sporadic cases and only 8% to 19% of familial cases.[1,4] In contrast, the presence of multiple CMs is strongly suggestive of familial CM; approximately 75% of all patients with multiple lesions are ultimately found to have affected relatives.[9] Only 10% to 25% of individuals with multiple lesions are sporadic cases, with the remainder of patients with multiple CMs often attributed to secondary effects of radiation therapy.[1,10–12]

ETIOLOGY

The cause of CMs remains under investigation. Recent advances have been made in the understanding of the contribution that specific mutations play in the development of these lesions. In particular, 3 genes have been associated with the formation of CMs: CCM1 (also known as *KRIT1*, found on chromosome 7q), CCM2 (also known as *malcaverin*, found on 7p), and CCM3 (also known as *Programmed Cell Death 10*, on 3p).[13–27] Molecular studies of CCM1 have revealed that this binding protein (Krev-1/rap 1a binding protein) is essential for normal embryonic vascular development and mutations in this gene, found in hereditary cases of CM, result in loss of function.[28] In patients with these CCM1 mutations, nearly all have radiographic evidence of multiple CMs, but only about 60% of patients develop symptoms.[29]

Department of Neurosurgery, Children's Hospital Boston, Harvard Medical School, 300 Longwood Avenue, Boston, MA 02115, USA
* Corresponding author.
E-mail address: edward.smith@childrens.harvard.edu

Neurosurg Clin N Am 21 (2010) 483–490
doi:10.1016/j.nec.2010.03.003
1042-3680/10/$ – see front matter

neurosurgery.theclinics.com

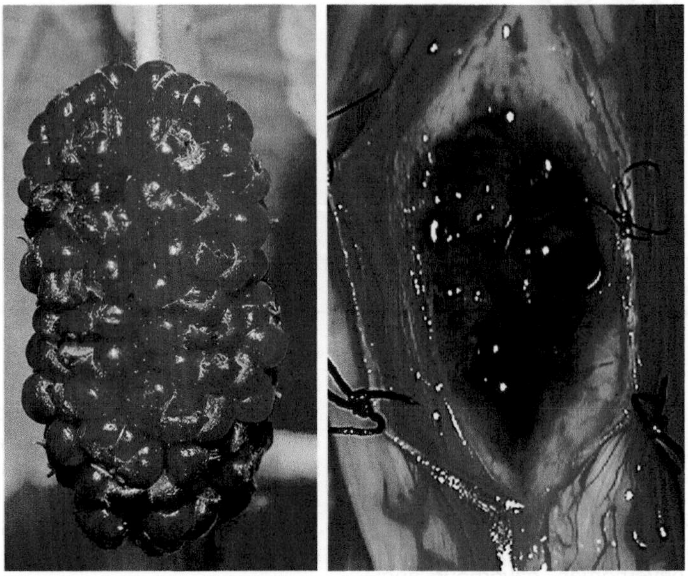

Fig. 1. Comparison between a cavernous malformation (same case depicted in the magnetic resonance imaging studies of spinal cord lesion in **Fig. 3**) and a mulberry. Note multiple lobules and variegated appearance of the lesion.

Patients with familial CMs are prone to developing new lesions throughout their lifetime. Periodic MRI studies are recommended to follow patients known to be affected. Screening of family members, genetically and radiographically, remains controversial, but may be helpful for genetic counseling and evaluating risk.[30,31] Other systems may be affected including skin, eyes, and visceral organs; with CCM1 found as the most commonly mutated gene in these patients.[32,33] It is our practice to refer patients with multiple CMs to the genetics service for mutational testing and counseling.

PRESENTATION

CMs may never cause symptoms and may be discovered only incidentally at autopsy or may be responsible for a variety of neurologic complaints. The neurologic signs and symptoms of symptomatic CMs correlate with the anatomic site of involvement and the age at presentation. CMs occur anywhere in the CNS, with symptomatic lesions most commonly presenting with hemorrhage, seizure, or focal neurologic deficit.[8,34–36] Intracranial CMs cause symptoms by (relatively) low-pressure hemorrhages that exert a mass effect on the surrounding brain. The extravasation of blood into brain parenchyma creates a hemosiderin ring that may predispose susceptible tissue to seizure. Children with CMs may also have headache as a symptom, presumably secondary to mass effect or irritation of dural nociceptors from hemorrhage products.

RADIOGRAPHIC FINDINGS

Radiographic evaluation of suspected CM usually begins with computerized tomography (CT) or MRI. CMs are generally poorly visualized with angiography; as such, this investigation is generally not indicated in the evaluation.[37] CMs are often undetectable on angiography and are therefore grouped with the heterogeneous group of angiographically occult vascular malformations. These lesions can range in size from microscopic to near-hemispheric with an average diameter of about 5 cm in children.[7]

The typical CT appearance is a well-defined collection of multiple rounded densities showing minor contrast enhancement and without a mass effect. Often, there are calcifications.[38] Recent hemorrhage may or may not be present, depending on the clinical setting. MRI studies are distinctive; typically, a popcorn appearance with an associated bloom on susceptibility imaging, suggesting hemosiderin deposition (**Fig. 2**).[8,39–41] Although the characteristics of CMs may vary considerably between children, attempts have been made to classify imaging findings and correlate them with pathology.[1] A grading system has been proposed that clusters CMs into 4 categories based on T1, T2, and susceptibility imaging characteristics.[1]

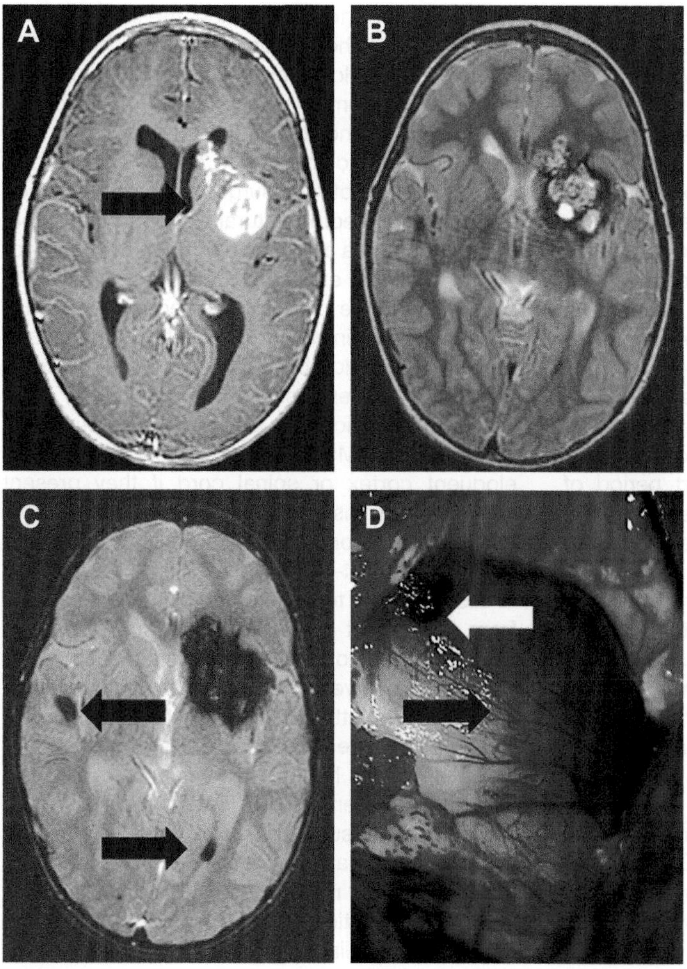

Fig. 2. MRI appearance of cavernous malformations. (*A*) Depicts T1 post-contrast axial study of left frontal lesion; note irregular enhancement and presence of associated developmental venous malformation (*arrow*). (*B*) T2 images demonstrating the popcorn appearance of a lesion with multiple small cysts and darker rim of hemosiderin on the periphery. (*C*) Susceptibility images reveal bloom of previous hemorrhages and highlight other lesions within this patient (*arrows*). (*D*) Operative correlation of radiographic studies with greenish, hemosiderin-stained surrounding tissue (*black arrow*) and darker, mulberry-like malformation (*white arrow*).

Of particular note is the high rate of finding a developmental venous anomaly (DVA) in association with a CM (see **Fig. 2**). DVAs have been reported with frequencies approaching 100% in young children with CMs.[7,42] This finding is of particular relevance with regard to surgical therapy as these DVAs provide venous drainage to normal brain, and should be preserved at surgery if possible.[43,44] Certain investigators have implicated DVAs in the cause of cavernomas.[45]

In a review of 163 previously published cases, 126 patients (76.8%) had supratentorial malformations, 34 (20.7%) were infratentorial, 4 (2.5%) were intraventricular, and 4 (2.5%) were multiple.[46] Calcifications were observed in 18 cases (11%). Among 31 patients studied by cerebral angiography, normal findings or an avascular mass were encountered. With the advent of MRI, increased imaging sensitivity has revealed a higher rate of patients with multiple CMs, with up to 21% of patients with CM found to have multiple lesions.[35] If multiple CMs are seen on imaging, then a familial or postradiation cause should be considered.[47]

In patients presenting with acute hemorrhage, it may be difficult to ascertain the diagnosis. Strong consideration must be given to the possibility of an arteriovenous malformation (AVM), which is found more commonly than CM in children. In this particular clinical scenario (unlike general screening as previously discussed) angiography is extremely helpful in distinguishing between these entities. In children presenting with cystic or calcified lesions, the differential diagnosis may include tumors and susceptibility imaging may aid in indentifying evidence of previous hemorrhage or other CMs.

NATURAL HISTORY AND SELECTION OF TREATMENT

Once a CM has been identified in a child, referral to a pediatric neurosurgeon is an appropriate first step. The surgeon must then weigh what is known about the risks of observation against the risks of intervention. The natural history of CMs can be difficult to predict. Depending on individual investigators' definitions of hemorrhage, annual rates from CMs vary between near undetectable to about 3% for lesions that are found incidentally and range between less than 4% to more than 23% for lesions that were found after a hemorrhage.[1,34,48–50] In general, hemorrhage from CMs is better tolerated with regard to mortality than from other high-flow lesions, such as AVMs. However, fatal hemorrhage from CM is a well-known entity, particularly if the lesion is in a high-risk location, such as the posterior fossa.[34,51]

Of those children who have symptomatic hemorrhage, many can be at risk for temporal clustering of hemorrhages in a short period of time with a rate of up to about 2% per lesion per month and 24% per year.[49,52] With repeated hemorrhage, the usual motif is that of progressive stepwise deficits. The child often presents with a profound decline in function at the time of hemorrhage, with subsequent partial recovery over several weeks to months. However, most children (63%) are unable to recover completely back to baseline.[7,49,51,53–55] With each subsequent hemorrhage, the ultimate level of function declines (**Fig. 3**).

Given this natural history, several investigators have advocated early treatment of CMs in children, as their long life span may favor a more aggressive approach.[36,49,56,57] Symptomatic lesions are considered for therapy. There has been debate regarding the usefulness of extirpation of asymptomatic lesions.[58] The decision to intervene is especially difficult in the patient who presents with symptoms and has multiple lesions. If the symptoms can be localized to a single lesion, which is amenable to surgical resection, then that lesion should generally be removed.[1,36] Nevertheless, in the child with multiple CMs, the family should be informed that other lesions may appear and could potentially cause symptoms in the future.

Outcomes of surgical therapy have been remarkably good, with most series reporting a near 0% mortality rate and a 4% to 5% rate of new permanent deficits.[53,58] Risks greatly increase in sensitive locations such as the brainstem with rates of new, permanent, postoperative deficits ranging from 12% to 25%, suggesting a need to approach lesions in these areas with caution.[54,55]

For CMs located in high-risk locations, such as the brain stem or eloquent cortex, there is controversy regarding the potential role of radiation as a possible treatment option.[53,54,59] Radiosurgery has been reported to reduce the frequency of hemorrhage in these lesions from 17.3% to 4.5% per year.[50,60] However, this decreased rate of hemorrhage comes at the cost of increased complications, including a 16% incidence of new permanent neurologic deficit and a 3% mortality rate.[60] The use of radiosurgery must be balanced against the expected natural history of the lesion. When these data are viewed through the perspective of a child's expected long life span and are coupled with the poorly quantified long-term risk of secondary injury from radiation exposure, resection should be considered as first-line therapy whenever possible.

At our institution, it is our practice to surgically resect single CMs when they are located in non-eloquent cortex or spinal cord if they present with symptoms, documented radiographic enlargement, or hemorrhage (usually after a minimum of 4–6 weeks following hemorrhage to allow swelling to resolve, unless there is urgency from significant mass effect). For lesions in eloquent cortex or in the brainstem, we commonly decide to observe the lesion initially to determine if it manifests a pattern of recurrent hemorrhage that would justify the risk of surgical intervention. If a subsequent hemorrhage occurs, then we frequently undertake an operation. For deep lesions that are surgically inaccessible, we usually observe and treat symptomatically with very few ever referred for radiosurgery.

We refer patients with multiple lesions for genetic counseling. If none of the lesions are symptomatic, we observe them with annual MRI studies. If individual lesions grow, become symptomatic, or manifest new hemorrhage on imaging, then we subject that individual lesion to the algorithm detailed earlier.

SURGICAL TECHNIQUE

Surgical management of CMs in children is similar to that in adults.[1,8,58,61] In addition to the general principles of removing the entire lesion and preserving normal surrounding vasculature (especially associated DVAs), resection of a CM may include the removal of the surrounding hemosiderin ring, if the lesion is cortical; associated with seizures, and in a low-risk location. In contrast, lesions in eloquent cortex, in the brain stem, or in the spinal cord should generally not have any non-lesional tissue resected to minimize injury to sensitive surrounding structures (see **Fig. 1**).

At our institution, we have routinely used frameless stereotaxy to aid in the localization of cranial lesions. This adjunct is particularly useful for deep lesions and we have found that placement

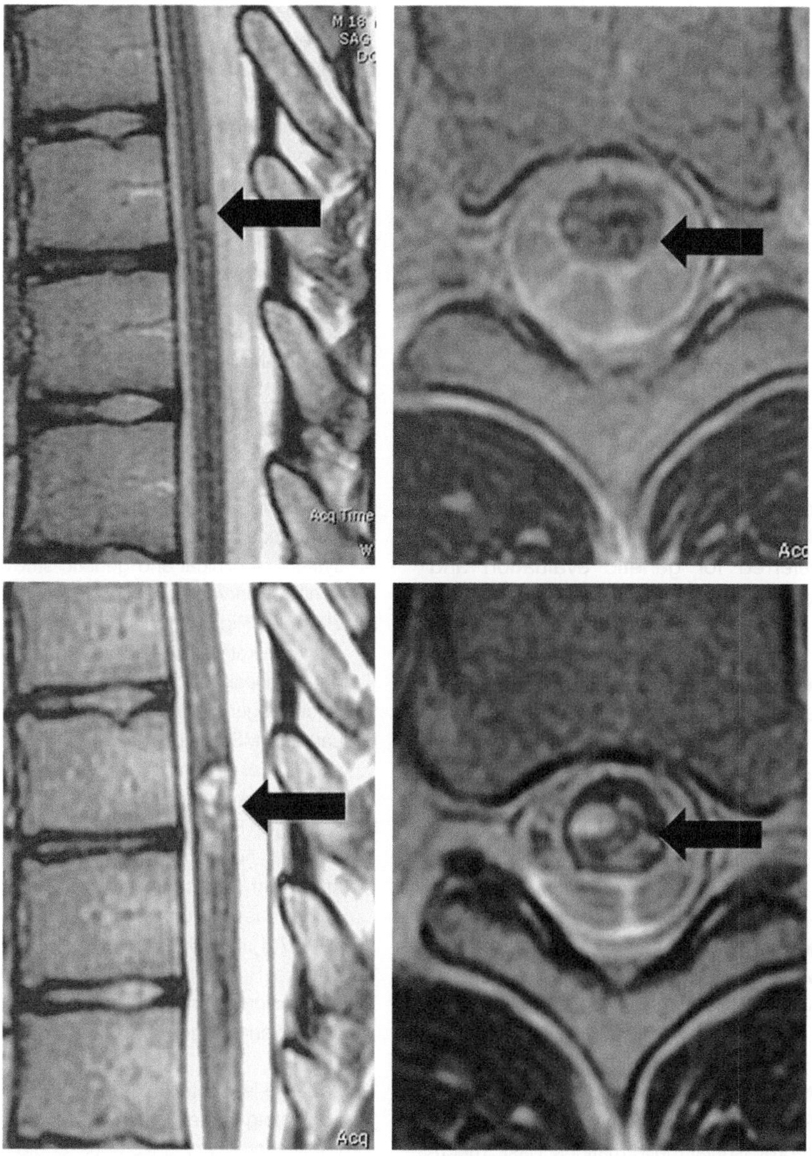

Fig. 3. Serial MRI studies of a spinal cord lesion showing progressive enlargement with serial hemorrhages. These images were taken 6 months apart, with 2 distinct presentations of lower extremity sensory changes, weakness, and urinary incontinence. Each time the child made a recovery from the presentation examination, but never returned to his neurologic baseline and worsened with subsequent hemorrhages (operative photograph in **Fig. 1**).

of a catheter along the planned trajectory of approach, after opening the dura, is helpful as a guide to the lesion during dissection. We have also found the use of intraoperative ultrasound of immense value for real-time localization and assessment of extent of resection.

POSTOPERATIVE ISSUES

Close follow-up is indicated in patients who have undergone surgical resection of a CM. CMs can recur if not excised completely and a generation of new lesions has been documented, particularly in the setting of radiation-induced lesions and in familial cases.[47,62] In most patients, a postoperative MRI is ordered, usually 6 weeks to 6 months postoperatively, to assess the extent of resection and to serve as a new baseline for comparison with future studies. It is the practice in our institution to obtain follow-up imaging at 1-year intervals for 2 to 5 years postoperatively.

Patients with multiple CMs should have annual imaging to ascertain if there is progression of any lesion because, in the pediatric population, there is a life-long risk for a lesion to bleed or grow, with surgery being subsequently required. It is less clear how to proceed with adults who have multiple lesions. Nevertheless, family members of patients with multiple lesions should be considered for screening studies. Candidates for screening include first-degree relatives with multiple CMs and/or family members with symptoms suggestive of intracranial disease (seizures, headaches, or neurologic deficits).

SUMMARY

The management of children with CMs requires a clear understanding of the natural history of these lesions and the risks of surgical intervention. Presentation is usually hemorrhage, seizure, focal neurologic deficit, or headache. Diagnosis is best made with MRI. Patients with multiple lesions should be referred for genetic evaluation and counseling. Individuals with symptomatic, growing, or hemorrhagic malformations should be considered for surgical resection. Close follow-up after diagnosis and treatment is helpful to identify lesion progression or recurrence.

REFERENCES

1. Zabramski JM, Wascher TM, Spetzler RF, et al. The natural history of familial cavernous malformations: results of an ongoing study. J Neurosurg 1994; 80(3):422–32.
2. Hang Z, Shi Y, Wei Y. A pathological analysis of 180 cases of vascular malformation of brain. Zhonghua Bing Li Xue Za Zhi 1996;25(3):135–8.
3. Barnes B, Cawley CM, Barrow DL. Intracerebral hemorrhage secondary to vascular lesions. Neurosurg Clin N Am 2002;13(3):289–97.
4. Gault J, Sarin H, Awadallah NA. Pathobiology of human cerebrovascular malformations: basic mechanisms and clinical relevance. Neurosurgery 2004; 55(1):1–17.
5. Al-Shahi R, Bhattacharya JJ, Currie DG, et al. Prospective, population-based detection of intracranial vascular malformations in adults: the Scottish Intracranial Vascular Malformation Study (SIVMS). Stroke 2003;34(5):1163–9.
6. Baumann SB, Noll DC, Kondziolka DS, et al. Comparison of functional magnetic resonance imaging with positron emission tomography and magnetoencephalography to identify the motor cortex in a patient with an arteriovenous malformation. J Image Guid Surg 1995;1(4):191–7.
7. Mottolese C, Hermier M, Stan H, et al. Central nervous system cavernomas in the pediatric age group. Neurosurg Rev 2001;24(2–3):55–71 [discussion: 72–3].
8. Fortuna A, Ferrante L, Mastronardi L, et al. Cerebral cavernous angioma in children. Childs Nerv Syst 1989;5(4):201–7.
9. Labauge P, Laberge S, Brunereau L, et al. Hereditary cerebral cavernous angiomas: clinical and genetic features in 57 French families. Societe Francaise de Neurochirurgie. Lancet 1998;352(9144): 1892–7.
10. Otten P, Pizzolato GP, Rilliet B, et al. 131 cases of cavernous angioma (cavernomas) of the CNS, discovered by retrospective analysis of 24,535 autopsies. Neurochirurgie 1989;35(2):82–3, 128–31.
11. Siegel AM, Andermann E, Badhwar A, et al. Anticipation in familial cavernous angioma: a study of 52 families from International Familial Cavernous Angioma Study. IFCAS Group. Lancet 1998; 352(9141):1676–7.
12. Siegel AM, Bertalanffy H, Dichgans JJ, et al. Familial cavernous malformations of the central nervous system. A clinical and genetic study of 15 German families. Nervenarzt 2005;76(2):175–80.
13. Zhang J, Rigamonti D, Dietz HC, et al. Interaction between krit1 and malcavernin: implications for the pathogenesis of cerebral cavernous malformations. Neurosurgery 2007;60(2):353–9.
14. Laurans MS, DiLuna ML, Shin D, et al. Mutational analysis of 206 families with cavernous malformations. J Neurosurg 2003;99(1):38–43.
15. Laberge S, Labauge P, Marechal E, et al. Genetic heterogeneity and absence of founder effect in a series of 36 French cerebral cavernous angiomas families. Eur J Hum Genet 1999;7(4):499–504.
16. Shenkar R, Elliott JP, Diener K, et al. Differential gene expression in human cerebrovascular malformations. Neurosurgery 2003;52(2):465–77 [discussion: 477–8].
17. Laberge-le Couteulx S, Jung HH, Labauge P, et al. Truncating mutations in CCM1, encoding KRIT1, cause hereditary cavernous angiomas. Nat Genet 1999;23(2):189–93.
18. Labauge P, Enjorals O, Bonerandi JJ, et al. An association between autosomal dominant cerebral cavernomas and a distinctive hyperkeratotic cutaneous vascular malformation in 4 families. Ann Neurol 1999;45(2):250–4.
19. Dupre N, Verlann DJ, Hand CK, et al. Linkage to the CCM2 locus and genetic heterogeneity in familial cerebral cavernous malformation. Can J Neurol Sci 2003;30(2):122–8.
20. Craig HD, Günel M, Cepeda O, et al. Multilocus linkage identifies two new loci for a mendelian form of stroke, cerebral cavernous malformation, at 7p15-13 and 3q25.2-27. Hum Mol Genet 1998; 7(12):1851–8.
21. Marchuk DA, Gallione CJ, Morrision LA, et al. A locus for cerebral cavernous malformations maps

to chromosome 7q in two families. Genomics 1995; 28(2):311–4.
22. Gil-Nagel A, Dubovsky J, Wilcox KJ, et al. Familial cerebral cavernous angioma: a gene localized to a 15-cM interval on chromosome 7q. Ann Neurol 1996;39(6):807–10.
23. Gunel M, Awad IA, Finberg K, et al. A founder mutation as a cause of cerebral cavernous malformation in Hispanic Americans. N Engl J Med 1996;334(15): 946–51.
24. Gunel M, Awad IA, Anson J, et al. Mapping a gene causing cerebral cavernous malformation to 7q11.2-q21. Proc Natl Acad Sci U S A 1995; 92(14):6620–4.
25. Dubovsky J, Zabramski JM, Kurth J, et al. A gene responsible for cavernous malformations of the brain maps to chromosome 7q. Hum Mol Genet 1995; 4(3):453–8.
26. Chen L, Tanriover G, Yano H, et al. Apoptotic functions of PDCD10/CCM3, the gene mutated in cerebral cavernous malformation 3. Stroke 2009;40(4): 1474–81.
27. Tanriover G, Boylan AJ, Diluna ML, et al. PDCD10, the gene mutated in cerebral cavernous malformation 3, is expressed in the neurovascular unit. Neurosurgery 2008;62(4):930–8.
28. Whitehead KJ, Plummer NW, Adams JA, et al. Ccm1 is required for arterial morphogenesis: implications for the etiology of human cavernous malformations. Development 2004;131(6):1437–48.
29. Hayman LA, Evans RA, Ferrell RE, et al. Familial cavernous angiomas: natural history and genetic study over a 5-year period. Am J Med Genet 1982; 11(2):147–60.
30. Nannucci S, Pescini F, Poggesi A, et al. Familial cerebral cavernous malformation: report of a further Italian family. Neurol Sci 2009;30(2):143–7.
31. Penco S, Ratti R, Bianchi E, et al. Molecular screening test in familial forms of cerebral cavernous malformation: the impact of the Multiplex Ligation-dependent Probe Amplification approach. J Neurosurg 2009;110(5):929–34.
32. Sirvente J, Enjolras O, Wassef M, et al. Frequency and phenotypes of cutaneous vascular malformations in a consecutive series of 417 patients with familial cerebral cavernous malformations. J Eur Acad Dermatol Venereol 2009;23(9):1066–72.
33. Toll A, Parera E, Giménez-Arnau AM, et al. Cutaneous venous malformations in familial cerebral cavernomatosis caused by KRIT1 gene mutations. Dermatology 2009;218(4):307–13.
34. Aiba T, Tanaka R, Koike T, et al. Natural history of intracranial cavernous malformations. J Neurosurg 1995;83(1):56–9.
35. Kim DS, Park YG, Choi JU, et al. An analysis of the natural history of cavernous malformations. Surg Neurol 1997;48(1):9–17 [discussion: 17–8].
36. Frim DM, Scott RM. Management of cavernous malformations in the pediatric population. Neurosurg Clin N Am 1999;10(3):513–8.
37. Kesava PP, Turski PA. MR angiography of vascular malformations. Neuroimaging Clin N Am 1998;8(2): 349–70.
38. Bartlett JE, Kishore PR. Intracranial cavernous angioma. AJR Am J Roentgenol 1977;128(4):653–6.
39. Rigamonti D, Drayer BP, Johnson PC, et al. The MRI appearance of cavernous malformations (angiomas). J Neurosurg 1987;67(4):518–24.
40. Imakita S, Nishimura T, Yamada N, et al. Cerebral vascular malformations: applications of magnetic resonance imaging to differential diagnosis. Neuroradiology 1989;31(4):320–5.
41. Sage MR, Blumbergs PC. Cavernous haemangiomas (angiomas) of the brain. Australas Radiol 2001;45(2):247–56.
42. Rigamonti D, Hadley MN, Drayer BP, et al. Cerebral cavernous malformations. Incidence and familial occurrence. N Engl J Med 1988;319(6):343–7.
43. Lasjaunias P, Terbrugge K, Rodesch G, et al. True and false cerebral venous malformations. Venous pseudo-angiomas and cavernous hemangiomas. Neurochirurgie 1989;35(2):132–9.
44. Ostertun B, Solymosi L. Magnetic resonance angiography of cerebral developmental venous anomalies: its role in differential diagnosis. Neuroradiology 1993;35(2):97–104.
45. Wurm G, Schnizer M, Fellner FA. Cerebral cavernous malformations associated with venous anomalies: surgical considerations. Neurosurgery 2005;57(Suppl 1):42–58.
46. Voigt K, Yasargil MG. Cerebral cavernous haemangiomas or cavernomas. Incidence, pathology, localization, diagnosis, clinical features and treatment. Review of the literature and report of an unusual case. Neurochirurgia (Stuttg) 1976;19(2):59–68.
47. Baumgartner JE, Ater JL, Ha CS, et al. Pathologically proven cavernous angiomas of the brain following radiation therapy for pediatric brain tumors. Pediatr Neurosurg 2003;39(4):201–7.
48. Moriarity JL, Clatterbuck RE, Rigamonti D. The natural history of cavernous malformations. Neurosurg Clin N Am 1999;10(3):411–7.
49. Porter PJ, Willinsky RA, Harper W, et al. Cerebral cavernous malformations: natural history and prognosis after clinical deterioration with or without hemorrhage. J Neurosurg 1997;87(2):190–7.
50. Kondziolka D, Lunsford LD, Kestle JR. The natural history of cerebral cavernous malformations. J Neurosurg 1995;83(5):820–4.
51. Fritschi JA, Reulen HJ, Spetzler RF, et al. Cavernous malformations of the brain stem. A review of 139 cases. Acta Neurochir (Wien) 1994;130(1–4):35–46.
52. Barker FG 2nd, Amin-Hanjani S, Butler WE, et al. Temporal clustering of hemorrhages from untreated

cavernous malformations of the central nervous system. Neurosurgery 2001;49(1):15–24 [discussion: 24–5].
53. Scott RM, Barnes P, Kupsky W, et al. Cavernous angiomas of the central nervous system in children. J Neurosurg 1992;76(1):38–46.
54. Scott RM. Brain stem cavernous angiomas in children. Pediatr Neurosurg 1990/1991;16(6):281–6.
55. Porter RW, Detwiler PW, Spetzler RF, et al. Cavernous malformations of the brainstem: experience with 100 patients. J Neurosurg 1999;90(1):50–8.
56. Mazza C, Scienza R, Beltramello A, et al. Cerebral cavernous malformations (cavernomas) in the pediatric age-group. Childs Nerv Syst 1991;7(3):139–46.
57. Giulioni M, Acciarri N, Padovani R, et al. Surgical management of cavernous angiomas in children. Surg Neurol 1994;42(3):194–9.
58. Amin-Hanjani S, Ogilvy CS, Ojemann RG, et al. Risks of surgical management for cavernous malformations of the nervous system. Neurosurgery 1998;42(6):1220–7 [discussion: 1227–8].
59. Di Rocco C, Iannelli A, Tamburrini G. Cavernous angiomas of the brain stem in children. Pediatr Neurosurg 1997;27(2):92–9.
60. Amin-Hanjani S, Ogilvy CS, Candia GJ, et al. Stereotactic radiosurgery for cavernous malformations: Kjellberg's experience with proton beam therapy in 98 cases at the Harvard Cyclotron. Neurosurgery 1998;42(6):1229–36 [discussion: 1236–8].
61. Di Rocco C, Iannelli A, Tamburrini G. Surgical management of paediatric cerebral cavernomas. J Neurosurg Sci 1997;41(4):343–7.
62. Larson JJ, Ball WS, Bove KE, et al. Formation of intracerebral cavernous malformations after radiation treatment for central nervous system neoplasia in children. J Neurosurg 1998;88(1):51–6.

Pediatric Intracranial Aneurysms

Brian J. Jian, MD, PhD[a], Steven W. Hetts, MD[b], Michael T. Lawton, MD[a], Nalin Gupta, MD, PhD[a,*]

KEYWORDS

• Intracranial aneurysm • SAH • Endovascular treatment
• Pediatric aneurysm

Intracranial aneurysms in children are rare; 0.5% to 4.6% of intracranial aneurysms occur in patients aged 18 years or younger.[1–7] In a cooperative study reported in 1966, only 41 of 6368 (0.6%) ruptured aneurysms were found in patients younger than 19 years.[8] Aneurysms occurring in very young children and infants are exceedingly rare. In adults, aneurysms are believed to form as a result of multiple risk factors (eg, family history, age older than 50 years, smoking, cocaine use, and hypertension) present over the course of an individual's life span. In childhood, most of these aneurysmal risk factors do not exist, and for this reason, the pathogenesis is believed to be different.[9–11] Some investigators have proposed that a vasculopathy predisposes regions of the cerebral vasculature to aneurysm formation.[12,13] In multiple case series, primarily since the 1970s, pediatric aneurysms have been reported to exhibit features that differ from those in adults, such as male predominance, a higher incidence in locations such as the posterior circulation and internal carotid bifurcation, and greater numbers of giant aneurysms.[2,14–17]

Discrepancies exist in the clinical description of pediatric aneurysms, likely related to the small numbers reported in most case series. Since the comprehensive review by Huang, other case series (including from the authors' institution) have been published.[18–20] Data from these larger series have confirmed some earlier findings and have contradicted others. It is likely that considerable heterogeneity exists with respect to the pathology, diagnosis, and treatment of these lesions.

The past 20 years have witnessed a gradual shift from exclusively surgical approaches toward endovascular treatment and multimodality therapeutic plans.[12,13,21] The increasing number of options available for the treatment of complex aneurysms suggest that treatment should be guided by the best available evidence and executed by centers with expertise in each of these therapeutic tools.

CLINICAL PRESENTATION

As in adults, children with intracranial aneurysms can present with subarachnoid hemorrhage (SAH), headache, direct compressive effects, focal neurologic deficits, or seizures. If SAH is present, nearly 60% of patients will have a cerebral aneurysm.[22] Fusiform aneurysms tend to present with nonhemorrhagic deficits.[19] Many patients (30%–85%) with SAH confirmed by radiographic imaging or lumbar puncture typically present good clinical function defined by a Hunt and Hess grade between 1 and 3. Patients with poor clinical function have a Hunt and Hess grade of 4 to 5, occurring 15% to 42% of the time (**Table 1**).[12,17,18,24,25] The reason for the better clinical grade at presentation is unclear but may be because of several factors, such as fewer comorbidities, clouding the initial diagnosis, and a greater tendency to refer cerebrovascular cases to tertiary centers. Specific biologic features such as the activity of

[a] Department of Neurological Surgery, University of California San Francisco, 505 Parnassus Avenue, Room M779, San Francisco, CA 94143-0112, USA
[b] Department of Radiology, University of California San Francisco, 505 Parnassus Avenue, Room L352, San Francisco, CA 94143-0628, USA
* Corresponding author.
E-mail address: guptan@neurosurg.ucsf.edu

Neurosurg Clin N Am 21 (2010) 491–501
doi:10.1016/j.nec.2010.03.005
1042-3680/10/$ – see front matter

Table 1
Summary of published reports describing pediatric intracranial aneurysms

Year	Authors	Cases (n)	Boys (%)[a]	Girls (%)[a]	SAH (%)	Good Grade (%)	Poor Grade (%)	Giant (%)	ICA Terminus (%)	Posterior Circulation (%)	Surgical or Endovascular Treatment (%)	Good Outcome (%)	Death (%)	Years of Follow-Up
1939	McDonald and Korb[40]	61	60	34	87	[a]	[a]	[a]	16	23	[a]	[a]	[a]	[a]
1940–64	Case reports	9	78	22	100	22	78	11	22	22	33	33	66	[a]
1963	Stehbens[41]	3	33	66	33	0	100	[a]	[a]	[a]	[a]	[a]	100	[a]
1965–1990	Case reports	35	[a]	[a]	[a]	[a]	[a]	[a]	[a]	[a]	67	25	75	[a]
1965	Matson[23]	13	92	8	92	[a]	[a]	[a]	8	15	92	62	23	0–12
1966	Locksley et al[8]	41	73	27	100	[a]	[a]	[a]	15	17	[a]	[a]	[a]	[a]
1971	Patel and Richardson[5]	58	55	45	100	69	31	0	34	5	64	52	31	1–22
1973	Sedzimir and Robinson[7]	50	56	44	100	[a]	[a]	[a]	36	4	50	70	28	2–15
1975	Amacher and Drake[42]	16	69	31	88	44	44	44	13	31	69	56	38	[a]
1977	Almeida et al[43]	11	55	45	91	82	18	0	55	9	91	64	27	0–15
1978	Batnitzky and Muller[44]	12	67	31	83	[a]	[a]	25	25	25	[a]	[a]	25	[a]
1980	Gerosa et al[2]	15	67	33	80	87	13	20	33	0	100	67	13	2–22
1981	Heiskanen and Vikki[16]	32	53	47	100	[a]	[a]	[a]	50	6	100	75	6	0.5–11
1981	Amacher et al[15]	26	62	38	65	96	4	[a]	[a]	[a]	96	92	4	[a]

1982	Storrs et al[45]	29	45	55	76	38	62	31	31	31	72	45	34	[a]
1983	Schauseil-Zipf et al[46]	15	67	33	60	20	[a]	[a]	[a]	7	80	13	33	1–17
1983	Ostergaard and Voldby[4]	43	58	42	77	72	28	5	44	7	81	53	30	0.25–14
1985	Humphreys et al[47]	35	[a]	[a]	74	11	63	29	26	20	66	40	40	[a]
1986	Pasqualin et al[48]	31	[a]	[a]	94	[a]	[a]	3	29	3	61	52	3	[a]
1988	Roche et al[6]	43	70	30	81	[a]	[a]	7	26	16	95	79	12	[a]
1989	Meyer et al[3]	24	71	25	54	50	4	54	8	46	100	92	4	1–7
1991–2002	Case reports	47	[a]	[a]	[a]	[a]	[a]	[a]	[a]	[a]	70	63	26	0–19
1991	Herman et al[49]	16	56	44	63	38	6	19	6	19	94	75	6	0.67–6
2001	Proust et al[17]	22	73	27	95	59	36	14	36	9	100	64	23	[a]
2004	Huang et al[50]	19	68	32	58	42	16	37	11	42	84	95	5	0.1–9
2005	Lasjaunias et al[12]	59	59	41	50	30	18		4	27	67	52	10	0–6
2005	Agid et al[24]	33	16	17	9	[a]	[a]	30	22	30	70	64	15	12
2005	Krishna et al[25]	22	64	36	91	68	32	13.6	20	24	77	82	10	0.1–2.5
2006	Sanai et al[20]	32	44	56	22	85	15	40	13	28	90	78	0	6
2008	Vaid et al[51]	36	52	48	92	58	42	21	18	30	75	78	11	0.1–3.5
2009	Hetts et al[19]	77	52	48	32	[a]	[a]	11	[a]	22	77	[a]	1	[a]
Total		965	60	37	74	51	34	21	24	19	79	62	24	

[a] Numbers do not sum to 100% in all cases, reflecting discrepancies in the original reports.

the nitric oxide synthase pathway and the robustness of leptomeningeal arterial collaterals may also play a role.[12,26]

Matson[23] originally noted that pediatric aneurysms occur slightly more commonly in men. This finding has been affirmed in multiple case series with male/female ratios ranging from 1:1 to 11:1.[1,17,23,27] In the larger case series, however, the male/female ratio is closer to 1.5:1 (see **Table 1**).[1,4–8,12,19] One possible explanation for this difference is that 14% to 39% of pediatric aneurysms are a result of trauma, which is substantially more common among men.[28,29] In situations in which behavior is less likely to influence the clinical presentation, Buis and colleagues[27] noted that the male/female ratio of aneurysms was 1.1:1 in children younger than 1 year.

DIAGNOSIS

With the increasing availability of multidetector computed tomographic (CT) scanners, magnetic resonance imaging (MRI), and 3-dimensional image processing, the identification of a cerebral aneurysm as a cause of SAH can occur not only in a tertiary referral center but also at a community hospital. Furthermore, the technical quality of catheter angiography has improved over the last decade with advances such as 3-dimensional rotational angiography and angio-CT. These technological improvements have allowed more detailed studies to be obtained in affected patients.

For a child with a suspected SAH, the diagnostic sequence begins with a noncontrast CT scan of the head. If this study is normal but the clinical story is consistent with an SAH, then a lumbar puncture is required. The presence of blood or xanthochromia should prompt a contrast-enhanced imaging study of the intracerebral vasculature. At this point, the diagnostic decisions may vary depending upon the age of the child, the clinical status, and availability of invasive imaging and interventional treatments. In adults, a CT angiogram (CTA) or MR angiogram (MRA) is usually performed after the noncontrast CT scan to quickly identify the source of the SAH. At the authors' institution, children older than 14 years receive a CTA immediately after the identification of subarachnoid blood on noncontrast CT. Some institutions, including the authors', proceed directly to catheter angiography after a noncontrast head CT, particularly because the false-negative rate of CTA exceeds 10% in some studies.[30] The choice of the imaging modality is made on a case-by-case basis with an effort to reduce radiation exposure while obtaining the necessary data needed to plan subsequent interventions and postoperative management. Although Hetts and colleagues'[19] and other studies have reported no delayed sequelae of radiation exposure to patients undergoing endovascular therapy, short follow-up times limit the ability to draw any definitive conclusions.[31]

For those young individuals with unruptured aneurysms that initially present with generalized headaches or even seizures, a postcontrast CT scan may miss the underlying pathology. It is notable that non-SAH headaches and seizures have been reported to be the presenting symptoms of pediatric aneurysm up to 40% of the time.[18,19] Consequently, MRI or MRA is a valuable tool for examining these individuals and following them in the years to come if conservative management is the chosen treatment strategy, as well as for surveillance for development of new or enlarging aneurysms that may require treatment at a later time.

ANEURYSM FEATURES

The overall location and size of aneurysms in children differ from those found in the adult population.[12,19,32,33] Aneurysms of the internal carotid artery (ICA) typically occur at similar frequencies in both populations. However, there is a greater preponderance of aneurysms at the ICA terminus in the pediatric patient compared with the adult (**Table 2**). Aneurysms of the middle cerebral artery (MCA) appear to occur in similar distributions between the 2 subgroups. Approximately 18% of identified aneurysms are found along the MCA in both adults and children. The distribution of aneurysms in the posterior and anterior circulation, however, appear to be different in the subgroups. In adults, anterior cerebral artery (ACA) (including anterior communicating artery) aneurysms occur approximately 34% of the time, whereas in children recent reviews have encountered ACA aneurysms only about 5% to 10% of the time. In contrast, children appear to be more prone to aneurysms of the posterior circulation. Aneurysms in this region appear approximately 25% of the time in children, whereas in the adult population they are less common (~8%).

In the most recent series from the authors' institution, 40 females (52%) and 37 (48%) males who ranged in age (at diagnosis) from 3 months to 18 years (mean, 12 ± 5 years) were included. This gender distribution differs from other reports in the literature in which an overall male predominance is noted. There were a total of 103 aneurysms, 11% of which were greater than 25 mm in diameter and were defined as giant aneurysms.

Table 2
Adult and pediatric aneurysms by location

Location	Pediatric Aneurysm (%)[a]	Adult Aneurysm (%)[b]
ICA terminus	39–51 (24[c])	38.1 (4[c])
Anterior cerebral artery (ACA)	5.4–10	34.6
Middle cerebral artery (MCA)	13.5–21	18.4
Posterior circulation	22–27	8.6

[a] *Data from* Refs.[12,19,32]
[b] *Data from* Locksley HB. Natural history of subarachnoid hemorrhage, intracranial aneurysms and arteriovenous malformations. Based on 6368 cases in the cooperative study. J Neurosurg 1966;25(2):219–39.
[c] ICA terminus data from **Table 1**.

About 22% of these aneurysms were found to be in the posterior circulation, which is in agreement with the other series in which a posterior circulation location occurred in 4% to 27% of patients.[7,19] In contrast, aneurysms in adults are seen in the posterior circulation only 8% of the time (see **Table 2**) and giant aneurysms are even rare.[12,18,19,24,32,34]

Three large case series have subdivided aneurysms into 4 categories: fusiform, saccular, infectious, and traumatic.[12,19,34] These studies have identified that the rate of hemorrhagic presentation differs considerably among aneurysm subtypes. Hemorrhage was more likely a result from saccular aneurysm rupture (**Fig. 1**) than from fusiform or infectious aneurysms (**Fig. 2**, **Table 3**). Furthermore, traumatic aneurysms, as expected, were seen closer to the skull base in the anterior and posterior circulations than in the distal MCA or ACA (**Fig. 3**).

TREATMENT

General Principles

It is clear that a multidisciplinary team consisting of stroke neurologists, cerebrovascular neurosurgeons, and neurointerventional radiologists is best able to treat complex intracranial aneurysms and achieve optimal results.[35] Treatment options include observation, endovascular therapy, or surgical clipping. Endovascular treatment includes the use of detachable coils with or without stents delivered through microcatheters after transfemoral selective catheterization of the involved intracranial arteries. Surgical treatment includes direct clipping, clip reconstructions, and aneurysm trapping with or without bypass procedures.

Aneurysm morphology and etiology have therapeutic implications. In the series by Lasjaunias and colleagues[12] and Hetts and colleagues,[19] saccular aneurysms were the most likely to rupture (>75%

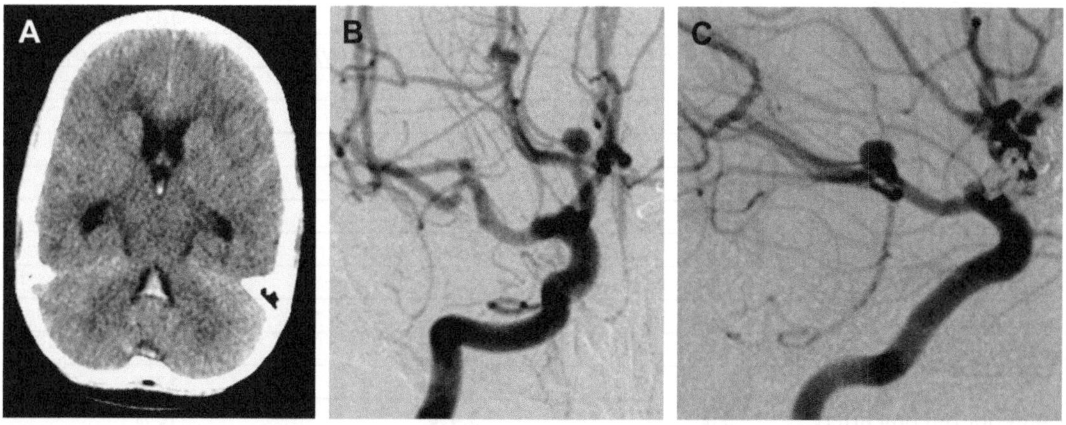

Fig. 1. Saccular aneurysm. A 17-year-old girl with Majewsky type II osteodysplastic dwarfism presented with headache. Subarachnoid and intraventricular hemorrhage was demonstrated on nonenhanced CT (*A*). Initial diagnostic catheter angiography demonstrated 10 saccular intracranial aneurysms, the majority and largest of which were associated with the left anterior circulation. The patient underwent a left pterional craniotomy with clipping of multiple aneurysms. A saccular right P1/P2 posterior cerebral artery (PCA) aneurysm, filling via a near-fetal PCA on anteroposterior (AP) (*B*) and lateral (*C*) right ICA angiograms, underwent endovascular coiling during the same admission.

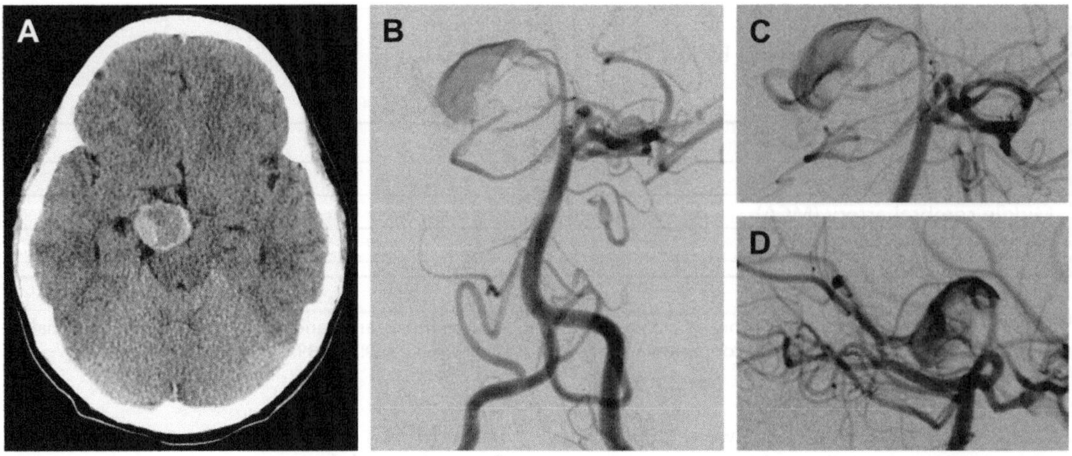

Fig. 2. Fusiform aneurysm. A 13-year-old otherwise healthy boy presented with 2 months of headache and right cranial nerve III palsy. A nonenhanced CT scan (*A*) demonstrates a hyperdense mass in the right suprasellar cistern with mass effect on the midbrain and interpeduncular fossa. Catheter angiography of the left vertebral artery in the AP (*B*), magnified Water (*C*), and magnified reverse Schuller (*D*) projections confirmed the presence of a giant partially thrombosed fusiform in the right P1/P2 posterior cerebral artery aneurysm. This lesion subsequently underwent endovascular coiling, with resolution of the patient's oculomotor palsy.

and >35%, respectively). Infectious aneurysms in both series ruptured at a relatively low rate (17% and 13%, **Fig. 4**). The behavior of fusiform aneurysms is unclear because these 2 studies report disparities in their rupture rates, 8% in the series by Hetts and colleagues and 40% in the series by Lasjaunias and colleagues. Some of these discrepancies may relate to the nature of the aneurysms themselves, as Lasjaunias and colleagues proposed that dissecting aneurysms be put in the fusiform group, whereas the authors proposed that only if a dissection can be demonstrated

Table 3
Recent studies demonstrating aneurysm location and features

	Lasjaunias et al[12]	Agid and Terbrugge[34]	Hetts et al[19]
Patient (n)	59	33	77
Number of Aneurysms	75	37	103
Age	7.6 y (8 d–15 y)	10.2 y (1 d–17 y)	12 y (3 mo–18 y)
Sex (% male)	59%	48%	48%
Morphology			
Fusiform	56%	19%	31%
Saccular	27%	46%	46%
Infectious	14%	8%	12%
Traumatic	3%	14%	14%
Giant (>25 mm)	1.3%	—	11%
Multiple	15%	—	16%
ICA Aneurysm	39%	40%	51%
MCA Aneurysms	21%	13.5%	17%
Anterior cerebral artery Aneurysms	9%	5.4%	10%
Posterior Circulation	27%	24%	22%
Hemorrhage	54%	30%	32%
Cerebral Infarction	3.1%–12.5%	12.1%	7.8%
Mortality	10.4%	15%	1.3%

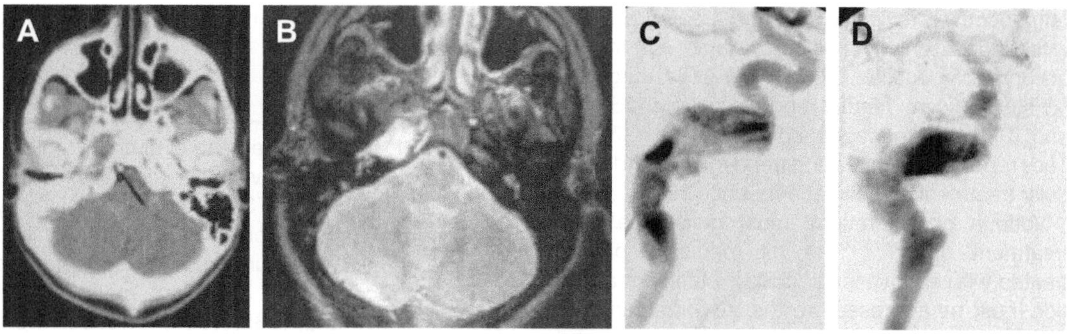

Fig. 3. Traumatic aneurysm. A 15-year-old girl presented with right-sided pulsatile tinnitus and a vascular mass behind the right tympanic membrane 3 years after a motor vehicle accident in which skull base fractures were sustained. A nonenhanced CT (*A*) and T2-weighted MRI (*B*) demonstrate a mass enlarging at the right petrous carotid canal. Catheter angiography of the right ICA in the lateral (*C*) and AP (*D*) projections confirms a fusiform dissecting traumatic aneurysm of the high cervical and petrous segments of the ICA. This lesion was treated with endovascular parent artery occlusion, with resolution of tinnitus.

(pathologically, from angiographic imaging with a dissection flap seen or from MRI with thrombus identified between layers of the artery wall) can an aneurysm be termed dissecting, whether it is fusiform or not.

Endovascular Treatment

Agid and colleagues[24] examined 33 patients younger than 18 years at their institution over a 12-year period (between 1992 and 2004), and they

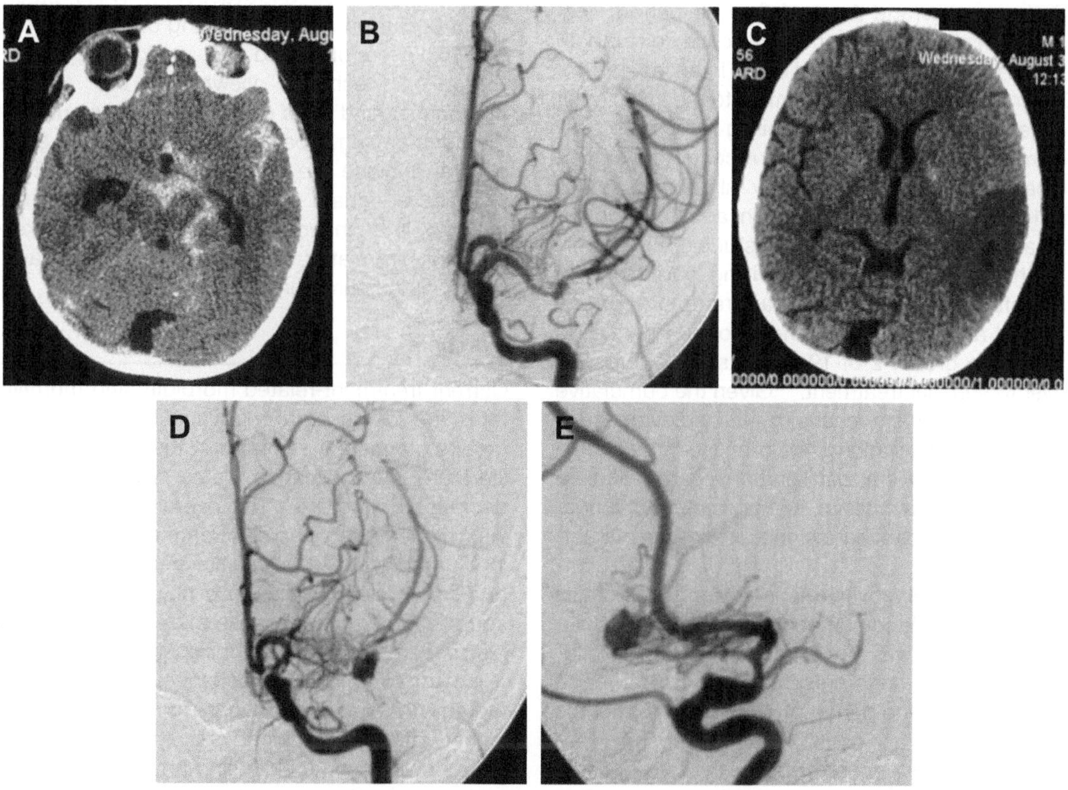

Fig. 4. Infectious aneurysm. A 12-year-old boy with trisomy 21 and enterococcus endocarditis and bacteremia presented with SAH (*A*). The initial angiogram showed evidence of a vasculopathy involving the left MCA (*B*). One week after the SAH, a left MCA distribution infarction was clearly visible (*C*). A follow-up angiogram done at that time showed evolution of the aneurysm with an increase in size and irregularity of the dome (AP [*D*], lateral [*E*]). The aneurysm was treated with superficial temporal artery to MCA bypass and trapping.

retrospectively reviewed surgically treated patients with endovascularly treated patients. Of the 37 aneurysms identified, 10 were treated surgically (27%), 13 were treated endovascularly (35.1%), and 14 were managed conservatively (37.8%). They reported an increasing trend toward endovascular treatment of their patients since 1997.

Various considerations must guide the best treatment option.[19,20] In the pediatric patient treated with endovascular coiling, sufficient attention must be addressed to the life expectancy of the child, the need for continued follow-up, and the possible need for retreatment. In the authors' series, a total of 103 aneurysms were identified in 77 patients over a 27-year period. Among the 77 patients, 19 underwent primary aneurysm coiling, 19 underwent primary surgical clipping, 11 were treated with carotid occulusion, 10 were treated with trapping and/or vascular bypass, and 18 with long-segment vascular dysplasia involving multiple territories were managed conservatively.

In the patients treated with coil embolization, discussions must be performed regarding the potential need to re-treat the coiled aneurysm. During an average 2-year follow-up period, 4 of 19 (21%) patients treated by selective coil embolization required retreatment of the index aneurysm. This recanalization rate is similar to the initial adult experience with aneurysm coiling using bare platinum detachable coils; more recently developed bioactive coils have typically shown closer to a 10% recanalization rate[36] in adults, although bioactive coils have not been studied extensively in children. No patients receiving coiling in the authors' pediatric cohort had rerupture of the treated aneurysm during the follow-up period. In this same group, 2 of 19 patients (10%) crossed over to surgical treatment.[19] Given the cumulative nature of aneurysm recanalization and evidence of delayed recanalization in children (such as an ICA terminus aneurysm with partial recanalization 6 years after initial coiling), it is possible that longer follow-up would reveal a higher proportion of treatment failure.

In the conservatively managed group, most of whom had long-segment fusiform vascular dysplasia that was not amenable to simple clipping or coiling, none presented with SAH over an average follow-up period of 41-months (6 months to 10 years). These patients underwent serial MRI studies to follow aneurysm growth. Two patients showed minimal aneurysm enlargement. One patient had significant enlargement and underwent primary stent coiling of a paraclinoid saccular component of a fusiform aneurysm 4 years into the observation period. No other patients required treatment. None of these patients had SAH during the follow-up period.

Surgical Treatment

Since 1981, there has been an evolution in microneurosurgical and endovascular techniques used at the authors' hospital. Separating the University of California San Francisco (UCSF) cohort into discrete time periods underscores the changes that have occurred in aneurysm management. Between 1981 and 1985, 100% of cases were treated surgically (clipping or bypass/trapping). From 1986 to 1990, 18% of cases were treated surgically, 73% were treated endovascularly (all being parent artery occlusions), and 9% were observed. Endovascular coiling of pediatric aneurysms at UCSF began in 1991; during the next 5 years, 33% of cases were treated surgically, 47% were treated endovascularly (57% by coiling and 43% by parent artery occlusion), and 20% were observed. From 1996 to 2000, 27% of cases were treated surgically, 33% were treated endovascularly (all coiling), and 40% were observed. Since 2001, 45% of cases were treated surgically, 45% were treated endovascularly (14% parent artery occlusion and 86% coiling or stent coiling), and 10% were observed.[19]

From a technical viewpoint, the surgical approaches and tools are similar to those used in the adult setting. Specific issues related to small children include the careful monitoring of blood loss and adequate volume replacement, the use of immobilization techniques that reduce the likelihood of pin-related complications, and the age-appropriate neuromonitoring techniques.

Outcome

Current treatment-related morbidity and mortality rates are low in both endovascular and surgical groups compared with rates in the earlier medical literature. Complication rates have generally decreased with time. The overall infarction rate was higher after surgical treatment (4 of 29 or 14%) than after endovascular treatment (2 of 30 or 7%).[19] Selection bias may play a role in these complication rates, because more complex aneurysms were likely referred for surgical treatment.

In the authors' experience, microsurgical therapy for pediatric aneurysms seems to have higher rates of complete obliteration and lower rates of recurrence, indicating an advantage over endovascular therapy in the areas of efficacy and durability.[20] The issue of treatment durability is particularly an issue with children, because in them life expectancy is measured in decades. Overall, clinical factors such as aneurysm configuration, surgical risks, and patient variables such as age and comorbidities should be discussed by the entire cerebrovascular team to achieve a treatment consensus. Finally, parental concerns should be addressed with serious discussions regarding durability of treatment, delayed complications, angiographic surveillance, and the potential for additional treatment later in life.

Posttreatment Management

SAH is generally considered better tolerated by children than by adults, although the mechanism for this better tolerance is uncertain. Although it has been reported that approximately 30% of SAH have radiographic evidence of vasospasm, most of these radiographic findings seem to lack any clinical significance. Several series have reported the low rate of clinically significant vasospasm in cases of ruptured pediatric intracranial aneurysms.[12,18,37] The authors' series confirmed this observation: 4 patients had imaging-proved vasospasm and only 1 required therapy to reverse an ischemic neurologic deficit. The basis for better tolerance of vasospasm in children, a leading cause of morbidity in adult patients with SAH, is unclear. Although it has been proposed that the leptomeningeal collateral supply to watershed areas may be more abundant in the pediatric patient, thereby making distal ischemic infarcts less frequent, proving this theory is challenging.

PROPOSED FOLLOW-UP GUIDELINES

Regardless of aneurysm treatment or observation, children with intracranial aneurysms require follow-up imaging and clinical surveillance, given their expected long life spans during which additional aneurysms could arise or treated aneurysms could recur. As suggested previously,[12] aneurysmal disease is both an acute and chronic condition and requires longitudinal management, with emphasis on the ongoing disease entity itself as opposed to just the mode of treatment when an aneurysm becomes acutely symptomatic. The fact that 6 patients in the authors' series developed de novo aneurysms or significant enlargement of previously untreated aneurysms between 6 months and 12 years after initial presentation underscores the need for careful follow-up.

Although some of these new aneurysms may have formed due to increased wall stresses on inherently dysplastic vessels in the setting of increased flow through remaining vessels after occlusion of a carotid or vertebral artery, other aneurysms grew despite preservation of parent artery flow. New and enlarging aneurysms developed in patients initially treated surgically and endovascularly, as has been reported previously by other investigators.[10,38,39] These findings suggest that a brain aneurysm in a child should be considered as a potentially chronic progressive condition. Vigilant long-term follow-up with appropriate clinical and minimally invasive imaging surveillance seems warranted and prudent. Consequently, the following is proposed:

- For endovascularly coiled aneurysms, an initial diagnostic and therapeutic catheter angiogram is done with a follow-up catheter angiogram in 6 months. If there is no evidence of recanalization at 6 months then an annual MRA is done, eventually decreasing to once every 5 years.
- For surgically clipped aneurysms, initial preoperative and postoperative catheter angiograms are done. If no residual aneurysm after clipping is noted then an annual MRA is done, eventually decreasing to once every 5 years.

SUMMARY

Intracranial aneurysms in children differ from those in adults in location, morphology, etiology, natural history, and, hence, management. Several series have been published detailing the experience of various institutions with pediatric intracranial aneurysms,[12,18,37] including the authors' institution.[19,20] Childhood aneurysms have a higher rate of posterior circulation, ICA terminus, fusiform, and giant aneurysms as compared with adult patients with aneurysms. Furthermore, improved short-term outcomes compared with those reported before surgical- and endovascular-treatment series are likely a reflection of continued improvements during the past 3 decades in endovascular and microsurgical techniques for aneurysm treatment and of improved early diagnosis of aneurysms and optimization of intensive care for pediatric patients.

REFERENCES

1. Locksley HB, Sahs AL, Knowler L. Report on the cooperative study of intracranial aneurysms and subarachnoid hemorrhage. Section II. General survey of cases in the central registry and characteristics of the sample population. J Neurosurg 1966; 24(5):922–32.
2. Gerosa M, Licata C, Fiore DL, et al. Intracranial aneurysms of childhood. Childs Brain 1980;6(6): 295–302.

3. Meyer FB, Sundt TM Jr, Fode NC, et al. Cerebral aneurysms in childhood and adolescence. J Neurosurg 1989;70(3):420–5.
4. Ostergaard JR, Voldby B. Intracranial arterial aneurysms in children and adolescents. J Neurosurg 1983;58(6):832–7.
5. Patel AN, Richardson AE. Ruptured intracranial aneurysms in the first two decades of life. A study of 58 patients. J Neurosurg 1971;35(5):571–6.
6. Roche JL, Choux M, Czorny A, et al. [Intracranial arterial aneurysm in children. A cooperative study. Apropos of 43 cases]. Neurochirurgie 1988;34(4): 243–51 [in French].
7. Sedzimir CB, Robinson J. Intracranial hemorrhage in children and adolescents. J Neurosurg 1973;38(3): 269–81.
8. Locksley HB, Sahs AL, Sandler R. Report on the cooperative study of intracranial aneurysms and subarachnoid hemorrhage. 3. Subarachnoid hemorrhage unrelated to intracranial aneurysm and A-V malformation. A study of associated diseases and prognosis. J Neurosurg 1966;24(6):1034–56.
9. Juvela S. Risk factors for multiple intracranial aneurysms. Stroke 2000;31(2):392–7.
10. Juvela S. Natural history of unruptured intracranial aneurysms: risks for aneurysm formation, growth, and rupture. Acta Neurochir Suppl 2002;82:27–30.
11. King JT Jr. Epidemiology of aneurysmal subarachnoid hemorrhage. Neuroimaging Clin N Am 1997; 7(4):659–68.
12. Lasjaunias P, Wuppalapati S, Alvarez H, et al. Intracranial aneurysms in children aged under 15 years: review of 59 consecutive children with 75 aneurysms. Childs Nerv Syst 2005;21(6):437–50.
13. terBrugge KG. Neurointerventional procedures in the pediatric age group. Childs Nerv Syst 1999; 15(11–12):751–4.
14. Allison JW, Davis PC, Sato Y, et al. Intracranial aneurysms in infants and children. Pediatr Radiol 1998; 28(4):223–9.
15. Amacher AL, Drake CG, Ferguson GG. Posterior circulation aneurysms in young people. Neurosurgery 1981;8(3):315–20.
16. Heiskanen O, Vilkki J. Intracranial arterial aneurysms in children and adolescents. Acta Neurochir (Wien) 1981;59(1–2):55–63.
17. Proust F, Toussaint P, Garnieri J, et al. Pediatric cerebral aneurysms. J Neurosurg 2001;94(5): 733–9.
18. Huang J, McGirt MJ, Gailloud P, et al. Intracranial aneurysms in the pediatric population: case series and literature review. Surg Neurol 2005; 63(5):424–32 [discussion: 432–3].
19. Hetts SW, Narvid J, Sanai N, et al. Intracranial aneurysms in childhood: 27-year single-institution experience. AJNR Am J Neuroradiol 2009;30(7):1315–24.
20. Sanai N, Quinones-Hinojosa A, Gupta NM, et al. Pediatric intracranial aneurysms: durability of treatment following microsurgical and endovascular management. J Neurosurg 2006;104(2 Suppl): 82–9.
21. Molyneux A, Kerr R, Stratton I, et al. International Subarachnoid Aneurysm Trial (ISAT) of neurosurgical clipping versus endovascular coiling in 2143 patients with ruptured intracranial aneurysms: a randomised trial. Lancet 2002;360(9342):1267–74.
22. Jordan LC. Assessment and treatment of stroke in children. Curr Treat Options Neurol 2008;10(6): 399–409.
23. Matson DD. Intracranial arterial aneurysms in childhood. J Neurosurg 1965;23(6):578–83.
24. Agid R, Souza MP, Reintamm G, et al. The role of endovascular treatment for pediatric aneurysms. Childs Nerv Syst 2005;21(12):1030–6.
25. Krishna H, Wani AA, Behari S, et al. Intracranial aneurysms in patients 18 years of age or under, are they different from aneurysms in adult population? Acta Neurochir (Wien) 2005;147(5):469–76 [discussion: 476].
26. Khurana VG, Meissner I, Sohni YR, et al. The presence of tandem endothelial nitric oxide synthase gene polymorphisms identifying brain aneurysms more prone to rupture. J Neurosurg 2005;102(3): 526–31.
27. Buis DR, van Ouwerkerk WJ, Takahata H, et al. Intracranial aneurysms in children under 1 year of age: a systematic review of the literature. Childs Nerv Syst 2006;22(11):1395–409.
28. Ventureyra EC, Higgins MJ. Traumatic intracranial aneurysms in childhood and adolescence. Case reports and review of the literature. Childs Nerv Syst 1994;10(6):361–79.
29. Yazbak PA, McComb JG, Raffel C. Pediatric traumatic intracranial aneurysms. Pediatr Neurosurg 1995;22(1):15–9.
30. Kallmes DF, Layton K, Marx WF, et al. Death by nondiagnosis: why emergent CT angiography should not be done for patients with subarachnoid hemorrhage. AJNR Am J Neuroradiol 2007;28(10):1837–8.
31. Liu HM, Wang YH, Chen YF, et al. Endovascular treatment of brain-stem arteriovenous malformations: safety and efficacy. Neuroradiology 2003; 45(9):644–9.
32. Agid R, Jonas Kimchi T, Lee SK, et al. Diagnostic characteristics and management of intracranial aneurysms in children. Neuroimaging Clin N Am 2007;17(2):153–63.
33. Locksley HB. Natural history of subarachnoid hemorrhage, intracranial aneurysms and arteriovenous malformations. Based on 6368 cases in the cooperative study. J Neurosurg 1966;25(2):219–39.
34. Agid R, Terbrugge K. Pediatric aneurysms. J Neurosurg 2007;106(Suppl 4):328 [author reply: 328–9].

35. Johnston SC. Effect of endovascular services and hospital volume on cerebral aneurysm treatment outcomes. Stroke 2000;31(1):111–7.
36. White PM, Lewis SC, Nahser H, et al. (HELPS trial): procedural safety and operator-assessed efficacy results. AJNR Am J Neuroradiol 2008; 29(2):217–23.
37. Aryan HE, Giannotta SL, Fukushima T, et al. Aneurysms in children: review of 15 years experience. J Clin Neurosci 2006;13(2):188–92.
38. Juvela S, Poussa K, Porras M. Factors affecting formation and growth of intracranial aneurysms: a long-term follow-up study. Stroke 2001;32(2): 485–91.
39. Koffijberg H, Buskens E, Algra A, et al. Growth rates of intracranial aneurysms: exploring constancy. J Neurosurg 2008;109(2):176–85.
40. McDonald CA, Korb M. Intracranial aneurysms. Arch Neurolo Psychiatry 1939;42:298–328.
41. Stehbens WE. Aneurysms and anatomical variation of cerebral arteries. Arch Pathol 1963;75:45–64.
42. Amacher LA, Drake CG. Cerebral artery aneurysms in infancy, childhood and adolescence. Childs Brain 1975;1(1):72–80.
43. Almeida GM, Pindaro J, Plese P, et al. Intracranial arterial aneurysms in infancy and childhood. Childs Brain 1977;3(4):193–9.
44. Batnitzky S, Muller J. Infantile and juvenile cerebral aneuryms. Neuroradiology 1978;16:61–4.
45. Storrs BB, Humphreys RP, Hendrick EB, et al. Intracranial aneurysms in the pediatric age-group. Childs Brain 1982;9(5):358–61.
46. Schauseil-Zipf U, Thun F, Kellermann K, et al. Intracranial arteriovenous malformations and aneurysms in childhood and adolescence. Eur J Pediatr 1983; 140(3):260–7.
47. Humphreys RP, Hendrick EB, Hoffman HJ, et al. Childhood aneurysms–atypical features, atypical management. Concepts Pediatr Neurosurg 1985;6: 213–29.
48. Pasqualin A, Mazza C, Cavazzani P, et al. Intracranial aneurysms and subarachnoid hemorrhage in children and adolescents. Childs Nerv Syst 1986; 2(4):185–90.
49. Herman JM, Rekate HL, Spetzler RF. Pediatric intracranial aneurysms: simple and complex cases. Pediatr Neurosurg 1991–1992;17(2):66–72.
50. Huang J, McGirt MJ, Gailloud P, et al. Intracranial aneurysms in the pediatric population: case series and literature review. Surg Neurol 2005; 63:424–32.
51. Vaid VK, Kumar R, Kalra SK, et al. Pediatric intracranial aneurysms: an institutional experience. Pediatr Neurosurg 2008;44(4):296–301.

Spinal Cord Vascular Malformations in Children

Debbie Song, MD[a], Hugh J.L. Garton, MD, MHSc[a], Daniel K. Fahim, MD[b], Cormac O. Maher, MD[a,*]

KEYWORDS

- Arteriovenous malformation • Arteriovenous fistula
- Cavernous malformation • Spinal cord
- Vascular malformation

Spinal vascular malformations comprise a diverse group of abnormalities, including arteriovenous malformations (AVMs), cavernous malformations, dural arteriovenous fistulas (AVFs), and capillary telangiectasias. These conditions each have distinct causes, presentations, radiologic appearances, natural histories, and treatments and are best considered separately. Although these lesions have been associated with a poor prognosis in the past, improvements in diagnosis and treatment have resulted in significantly better outcomes over the past 2 decades.[1,2] All of these lesion types may be found in the pediatric age range. This article explores the presentation, natural history, investigation, and treatment of spinal AVMs, spinal AVFs, and spinal cavernous malformations.

Various classification schemes exist to characterize arteriovenous lesions in the spinal cord. In any system of classification, a distinction should be made between AVFs and true AVMs. In 1993, Anson and Spetzler[3] attempted to classify spinal AVMs into 4 types. In this classification system, a type I AVM is actually a dural AVF, and types II, III, and IV are intradural lesions. A type II spinal AVM is an intramedullary glomus AVM characterized by a compact nidus of abnormal blood vessels within the spinal cord. Juvenile or metameric AVMs, referred to as type III lesions, are more extensive vascular lesions that can occupy the entire spinal canal at multiple levels and often extend into the paraspinal space.[4] Type IV malformations are perimedullary AVFs in which the transition from feeding artery to draining vein occurs without an intervening nidus of abnormal vessels.[4,5] Perimedullary fistulas can be further divided into 3 subtypes: a type IVa lesion, which is a small extramedullary fistula fed by a single arterial branch; a type IVb lesion, which is an intermediate-sized lesion supplied by multiple dilated arterial feeders; and a type IVc fistula, which is a high-flow, large-caliber, multipediculated fistula associated with dilated and tortuous vessels and a large shunt volume.[6]

The tendency for the classification system of Anson and Spetzler[3] to link AVFs with AVMs led Spetzler and colleagues[7] to propose a new classification system that draws a clearer distinction between these 2 distinct entities. This new classification system emphasizes the distinction between lesion type (eg, AVF or AVM) as well as location of the lesion within the spinal axis (eg, extradural, intradural extramedullary, and intradural intramedullary).[5] Intramedullary lesions may be further divided according to nidus type (eg, compact or diffuse). Intradural extramedullary fistulae are divided according to location (eg, ventral or dorsal).

[a] Department of Neurosurgery, University of Michigan, 1500 East Medical Center Drive, Room 3552, Ann Arbor, MI 48109-5338, USA
[b] Department of Neurosurgery, Baylor College of Medicine, One Baylor Plaza, Mail Stop BCM650, Houston, TX 77030, USA
* Corresponding author.
E-mail address: cmaher@med.umich.edu

Neurosurg Clin N Am 21 (2010) 503–510
doi:10.1016/j.nec.2010.03.004
1042-3680/10/$ – see front matter

SPINAL CORD AVMS

Pial spinal AVMs are lesions with a vascular nidus present within the spinal cord parenchyma. These lesions can be compact or diffuse. Compact glomus AVMs account for approximately 90% of all intramedullary spinal AVMs and are supplied by multiple feeders from the anterior and posterior spinal arteries.[3–5,8] The venous outflow of these lesions is usually diffuse, occurring in the rostral and caudal directions and on the dorsal and ventral surfaces of the spinal cord.[3] Glomus AVMs are most commonly seen at the dorsal cervicomedullary junction.[8,9] As with cerebral AVMs, associated aneurysms may increase the risk of hemorrhage.[3,4] Surgical resection is the mainstay of treatment of such lesions, and preoperative embolization is useful in select cases.

Juvenile or metameric AVMs are extensive lesions that typically have an intramedullary component and extend into the extramedullary and extradural space. These complex vascular lesions can occupy the entire spinal canal and extend into the paraspinal space.[4,5] They may involve multiple spinal levels and are supplied by several large medullary arterial feeders.[4] Diffuse intramedullary AVMs can involve the subarachnoid space, pia, and parenchyma of the spinal cord. Normal intervening neural tissue may be contained between the intraparenchymal portions of the AVM.[5] Secondary bony remodeling changes that can be seen in patients with juvenile AVMs include enlargement of the spinal canal with a widened interpedicular distance and erosion of the laminae and pedicles.[9] These lesions typically affect children and young adults and may involve the bone, muscle, skin, spinal canal, spinal cord, and nerve roots of an entire somite level, as seen in disorders such as Cobb syndrome.[5,8] These extensive lesions are difficult to treat, with the goals of therapy being to reduce mass effect, venous hypertension, and vascular steal. Endovascular embolization is the treatment of choice, but open surgical treatment may be required for decompressive purposes as well.[5] Surgical resection of diffuse lesions involves ligating the vascular loops at the pial surface rather than following the lesions into the parenchyma of the spinal cord.[5]

Demographics and Incidence

Spinal AVMs are one-tenth as common as intracranial AVMs.[8] Spinal AVMs are rare entities in children. In a recent review of 267 patients who presented with a spinal AVM in a single year, 22% of patients were 18 years or younger.[10] Intradural spinal AVMs are more likely to affect children and young adults, whereas dural AVFs are more likely to occur in patients older than 40 years.[4] In a study of 81 patients with spinal AVMs, the average age of patients with a symptomatic dural AVF was 49 years, whereas the average age for patients with symptomatic spinal cord AVM was 27 years.[4] Almost two-thirds of patients with an intradural spinal AVM were younger than 25 years.[4] Among intradural spinal AVMs, glomus-type AVMs are most common.[3,11] Syndromes associated with spinal cord AVMs include hereditary hemorrhagic telangiectasia, neurofibromatosis type I, Klippel-Trénaunay-Weber syndrome, and Cobb syndrome.[3,11,12]

Clinical Presentation and Pathophysiology

Children with spinal AVMs can present with acute, subacute, or chronic symptoms of back or radicular pain, sensorimotor deterioration, bowel or bladder dysfunction, and myelopathy. Most patients with a spinal AVM are diagnosed as young adults; however, patients often become symptomatic during childhood.[4,13] Thus, a spinal AVM should be included in the differential diagnosis for any child who presents with slowly progressive or acute symptoms of radiculopathy or myelopathy.

Sudden focal pain with a neurologic deficit is thought to reflect an acute hemorrhage and is the most common presentation of a spinal AVM in children; 40% of patients younger than 14 years present with acute symptoms.[6,14] Children may also present in a subacute fashion with recurrent events associated with a neurologic deficit from which there is some element of recovery; with time, however, there is a gradual deterioration in baseline neurologic function because of repeated hemorrhages and alterations of blood flow associated with the malformation.[14]

Subarachnoid and/or intramedullary hemorrhage is associated with intradural AVMs and produces acute symptoms. In the series reported by Rosenblum and colleagues,[4] 52% of patients with an intradural spinal AVM experienced a subarachnoid hemorrhage (SAH), whereas none of the patients with a dural AVF suffered SAH. SAH was the initial presenting symptom in 31% of patients with an intradural spinal AVM; among intradural AVMs, SAH most commonly occurred in patients with glomus malformations.[4] Thus, for patients who present with nontraumatic SAH and who have a negative cerebral angiogram, obtaining cervical spine magnetic resonance imaging (MRI) is imperative for evaluation of a spinal cord vascular malformation. An acute onset of neurologic deficit is more often found in children with glomus lesions, reflecting the higher incidence of SAH in these patients.[4] Less commonly, patients with glomus AVMs may present with progressive myelopathy due to mechanical compression or venous obstruction.[8]

High-pressure, high-volume, turbulent blood flow through intradural spinal AVMs can also lead to an arterial steal phenomenon that diverts blood away from the spinal cord parenchyma and results in ischemia.[4,14] Venous hypertension can also contribute to spinal cord ischemia, associated with progressive distention and engorgement of veins that drain intramedullary AVMs.[4,14] Progressive weakness is the most common initial symptom in patients with juvenile AVMs and perimedullary AVFs.[4,13] A sensory level may also be present in patients with spinal AVMs and reflects the spinal localization of the AVM nidus.[4] High-flow AVMs may also be associated with a spinal bruit or heart failure.[3,4]

Imaging

MRI is a sensitive modality for detecting spinal AVMs. Common findings include intradural signal voids reflecting dilated arteries or ectatic veins in or on the surface of the spinal cord, thrombosed veins, hematomyelia, spinal cord edema, syringomyelia, or spinal cord myelomalacia.[8] Intramedullary flow voids that are present in spinal cord AVMs appear as areas of hypointensity within the center of the spinal cord on axial T1-weighted images and as areas of hyperintensity on T2-weighted images (**Fig. 1**).[15] In addition, ectatic perimedullary veins and prominent flow voids in the subarachnoid space around the spinal cord are often visualized.[8]

Spinal angiography is the gold standard for diagnosing and defining the anatomy and angioarchitecture of spinal AVMs. The nidi of intradural AVMs are most commonly present within the spinal cord (80% of cases) but may less frequently be present on either the dorsal or ventral surface of the spinal cord.[3] Intradural spinal AVMs are often fed by multiple arterial feeders, are high-flow lesions, and can have single or multiple aneurysms associated with the arterial feeders or draining veins.

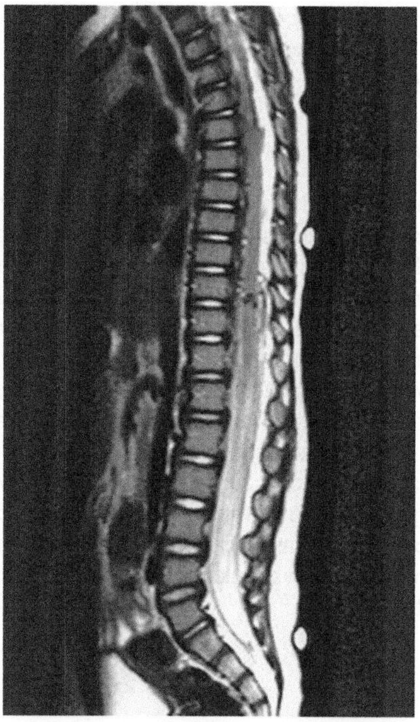

Fig. 1. Sagittal T2-weighted MRI illustrating the typical appearance of an intramedullary pial AVM of the spinal cord with dilated surface veins.

Treatment and Outcomes

Given the risk of hemorrhage and the cumulative risk of progressive neurologic deficit, treatment of spinal AVMs in the pediatric population is indicated in cases in which the estimated morbidity from treatment is acceptably low. Neurologic outcome after treatment has been directly correlated to preoperative motor function.[4] Other variables such as the age at symptom onset, degree of preoperative sensory loss, and rate of progression of neurologic deficit have not been shown to correlate with outcome.[4]

Surgical removal of glomus AVMs may be performed with similar principles that guide resection of intracranial AVMs.[16] Specifically, care is taken to identify and preserve draining veins until after the nidus is separated from the feeding vessels and surrounding parenchyma.[3] Intraoperative angiography can be technically challenging to perform for spinal malformations but may have a role in carefully selected cases.[17] Preoperative endovascular embolization may have a role in select cases.[18] Arterial side embolization as a treatment of intramedullary spinal AVMs is usually palliative at best and is rarely recommended as a primary treatment.[19] For endovascular treatment of spinal cord malformations, liquid embolic agents such as *n*-butylcyanoacrylate (NBCA) are preferred because they allow for easier filling of the distal nidus of a vascular malformation, they can be deposited in a more precise fashion, and they have a lower recanalization rate.[8] Complications from endovascular therapy can arise from inadvertent occlusion of arterial feeders supplying the spinal cord or venous branches draining the spinal cord. Intraoperative monitoring of somatosensory evoked potentials and motor evoked potentials is routinely performed during both open microsurgical excision and endovascular embolization of spinal cord AVMs.

SPINAL AVFS

Spinal AVFs, which lack an intervening nidus of vessels in the transition between arterial feeders and draining veins, can be further divided into extradural and intradural AVFs. An extradural AVF is a rare, abnormal communication between an extradural arterial branch that arises from a radicular artery and an epidural venous plexus.[5] This can result in venous engorgement with subsequent mass effect on adjacent nerve roots and the spinal cord (**Figs. 2** and **3**). On spinal angiography, slow retrograde venous drainage of the lesion can be demonstrated in association with enlarged medullary veins.[4] Endovascular embolization is often an effective therapy.[5]

Intradural AVFs can be further divided into dorsal or ventral AVFs. Intradural dorsal AVFs have a radicular feeding artery that communicates with an intradural medullary vein in the dural sleeve of a proximal nerve root and adjacent spinal dura.[4,5] These lesions are most often fed by a single arterial feeder originating in the thoracic or lumbar region. Dilated tortuous veins that drain in a rostral direction are usually seen on the dorsal aspect of the spinal cord, and in some cases, along the ventral aspect of the spinal cord as well.[4] Patients often present with myelopathy that is due in part to venous hypertension and vascular steal. Progressive sensorimotor myelopathy with lower-extremity weakness is the most common presentation.[5] Symptoms may be exacerbated by activity.[3,4] Chronic venous hypertension is thought to play a critical role in producing neurologic deterioration. Elevated venous pressures occur as arterial blood passes through the

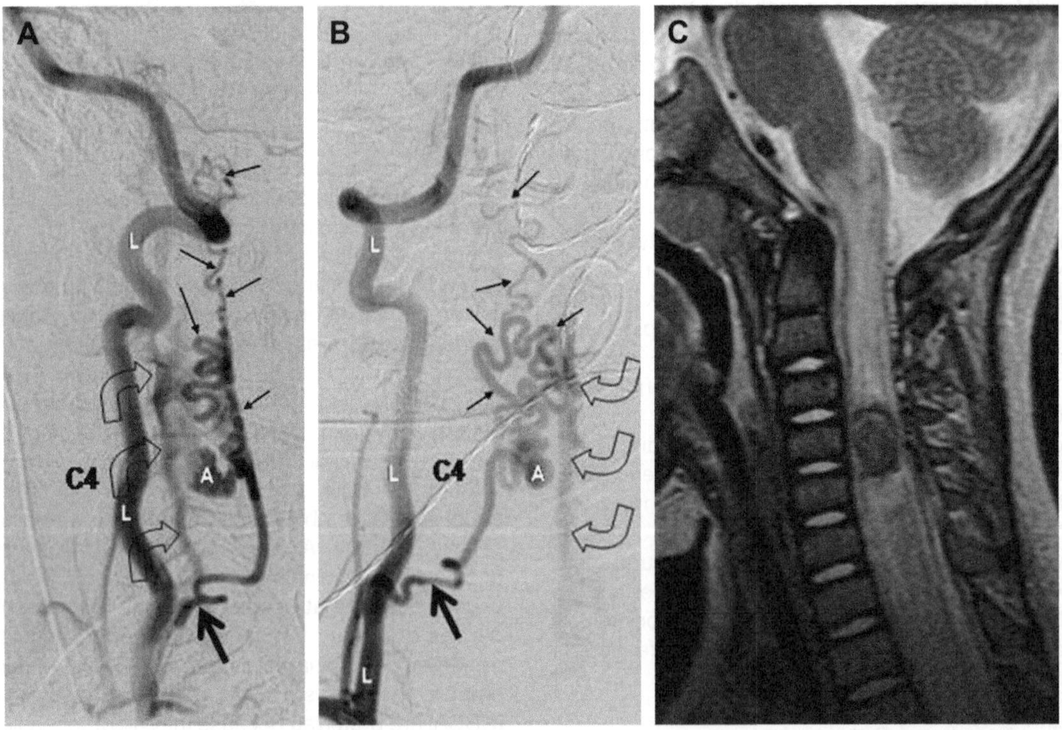

Fig. 2. Lateral (*A*) and anteroposterior (*B*) left subclavian or thyrocervical trunk angiograms (subtracted images; early arterial phase) reveal an enlarged radiculomeningeal branch of the left thyrocervical trunk entering the spinal canal at the C6-7 level (*large arrow*), which ascends to the C4-5 level. At the C4-5 level, an anteriorly oriented aneurysm (A) is identified. Further extending superiorly from the C4-5 level to the level of the foramen magnum are multiple serpiginous vessels representing engorged arterialized veins (*small arrows*). Finally, early filling of normal-appearing epidural venous structures is seen initially at the C3 and C4 levels with caudal drainage (*curved arrows*). The observed constellation of findings suggest an atypical perimedullary fistula at the C4 level giving rise to an aneurysm, arterialized veins extending cephalad, and early filling of epidural venous structures. Incidentally noted is transient reflux of contrast material into the left vertebral artery (L). Sagittal MRI (*C*) illustrating an aneurysm within the cervical cord.

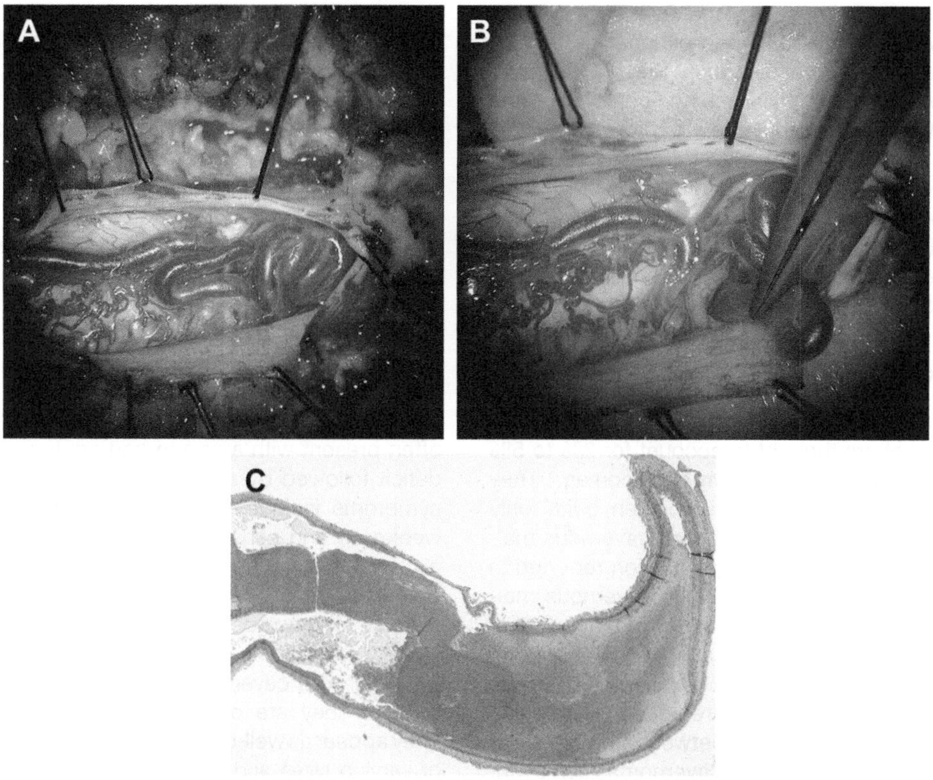

Fig. 3. Intraoperative views (*A* and *B*) of the patient represented in **Fig. 2**. The large aneurysm is removed and the arterialized vein is disconnected. The junction between the arterial and venous segments may be appreciated in the histologic specimen (*C*).

fistula into a draining medullary vein and transmits relatively high pressure to the valveless venous plexus and radial veins associated with the spinal cord.[4] These lesions may arise spontaneously or after trauma.[4,8,10]

Although spinal angiography remains the gold standard, magnetic resonance angiography is useful for predicting the level of the fistula before angiography, leading to decreased radiation and contrast dose.[20] For these reasons, preangiographic magnetic resonance investigation is especially useful in the pediatric age group. Intradural dorsal AVFs are best treated via surgical disruption of the fistula.[5,21] From a posterior approach, the arterialized vein should be isolated, cauterized, and ligated at its exit point from the margin on the dural nerve root sleeve.[5] This operation is straightforward, curative, and associated with minimal morbidity.[21]

An intradural ventral AVF is usually located in the midline and consists of a fistulous communication between the anterior spinal artery and an enlarged venous network in the subarachnoid space.[5] Intradural ventral AVFs can be small with a single feeder or they can be giant lesions with large, multipediculated feeders from the anterior spinal artery that communicates with dilated venous channels.[5,10] Smaller-sized lesions may be treated surgically via anterior or posterior approaches, with care taken to preserve anterior spinal artery branches.[5]

PARASPINAL AVMs

Paraspinal AVMs in children are rare, with less than 2 dozen reported cases in the literature.[22–24] These lesions can involve the paravertebral musculature, intervertebral foramen, or paravertebral region. Although such lesions may occur at any spinal cord level, in children they are most commonly found in the thoracic spine.[24] They can cause spinal cord dysfunction by spinal venous hypertension that leads to progressive myelopathy or by hemorrhage into the spinal canal that is associated with acute paraplegia. Paraspinal AVMs may manifest with a bruit or murmur, weakness, congestive heart failure secondary to arteriovenous shunting, myelopathy from mass effect of enlarged venous varices, or low back pain.[24] These lesions may be congenital or have a posttraumatic cause. Among children with paraspinal AVMs, presentation is bimodal, with most children presenting either before the age of 4 years or after 10 years.[24] Spinal angiography is the modality of choice in evaluating paraspinal AVMs, with MRI being a useful adjunct that can reveal engorged intrathecal and paraspinal veins (**Fig. 4**).[24] Successful obliteration of paraspinal AVMs in children can be performed via endovascular embolization with liquid embolic agents such as NBCA.[22–24]

CAVERNOUS MALFORMATIONS

Spinal cord cavernous malformations are rare lesions that are thought to account for 3% to 5% of all central nervous system cavernomas.[3] They are even more unusual in children, with only a handful of cases of spinal cord cavernous malformations in the pediatric population reported in the literature.[25–29] Histologically, cavernous malformations are characterized by thin-walled, dilated, sinusoidal endothelial channels lined with a subendothelial stroma that lacks smooth muscle and elastic tissue.[8,28] There is no intervening spinal cord parenchyma between the vascular channels in such lesions.[28] Cavernomas can occur throughout the neuraxis and often contain hemosiderin-laden macrophages, indicating hemorrhages of varying ages.

Despite the scarcity of cases of spinal cord cavernomas in children reported in the literature, differences exist in the clinical presentations of adults and children with such lesions. Whereas spinal cord cavernomas have a 2:1 predilection for women among adults, they are more common in boys than girls in the pediatric population.[3,28] Among children with spinal cord cavernous malformations, the mean age at which an initial symptomatic hemorrhage occurs is around 13 years.[28] Spinal cord cavernous malformations in children are evenly distributed throughout the thoracic and lumbar spinal cord, whereas they are most commonly located in the thoracic spinal cord in adults.[28] Adults with spinal cord cavernous malformations present with a slow, progressive myelopathy or with an acute deficit followed by a stuttering pattern of deterioration with intervening periods of clinical improvement. This is thought to reflect multiple hemorrhages or thromboses within the cavernoma.[28] In contrast, children with symptomatic spinal cord cavernomas often present with a severe and acute neurologic deficit followed by a rapid decline.[10,26] Common symptoms include radiating low back pain with weakness and sensory changes. Although these clinical features have been reported in a series of pediatric spinal cavernous malformations, it is difficult to draw definitive conclusions from the paucity of available data.

Spinal cord cavernomas are best visualized on MRI, as they are occult on spinal angiography. They appear as well-defined, intramedullary masses of varying sizes and mixed signal intensity on T1- and T2-weighted spin echo sequences.[3,8,28] Cavernous malformations have hyperintense areas on T1- and T2-weighted images with a peripheral rim of hypointensity on gradient echo sequences, which reflects the hemosiderin ring. Spinal cord cavernous malformations may be associated with multiple cavernomas elsewhere in the neuraxis or with familial cavernoma syndromes.[30] Thus, MRI of the entire neuraxis is indicated when a spinal cord cavernous malformation is identified in isolation.

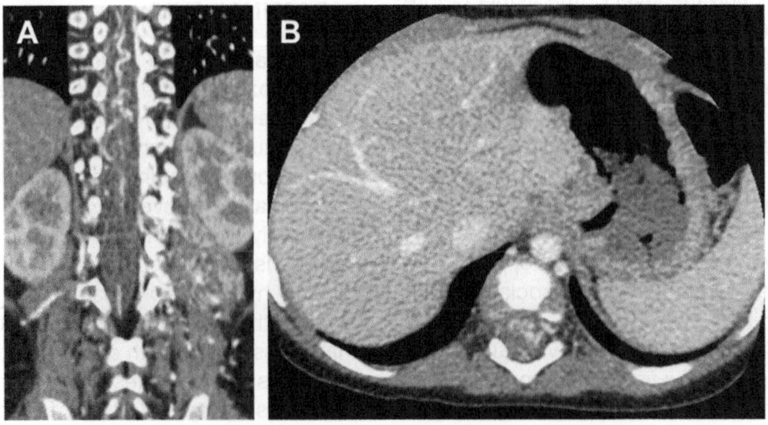

Fig. 4. Coronal (*A*) and axial (*B*) CT angiography illustrating a paraspinal AVM with multiple arterial feeders from the abdominal aorta and a nidus in the paraspinal musculature. The perimedullary venous plexus is dilated as a consequence of the fistula.

Spinal cord cavernous malformations have a higher risk of hemorrhage that has a greater potential for causing significant morbidity compared with supratentorial cavernomas. The actuarial risk of hemorrhage for a supratentorial cavernous malformation has been estimated to be 0.2% to 0.7% per year; the risk is 1.6% per year for spinal cord cavernomas and 2.7% per year for brainstem cavernomas.[3,28] Given the cumulative risk and greater morbidity of hemorrhage that is faced by children with spinal cord cavernous malformations, treatment via microsurgical excision is typically favored for those lesions that have bled or for asymptomatic lesions that present with an accessible pial surface. Surgical treatment is generally not recommended for asymptomatic spinal cord cavernomas that do not present to a pial surface. Typically, such lesions may be followed expectantly, with regular clinical and imaging surveillance. Microsurgical excision is the only means of curing a cavernous malformation. Radiosurgery is not an acceptable method of treatment. Most lesions can be surgically approached via dorsal laminectomy, but a posterolateral transpedicular approach may be required for more ventrally located lesions.[3] In children, laminoplasty with replacement of the bone and preservation of the supraspinous ligament is preferred to prevent long-term postoperative spinal deformities. For lesions that present at the pial surface, dissection can be performed directly over the lesion. For deeper lesions, a midline myelotomy or myelotomy in the dorsal root entry zone is performed. Dissection is performed in the thin plane of hemosiderin-laden gliosis around the cavernoma to limit trauma to the normal surrounding spinal cord tissue. Grossly, cavernous malformations have a distinctive purple mulberry appearance with a surrounding rim of yellow-brown discoloration from hemosiderin deposits. In contrast to cerebral cavernomas, the thin rim of hemosiderin-stained perilesional gliosis should not be removed in spinal cord cavernous malformations.[3,28] Complete excision of spinal cord cavernous malformations can usually be achieved safely, and generally, it has a good long-term outcome. As with spinal cord AVMs, the most predictive factor of surgical outcome is the patient's pretreatment neurologic status.[3]

SUMMARY

Spinal cord and paraspinal vascular malformations are rare entities in the pediatric population. Each of these lesion types has distinct clinical presentations and treatments. In general, the most common predictor of neurologic outcome after treatment is the pretreatment neurologic function.

REFERENCES

1. Aminoff MJ, Barnard RO, Logue V. The pathophysiology of spinal vascular malformations. J Neurol Sci 1974;23:255–63.
2. Aminoff MJ, Logue V. Clinical features of spinal vascular malformations. Brain 1974;97:197–210.
3. Anson JA, Spetzler RF. Surgical resection of intramedullary spinal cord cavernous malformations. J Neurosurg 1993;78:446–51.
4. Rosenblum B, Oldfield EH, Doppman JL, et al. Spinal arteriovenous malformations: a comparison of dural arteriovenous fistulas and intradural AVM's in 81 patients. J Neurosurg 1987;67:795–802.
5. Kim LJ, Spetzler RF. Classification and surgical management of spinal arteriovenous lesions: arteriovenous fistulae and arteriovenous malformations. Neurosurgery 2006;59:S195–201.
6. Padovani R, Tognetti F, Laudadio S, et al. Arteriovenous malformations of the spinal cord in the pediatric age group. Case report and review of the literature. Spine (Phila Pa 1976) 1986;11:23–5.
7. Spetzler RF, Detwiler PW, Riina HA, et al. Modified classification of spinal cord vascular lesions. J Neurosurg 2002;96:145–56.
8. Veznedaroglu E, Nelson PK, Jabbour PM, et al. Endovascular treatment of spinal cord arteriovenous malformations. Neurosurgery 2006;59:S202–9.
9. Zozulya YP, Slin'ko EI, Al Q II. Spinal arteriovenous malformations: new classification and surgical treatment. Neurosurg Focus 2006;20:E7.
10. Lad SP, Santarelli JG, Patil CG, et al. National trends in spinal arteriovenous malformations. Neurosurg Focus 2009;26:1–5.
11. Niimi Y, Berenstein A, Song J. Spinal vascular malformations. In: Albright AL, Pollack IF, Adelson PD, editors. Principles and practice of pediatric neurosurgery. 2nd edition. New York: Thieme; 2007. p. 1029–41.
12. Poisson A, Vasdev A, Brunelle F, et al. Acute paraplegia due to spinal arteriovenous fistula in two patients with hereditary hemorrhagic telangiectasia. Eur J Pediatr 2009;168:135–9.
13. Sure U, Wakat JP, Gatscher S, et al. Spinal type IV arteriovenous malformations (perimedullary fistulas) in children. Childs Nerv Syst 2000;16:508–15.
14. Eldridge PR, Holland IM, Punt JA. Spinal arteriovenous malformations in children. Br J Neurosurg 1989;3:393–7.
15. da Costa L, Dehdashti AR, terBrugge KG. Spinal cord vascular shunts: spinal cord vascular malformations and dural arteriovenous fistulas. Neurosurg Focus 2009;26:E6.

16. Connolly ES Jr, Zubay GP, McCormick PC, et al. The posterior approach to a series of glomus (Type II) intramedullary spinal cord arteriovenous malformations. Neurosurgery 1998;42:774–86.
17. Schievink WI, Vishteh AG, McDougall CG, et al. Intraoperative spinal angiography. J Neurosurg 1999;90:48–51.
18. terBrugge KG. Neurointerventional procedures in the pediatric age group. Childs Nerv Syst 1999;15:751–4.
19. Mullan S. Reflections upon the nature and management of intracranial and intraspinal vascular malformations and fistulae. J Neurosurg 1994;80:606–16.
20. Luetmer PH, Lane JI, Gilbertson JR, et al. Preangiographic evaluation of spinal dural arteriovenous fistulas with elliptic centric contrast-enhanced MR angiography and effect on radiation dose and volume of iodinated contrast material. AJNR Am J Neuroradiol 2005;26:711–8.
21. Atkinson JL, Miller GM, Krauss WE, et al. Clinical and radiographic features of dural arteriovenous fistula, a treatable cause of myelopathy. Mayo Clin Proc 2001;76:1120–30.
22. Cognard C, Semaan H, Bakchine S, et al. Paraspinal arteriovenous fistula with perimedullary venous drainage. AJNR Am J Neuroradiol 1995;16:2044–8.
23. Hui F, Trosselo MP, Meisel HJ, et al. Paraspinal arteriovenous shunts in children. Neuroradiology 1994;36:69–73.
24. Kitagawa RS, Mawad ME, Whitehead WE, et al. Paraspinal arteriovenous malformations in children. J Neurosurg Pediatr 2009;3:425–8.
25. Bakir A, Savas A, Yilmaz E, et al. Spinal intradural-intramedullary cavernous malformation. Case report and literature review. Pediatr Neurosurg 2006;42:35–7.
26. Deutsch H, Jallo GI, Faktorovich A, et al. Spinal intramedullary cavernoma: clinical presentation and surgical outcome. J Neurosurg 2000;93:65–70.
27. Nagib MG, O'Fallon MT. Intramedullary cavernous angiomas of the spinal cord in the pediatric age group: a pediatric series. Pediatr Neurosurg 2002;36:57–63.
28. Noudel R, Litre F, Vinchon M, et al. Intramedullary spinal cord cavernous angioma in children: case report and literature review. Childs Nerv Syst 2008;24:259–63.
29. Scott RM, Barnes P, Kupsky W, et al. Cavernous angiomas of the central nervous system in children. J Neurosurg 1992;76:38–46.
30. Cohen-Gadol AA, Jacob JT, Edwards DA, et al. Coexistence of intracranial and spinal cavernous malformations: a study of prevalence and natural history. J Neurosurg 2006;104:376–81.

Cerebral Venous Sinus (Sinovenous) Thrombosis in Children

Nomazulu Dlamini, MBBS, MRCPCH, MSc[a,b],
Lori Billinghurst, MD, MSc, FRCPC[a],
Fenella J. Kirkham, MD, FRCPCH[b,*]

KEYWORDS

• Cerebral sinovenous thrombosis • CSVT
• Pediatric • Neonatal • Stroke

Cerebral venous sinus (sinovenous) thrombosis (CSVT) is an increasingly recognized cause of childhood and neonatal stroke. Recent developments in the field highlight the expanding spectrum of perinatal brain injury associated with neonatal CSVT. Although there is considerable overlap in risk factors for neonatal and childhood CSVT, specific differences exist between the groups. Management remains controversial, unlike in adult sinovenous thrombosis. However, morbidity and mortality are significant, highlighting the continued need for high-quality studies within this field. This article reviews the literature on childhood CSVT (**Table 1**) and highlights developments in our understanding of neonatal CSVT.

EPIDEMIOLOGY

More than 40% of childhood CSVT occurs within the neonatal period, with an incidence of 2.6 per 100,000 children per year in one series.[5] The incidence of childhood CSVT varies between 0.4 and 0.7 per 100,000 children per year.[12,14] These figures are probably underestimates of the true incidence for several reasons. Children with CSVT, particularly neonates, often present with nonfocal neurologic signs and symptoms, and the diagnosis may not be suspected.[12] Old imaging techniques, the variable anatomy of sinovenous channels and rapid recanalization are all factors which may contribute to underdiagnosis. The lack of evidence supporting treatment and anxieties about safety of anticoagulation may also have reduced the impetus to make a diagnosis, particularly in suspected CSVT associated with hemorrhage.

ANATOMY AND PHYSIOLOGY OF THE VENOUS SYSTEM IN NEONATES AND CHILDREN

The venous sinuses and veins lie within the subarachnoid space. Arachnoid villi project into the venous sinuses of the dura and are concentrated on the superior sagittal sinus, which is important for absorption and drainage of cerebrospinal fluid. Venous drainage is achieved by 2 systems: the superficial and the deep. The superficial drainage system is composed of the superficial cortical veins, superior sagittal sinus (SSS), torcula or confluence of veins, right transverse sinus (dominant in the majority of individuals), sigmoid sinus, and internal jugular vein. The deep venous system consists of the basal veins, which drain blood from the basal ganglia and germinal matrix in preterm neonates, the Galenic system with the 2 internal cerebral veins that form the vein of Galen, the straight sinus, the basal vein of Rosenthal, the torcula, and the typically

[a] The Hospital For Sick Children, 555 University Avenue, Toronto, ON M5G 1X8, Canada
[b] Neurosciences Unit, UCL Institute of Child Health, 30 Guilford Street, London WC1N 1EH, UK
* Corresponding author. Neurosciences Unit, The Wolfson Centre, Mecklenburgh Square, London WC1N 2AP, UK.
E-mail address: F.Kirkham@ich.ucl.ac.uk

Neurosurg Clin N Am 21 (2010) 511–527
doi:10.1016/j.nec.2010.03.006
1042-3680/10/$ – see front matter

Table 1
Pediatric CSVT literature summary

Study	No. of patients	Demographics, N (%) Country	Males	Neonate	Risk Factors None, N (%)	Systemic (N or %)	Infection (%)	PT (%)	Infarction (%)	Treatment (%) Acute ACT	Chronic ACT	Outcome (%) Follow-up (y)	Death	Abnormal
Mallick et al, 2009[1]	21	UK	10 (48)	0	2 (10)	Nephrotic syndrome (3) CNS tumor (1) OCP (2) Dehydration (14) Anemia (19)	Any infection (71) OM/Mastoiditis (62) Sepsis (10)	25	14 Bland (100) Hemorrhagic (0)	100 UFH (100) LMWH (14)	67 Coumadin (100) LMWH (19)	0.42–6	10	29
Vieira et al, 2009[2]	53	Portugal	30 (57)	6 (11)	7 (13)	Nephrotic syndrome (2) CNS tumor (1) SLE (1) Head trauma (1) Diabetes (1) Chemotherapy (5) Dehydration (4)	Any infection (57) Mastoiditis (43) Meningitis (13)	40	NR	68	100 Coumadin (100)	1.1–6	0	43
Wasay et al, 2008[3]	70	USA	28 (40)	25 (36)	7 (10)	Nephrotic syndrome (1) SLE (2) SCD (1) Homocystinuria (3) Leukemia (2) OCP (1) Chemotherapy (1) Dehydration (4) Anemia (10) Fever (33)	Any infection (40) OM/MA/Sinusitis (24) Meningitis (3) Sepsis (13)	56	NR	21	12 Coumadin (100)	NR	13	46
Kenet et al, 2007[4]	396	Germany Israel UK Belgium	236 (60)	75 (19)	NR	NR	NR	NR	10 Bland (10) Hemorrhagic (90)	63 UFH (51) LMWH (48)	42 LMWH (76)	0–7.1	3	NR
Fitzgerald et al, 2006[5]	42	USA	24 (57)	42 (100)	NR	Cardiac condition (11) Dehydration (26)	Any infection (17) Meningitis (10) Sepsis (7)	64	60 Bland (12) Hemorrhagic (88) IVH (20)	7	0	0.2–15	3	79

Bonduel et al, 2006[6]	38	Argentina	27 (71)	NR	3 (8)	SLE (1) CNS tumor (2) Leukemia (8) Lymphoma (2) Head trauma (2) Chemotherapy (7) Dehydration (5)	Any Infection (50)	NR	NR	68 LMWH (68)	68 Coumadin (100)	0.25–11.5	23	32
Sébire et al, 2005[7]	42	UK	27 (64)	NR	0	Cardiac condition (2) IBD (1) Nephrotic syndrome (3) SLE (2) SCD (2) Thalassemia (1) CNS tumor (2) Leukemia (2) Dehydration (19) Anemia (19)	Any infection (55) OM (41) MA (26)	62	60 Bland (52) Hemorrhagic (48)	43 UFH (83) LMWH (17)	43	0.5–10	12	62
Kenet et al, 2004[8]	46	Israel	29 (63)	8 (17)	7 (15)	Cardiac condition (4) IBD (1) SLE (2) Homocystinuria (1) OCP (1) Head trauma (4)	Any infection (39) MA/Sinusitis (35)	42	NR	88	NR	NR	4	17
Barnes et al, 2004[9]	16	Australia	8 (50)	0	NR	NR	Any infection (88) OM/MA (44) Meningitis/Abscess (44)	31	NR	63 UFH (30) LMWH (80) Coumadin (30)	NR	0.02–5	NR	38
Heller et al, 2003[5]	149	Germany	84 (56)	40 (27)	44 (30)	IBD (1) Nephrotic syndrome (1) Steroid use (3) OCP (4) Head trauma (10)	Any infection (44) OM (3) MA (9) Meningitis (4) Sepsis (5) Sinusitis (3) Varicella (1) Gastroenteritis (3)	56	NR	88 UFH (47) LMWH (40)	73 LMWH (100)	NR	0	NR
Wu et al, 2002[10]	30	USA	NR	30 (100)	4 (13)	Cardiac condition (7) Dehydration (3)	Any infection (13) Sepsis (10) Pneumonia (3)	57	NR	NR	NR	NR	NR	NR

(continued on next page)

Table 1
(*continued*)

		Demographics, N (%)			Risk Factors				Infarction (%)	Treatment (%)		Outcome (%)		
Study	No. of patients	Country	Males	Neonate	None, N (%)	Systemic (N or %)	Infection (%)	PT (%)		Acute ACT	Chronic ACT	Follow-up (y)	Death	Abnormal
Huisman et al, 2001[11]	19	Switzerland	9 (47)	0	NR	Head trauma (9)	Any infection (37) MA (32) Meningitis (5)	NR	11	NR	NR	NR	11	NR
DeVeber et al, 2001[12]	160	Canada	87 (57)	69 (43)	4 (3)	Cardiac condition (8) Dehydration (25)	Any infection (27) Sepsis (18)	24	41 Bland (32) Hemorrhagic (68)	53 LWMH (59) UFH (41) Coumadin (46)	NR	0.05–5.2	8	38
Carvalho et al, 2000[13]	31	USA	21 (68)	19 (61)	NR	Cardiac condition (4) CNS tumor (1) Chemotherapy (1) Dehydration (13)	Any infection (39) MA (23) Meningitis (10) Sepsis (7)	NR	48	0	0	NR	13	52

All studies with more than 10 patients published since 2000 are included.

Abbreviations: ACT, anticoagulation; APTT, activated partial thromboplastin time; CNS, central nervous system; IBD, inflammatory bowel disease; IVH, intraventricular hemorrhage; LMWH, low molecular weight heparin; MA, mastoiditis; NR, not reported; OCP, oral contraceptive use; OM, otitis media; PT, prothrombotic tendency; SCD, sickle cell disease; SLE, systemic lupus erythematosus; UFH, unfractionated heparin.

nondominant left transverse sinus, which drains into the left sigmoid sinus and the left internal jugular vein.

The major venous outflow tracts include the internal jugular veins (IJV) and extrajugular collateral venous pathways such as the venous vertebral plexus and the extracranial emissary veins. In the supine position assumed by neonates, the IJV is the major venous outflow tract. However, in adult studies have shown that, in standing, the venous vertebral plexus is the main outflow tract. The extracranial emissary veins, are small, few, and not thought to play a major role in normal venous drainage. However, in certain conditions where there is congenital chronic venous outflow obstruction, such as craniosynostosis, they assume a central role providing an extracranial outflow pathway.[15,16] In most infants, the cavernous sinus is not yet connected to the cerebral veins, resulting in less reserve and increased vulnerability within the venous drainage system.[15,17]

Positioning of the neonate has been shown to have a major influence on venous outflow. Neck flexion and compression of the SSS by the occipital bone have been implicated in the etiology of venous stasis and thrombosis,[18–20] and is an area requiring further study.[21]

PATHOPHYSIOLOGICAL MECHANISMS

Thrombosis within the venous system results in outflow obstruction, venous congestion, and a consequent increase in capillary hydrostatic pressure, driving fluid into the interstitium and producing edema. A persistent increase in hydrostatic pressure may result in red blood cell diapedesis, and if in excess of arterial pressure, a reduction of arterial inflow and arterial ischemia can occur.

SPECTRUM OF BRAIN INJURY IN CSVT

The spectrum of brain injury in CSVT varies from venous congestion, which may or may not be appreciable on neuroimaging (**Fig. 1**), to the more recognized parenchymal ischemic injury, which may be cortical or subcortical, and involve deep gray matter (see **Fig. 1; Fig. 2**). The majority of the parenchymal infarcts are hemorrhagic. Less well appreciated is CSVT-related primary subarachnoid and subdural hemorrhage. In preterm and term neonates there is also an association between intraventricular hemorrhage (IVH) and CSVT.[22] Several studies demonstrate that CSVT is the most frequently recognized cause of symptomatic IVH, and is associated with basal ganglia and thalamic hemorrhage in term neonates. Deep venous thrombosis can be accompanied by hemorrhage into the ventricles as a result of blockage and hypertension in the deep venous drainage system.[10,23] Presumed perinatal ischemic stroke is a subgroup of perinatal stroke and encompasses imaging-confirmed focal infarction, which may be venous or arterial, presenting after the neonatal period. Perinatal venous infarction (PVI) is one of these periventricular infarction syndromes, and is an underrecognized cause of congenital hemiplegia.[24]

RISK FACTORS FOR CSVT DEVELOPMENT

As is the case in adults, CSVT in neonates, infants, and children is often multifactorial in etiology, with a predisposing comorbid condition or infirmity identified in up to 95% of those affected (see **Table 1**). These conditions include common childhood illnesses such as fever, infection, dehydration, and anemia, as well as acute and chronic medical conditions such as congenital heart disease, nephrotic syndrome, systemic lupus erythematosus, and malignancy (**Table 2**). As well as the maternal, there are neonatal risk factors for sinovenous thrombosis in the perinatal period (**Table 3**), which parallel those in older children.

In addition to these systemic risk factors, thrombosis can develop and propagate in response to local venous stasis. A large number of children have coincident local head and/or neck pathology, including head trauma, central nervous system tumors, or recent intracranial surgery. Historically, CSVT was a well-recognized complication of otitis media and mastoiditis, and while less attention has been paid recently to this important risk factor, otitis media or mastoiditis has been identified in 24% to 62% of all childhood CSVT case series and cohorts published in the last decade.[1,5,7,13,27,28] Indeed, in terms of observed frequency, infection appears to be the most common condition associated with CSVT in children outside of the neonatal period.

Anemia is frequently observed in children with CSVT, though mechanisms for its contribution to thrombus development are incompletely understood. Iron deficiency anemia and microcytosis are most commonly described[7,25,29–33] sometimes in association with thrombocytosis, but only one study with parallel controls is currently available.[25] CSVT has also been reported in chronic anemias, such as hemolytic anemia and Evans syndrome,[34] β-thalassemia major,[35] and sickle cell disease.[36–40] The diagnosis of anemia may be obscured by relative hemoconcentration (particularly if dehydration is also present) and a falsely elevated ferritin in the

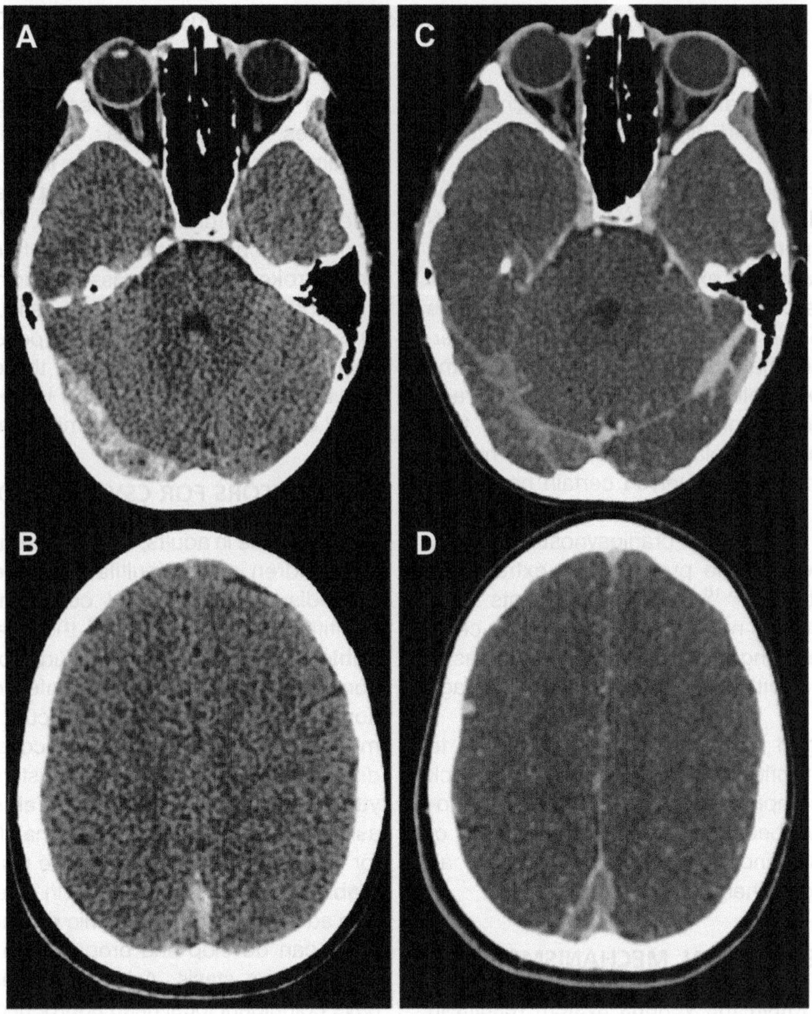

Fig. 1. Case synopsis. A previously healthy 8-year-old girl was admitted with a 3-week history of, intermittent emesis and a 4-day history of occipital headache, and photophobia. Examination revealed severe dehydration, mild hypertension, and tachycardia. Extensive thrombosis of both deep and superficial cerebral sinovenous systems was diagnosed on head CT and anticoagulation therapy was initiated. Progressive encephalopathy developed on hospital day 5, necessitating admission to the intensive care unit. Unexplained tachycardia (heart rate >200) developed on hospital day 15 and Graves disease was ultimately diagnosed (thyrotropin <0.01 mIU/L and free T4 >77.2 pmol/L.) The patient was then started on methimazole. Comprehensive prothrombotic testing uncovered a heterozygous mutation in the Factor V Leiden gene. She completed 6 months of anticoagulation with subcutaneous low molecular weight heparin. Follow-up neurologic examination revealed mild left incoordination and bilateral kinetic tremor (left > right), perhaps secondary to hemorrhagic venous infarction of the right thalamus. (*A*, *B*) Non-contrast axial head CT done at admission revealed heterogeneous attenuation within the right transverse and sigmoid sinuses (*A*) and posterior aspect of the superior sagittal sinus (*B*), suggesting acute and subacute components of the thrombus. (*C*, *D*) Contrast CT reveals filling defects within these same sinuses. (*E*, *F*) Initial axial fluid-attenuated inversion recovery (FLAIR) (*E*), T1 and T2 (not shown) MRI sequences as well as diffusion-weighted imaging (DWI) (*F*) showed normal brain parenchyma. (*H*, *I*) A repeat MRI done in the subacute period after the patient's clinical deterioration showed increased signal within the thalami bilaterally on FLAIR (*H*) and T2 (not shown). Corresponding areas of diffusion restriction on DWI (*I*) suggested venous congestion and infarction secondary to thalamostriate venous occlusion. Peripheral blooming was seen in the right thalamus on gradient echo sequences (not shown), evidence of petechial hemorrhage. (*K*, *L*) Follow-up MRI done 6 months after diagnosis showed low FLAIR (*K*) and T2 signal (not shown) in the right thalamus, corresponding to hemosiderin deposits from hemorrhagic infarction. DWI (*L*) similarly showed low signal. (*G*, *J*, *M*) Three-dimensional phase contrast MR venograms performed acutely (*G*) and subacutely (*J*) showed extensive sinovenous thrombosis, involving the right transverse and sigmoid sinuses (*black arrow*), right internal jugular vein, posterior superior and inferior sagittal sinuses, torcula, vein of Galen, basal vein of Rosenthal, and internal cerebral and thalamostriate veins. Left parietal cortical veins were also thrombosed (*white arrowheads*). The left transverse and sigmoid sinuses were spared (*white arrow*). Interval recanalization of the left internal cerebral vein and basal vein of Rosenthal was seen subacutely (*J*). A 2-dimensional time-of-flight MR venogram done 6 months post diagnosis (*M*) showed persistently absent flow within the right transverse sinus, but partially visualized flow within the right sigmoid sinus and jugular bulb (*black arrow*), evidence of either partial recanalization or slow flow within these sinuses. There was complete recanalization of the superior sagittal sinus, deep venous system, and left parietal cortical veins.

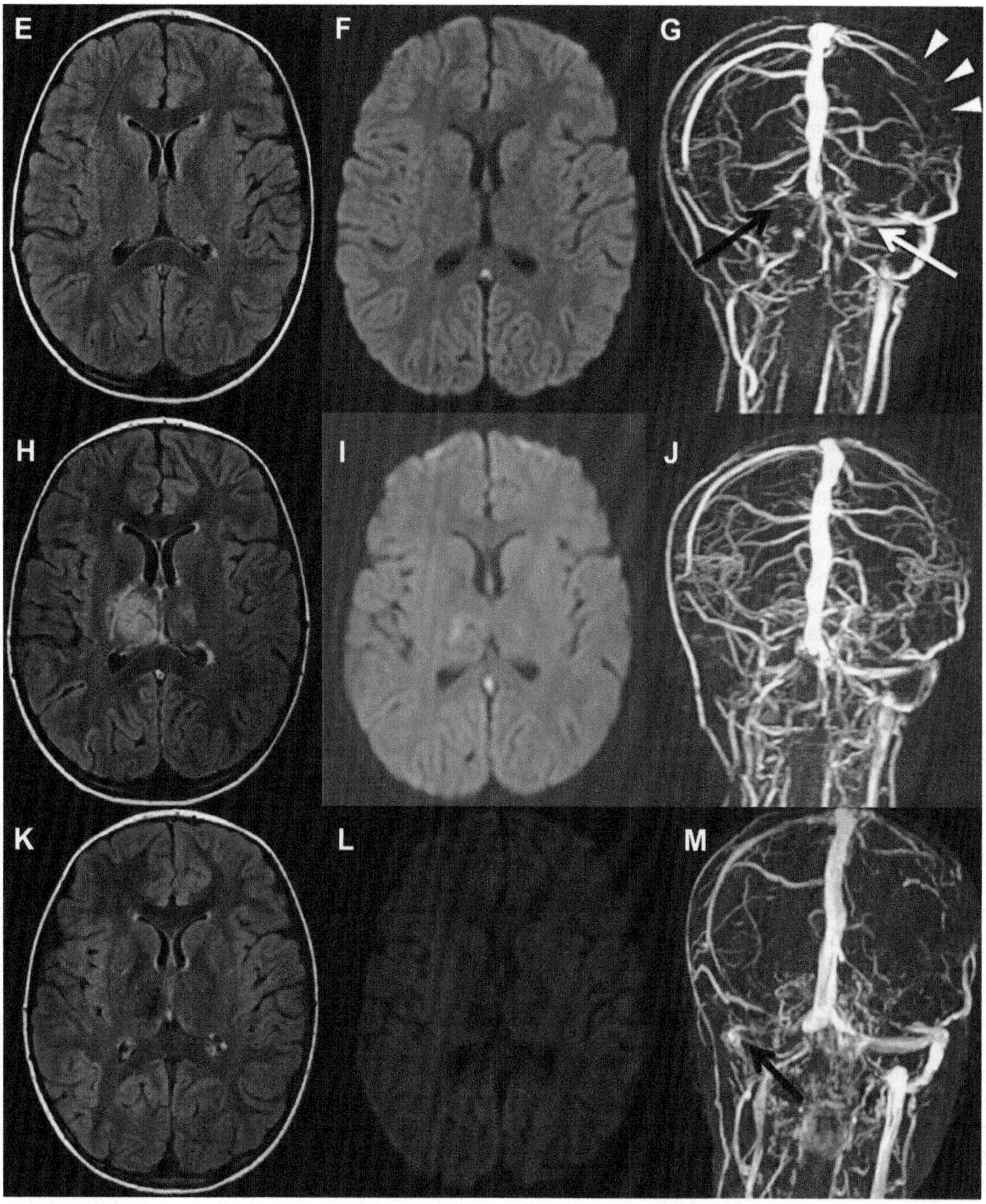

Fig. 1. (*continued*)

acute setting, so it is important that the diagnosis of anemia and iron deficiency should be comprehensively excluded or treated in all children with CSVT.

Dehydration is another important treatable risk factor for pediatric CSVT, secondary either to increased fluid losses from nephrotic syndrome[30] or gastroenteritis, or poor oral intake with infection or systemic medical illness. Dehydration and hypovolemia should always be carefully assessed and corrected to prevent thrombus propagation and promote recanalization of the affected vessel.

Other common illnesses, including meningitis[41] and diabetes,[29] may be complicated by CSVT, which can be difficult to diagnose so that data for incidence remain a minimum estimate.[28] Although occasionally recognized, there are few data on the prevalence of CSVT in convulsive and nonconvulsive seizures and status epilepticus[42] and otherwise unexplained hydrocephalus.[43]

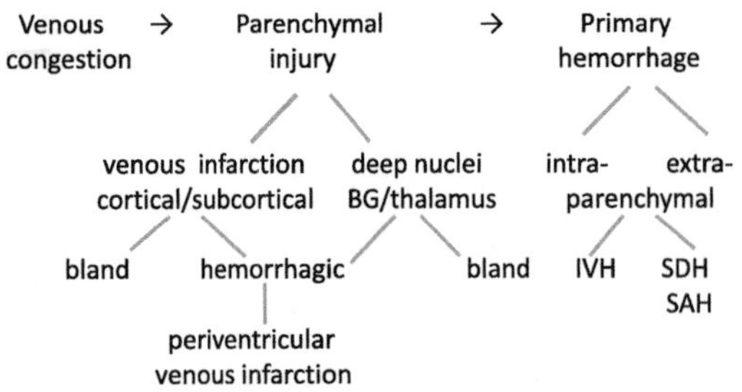

Fig. 2. Spectrum of CSVT related brain injury. BG, basal ganglia; SDH, subdural hemorrhage; IVH, intraventricular hemorrhage; SAH, subarachnoid hemorrhage.

CSVT may also be an important determinant of outcome in minor head injury,[44,45] and in traumatic[11,46,47] and nontraumatic coma (eg, secondary to cerebral malaria).[48] Other infections more commonly seen in tropical countries (eg, neurocystercercosis), may also be associated with CSVT.[49]

Certain chronic conditions such as inflammatory bowel disease,[50] systemic lupus erythematosus,[51] Cushing syndrome,[52] and thyrotoxicosis[53] (see **Fig. 1**) appear to predispose to CSVT, which may present in unusual ways, including psychiatric manifestations.[54]

PROTHROMBOTIC DISORDERS THAT MAY BE RISK FACTORS FOR CSVT IN CHILDREN

Prothrombotic states have been identified in 24% to 64% of children[5,7,28,55,56] and in 20% of neonates[10] with CSVT in recent series (see **Table 1**). However, these data are difficult to interpret as (1) the number and types of available prothrombotic tests have varied over the past 2 decades and vary between centers, (2) not all children have full prothrombotic profiles assessed, and (3) results may depend on the timing of testing. Indeed, acquired prothrombotic tendencies, such as protein C, protein S, and/or antithrombin deficiency secondary to infection or protein loss (eg, in nephrotic syndrome), may normalize on repeat investigation with resolution of the acute process. High factor VIII levels, which may be determined by genetic and acquired factors, are also common[7,57] but there are currently no controlled data. Although there is evidence for an excess of genetic polymorphisms, the relative importance of the Factor V Leiden mutation is less clear in children than in adults.[5,56,58] While uncommon, the prothrombin 20210 mutation does appear to be a risk factor for recurrence and should be excluded.[4]

Homocystinuria is a rarely described association,[59] and homozygotes for the thermolabile variant of the methylene tetrahydrofolate reductase (MTHFR) gene may have an increased risk of CSVT.[60] Hyperhomocysteinemia (which has been shown to be a risk factor in 2 case-controlled series in adults[61,62]) and its genetic determinants may be worth excluding or treating with folic acid and vitamin B_6 and B_{12} supplementation, as this has few risks, but further studies will be important.

Apart from those with the prothrombin 20210 mutation, who should probably be anticoagulated in high-risk situations,[4] there are few data on whether long-term treatment of any of the other prothrombotic disorders reduces the recurrence risk.[5,28] Investigation for prothrombotic disorders is expensive and may not guide management except in certain circumstances, such as determining the risks of using oral contraception (see later discussion). Nevertheless, full prothrombotic profiles should be considered in all affected children, to better counsel parents of patients and also contribute data that may improve our understanding of mechanisms underlying CSVT development.

CLINICAL PRESENTATION

The clinical manifestations of CSVT are nonspecific, and may be subtle in neonates and children (**Table 4**). Although rare, cerebral sinovenous thrombosis can occur antenatally as early as the second trimester and is detectable by fetal real-time and color Doppler ultrasound.[63] Reported cases are likely an underestimation of frequency, as the imaging characteristics mimic those of an intracranial tumor. Thrombosis often occurs within the posterior fossa and may occur in association with dural malformations such as dural arteriovenous shunts. Spontaneous regression of the thrombosis may occur, with a favorable outcome. Diagnosis is important, as therapeutic terminations of pregnancy have resulted in misdiagnosis.[64] The fetal venous drainage system may be less susceptible to thrombosis compared with the neonate, as fetal anastomoses may result in the fetus being able to redirect venous blood flow.[65]

Outside of the antenatal period most of the clinical scenarios occur at all ages, and the clinician requires a high index of suspicion to make the diagnosis. The clinical manifestations of CSVT are nonspecific, may be subtle (see **Table 4**), and may overlap with predisposing conditions such as infection and dehydration.[7,12] Seizures, altered levels of consciousness and encephalopathy, focal neurologic deficits (cranial nerve palsies, hemiparesis, hemisensory loss), and diffuse neurologic symptoms (headache, nausea, emesis) may result. While most of the clinical symptoms can occur at any age, seizures are more common in neonates, and focal and diffuse

Table 2
Conditions associated with pediatric cerebral sinovenous thrombosis

General
Dehydration
Infection
Fever
Hypoxic-ischemic injury
Post lumbar puncture
Head and neck infections
Otitis media and mastoiditis
Meningitis
Sinusitis
Upper respiratory tract infection
Other head and neck disorders
Head injury
Post intracranial surgery
Hydrocephalus (±ventriculoperitoneal shunt)
Anemia
Iron deficiency
Sickle cell disease
Thalassemia
Autoimmune hemolytic anemia
Paroxysmal nocturnal hemoglobinuria
Autoimmune disorders
Behçet disease
Systemic lupus erythematosus
Antiphospholipid antibody syndrome
Inflammatory bowel disease (ulcerative colitis, Crohn disease)
Thyrotoxicosis
Cushing syndrome
Idiopathic thrombocytopenic purpura
Malignancy
Leukemia
Lymphoma
Central nervous system tumors
Cardiac disease
Cyanotic congenital heart disease[25,26]
Post-operative
Postcatheterization
Renal disease
Nephrotic syndrome
Hemolytic-uremic syndrome
Drugs
L-Asparaginase
Oral contraceptives
Corticosteroids
Epoetin-α
Chromosomal disorders
Down syndrome
Metabolic conditions
Diabetic ketoacidosis
Homocystinuria

neurologic signs are more common in older infants and children.[12] The clinician should consider this diagnosis in a wide range of acute neurologic presentations in childhood, including those accompanied by neuroimaging evidence of hydrocephalus,[43] subdural effusion or hematoma,[66] subarachnoid hemorrhage,[67] or intracerebral hemorrhage or infarction, particularly in the parietal or occipital regions.[7] Presentation with pseudotumor cerebri[68] and isolated headache[69] have been well documented. A high index of suspicion is necessary to effect earlier detection and therapeutic strategies.

DIAGNOSIS

Neuroimaging Techniques

The keys to neuroradiological diagnosis (**Table 5**) are (1) a high index of suspicion of the diagnosis in the acute phase so that imaging is performed early, as the venous sinuses may recanalize before detection,[4,7,70] and (2) a good working relationship between treating clinicians and neuroradiologists

Table 3
Conditions associated with neonatal cerebral sinovenous thrombosis

Maternal conditions
Chorioamnionitis
Diabetes
Hypertension
Perinatal conditions
Meconium aspiration
Apgar <7 at 5 min
Intubated at birth
Neonatal infection
Polycythemia
Severe dehydration
Pneumonia
ECMO treatment
Congenital heart disease
Disseminated intravascular coagulation
Congenital diaphragmatic hernia

Abbreviation: ECMO, extracorporeal membrane oxidation.

Table 4
Symptoms and signs of cerebral sinovenous thrombosis in older children

Seizures (focal, generalized)
Depressed level of consciousness and coma
Lethargy
Nausea
Vomiting
Headache
Visual impairment (transient obscurations, reduced acuity, blindness)
Papilledema
Hemiparesis
Hemisensory loss
Ataxia
Speech impairment, mutism
Cranial nerve palsies (VI)
Acute psychiatric symptoms
Respiratory failure (in neonates)
Jittery movements (in neonates)

so that definitive neuroimaging and investigations are pursued if necessary.

Anatomic and clinical studies demonstrate a link between venous drainage and location of parenchymal infarcts.[71,72] Unenhanced computed tomography (CT) scans may detect deep venous thrombosis as linear densities in the expected locations of the deep and cortical veins (see **Fig. 1**A, B).[11,73] As the thrombus becomes less dense, contrast may demonstrate the "empty delta" sign, a filling defect, in the posterior part of the sagittal sinus (see **Fig. 1**C, D).[11,28] However, CT scan with contrast misses the diagnosis of CSVT in up to 40% of patients.[9,27,28] Diffusion and perfusion magnetic resonance imaging (MRI) may play a role in detecting venous congestion in cerebral venous thrombosis (see **Fig. 1**H, I) and in the differentiation of cytotoxic and vasogenic edema, but does not differentiate venous from arterial infarction. CT venography or MRI with venography (MRV) are now the methods of choice for investigation of CSVT.[7,9,71,74] The diagnosis is established by demonstrating a lack of flow in the cerebral veins (see **Fig. 1**G,J,M) with or without typical images of brain infarction (see **Fig. 1**E, F, H, I).

Table 5
Diagnosis of sinovenous thrombosis

	Level of Evidence
High index of suspicion in children with associated pre-existing disorder	IC
High index of suspicion in children presenting with headache, seizures, coma	IC
Plain CT	IC
MRI (T1-, T2-weighted, T2*, FLAIR)	IC
MRI with contrast	IIC
Diffusion-weighted MRI	IIC
CT venography	IIC
MR venography	IIC
Contrast MR venography	IIC
Transcranial Doppler	IIC
Conventional digital subtraction angiography	IIC

Abbreviations: CT, computed tomography; FLAIR, fluid-attenuated inversion recovery; MR, magnetic resonance; MRI, magnetic resonance imaging.

The superficial venous system is more frequently involved than the deep system, and the most common sites of CSVT are the transverse, superior sagittal, sigmoid, and straight sinuses. Between one- and two-thirds of children with CSVT may have parenchymal brain lesions such as venous infarction and hemorrhage.[71] MRI and MRV are important in both the demonstration of the infarct and the clot within the vessels.[71] On MRI, the thrombus is readily recognizable in the subacute phase, when it is of high signal on a T1-weighted scan, and MRV may not be required. In the acute phase, the thrombus is isodense with brain on T1-weighted imaging and of low signal on T2-weighted imaging. This appearance can be mistaken for flowing blood, but MRV will demonstrate an absence of flow in the thrombosed sinus. T2*-weighted MRI seems to be more sensitive than T1- or T2-weighted or fluid-attenuated inversion recovery (FLAIR) imaging in demonstrating venous thrombosis and associated hemorrhage.[75,76] However, MRI and MRV are techniques prone to flow artifacts (see **Fig. 1**M) and in equivocal cases, particularly if deep venous infarction or cortical venous thrombosis is suspected, an endoluminal technique such as high-resolution CT venography or conventional digital subtraction angiography may be required as a final arbiter.

INVESTIGATION, MONITORING, AND MANAGEMENT

Laboratory investigation of adult and pediatric CSVT is similar (**Table 6**). Treatment of CSVT (**Table 7**) has historically involved general supportive care or symptomatic measures, such

Table 6
Laboratory investigations in cryptogenic cerebral venous sinus thrombosis

	Level of Evidence
Essential	
Blood culture	IC
Full blood count	IC
Iron studies	IC
Thyroid function	IC
Antinuclear antibody or DNA binding	IC
Potentially useful	
Homocysteine	IIB
Vitamin status, ie, folate, B_6, B_{12}	IIB
Full prothrombotic screen (DNA and citrated samples)	IIB

as correction of dehydration and hypovolemia, antibiotics for cases involving infection, control of seizures with anticonvulsants, and medical and surgical measures aimed at decreasing intracranial pressure. In cases of otitis media-related and mastoiditis-related CSVT, many children receive parenteral antibiotic therapy, with either second- or third-generation cephalosporins (**Table 8**). Antibiotic choice and treatment duration in children with head and neck infections should be discussed with a local infectious disease specialist and consideration given to coverage with metronidazole, clindamycin, or vancomycin when anaerobic organisms are implicated (ie, *Fusobacterium necrophorum* in Lemierre syndrome or jugular venous thrombophlebitis).[42] The role of surgery, such as mastoidectomy, myringotomy, and/or tympanostomy tube insertion, in otitis media-related and mastoiditis-related CSVT is unclear,[77] but is often performed based on the preference of the treating otolaryngologist. Some patients develop intracranial hypertension within the clinical spectrum previously described as "pseudotumor cerebri" or "otitic" communicating hydrocephalus, and may require long-term acetazolamide therapy, serial lumbar punctures, or lumboperitoneal shunting (see section on Follow-up).

Pediatric case series published in the last decade differ in their reported use of antithrombotic agents after the diagnosis of CSVT is established. Treatment regimens vary between centers, but many older infants and children receive anticoagulation in the acute setting with either parenteral unfractionated heparin, subcutaneous low molecular weight heparin (LMWH), or oral warfarin (Coumadin; Bristol Myers-Squibb) (see **Table 1**). Some centers prefer to use unfractionated heparin acutely, as the effects of heparin can be reversed if intracranial

Table 7
Acute management

	Level of Evidence
Supportive treatment	
Rehydration	IC
Treat infection, eg, antibiotics for meningitis/mastoiditis/pharyngitis	IC
Treat cause, eg, mastoidectomy, steroids for SLE, inflammatory bowel	IC
Treat seizures	IC
Treat iron deficiency	IIB
Anticoagulate/monitor for 4 months whether or not there is hemorrhage	
IV heparin/APTT	IIB
SC heparin/Factor Xa	IIC
Warfarin/INR	IIC
Thrombolysis	IIC
Thrombectomy	IIC
Surgical decompression	IIC

Abbreviation: INR, international normalized ratio.

Table 8
Monitoring of child with acute sinovenous thrombosis

	Level of Evidence
Clinical seizures (duration, semiology)	IC
Level of consciousness (Glasgow Coma Scale adapted for children)	IC
Focal neurologic signs, eg, hemiparesis	IC
Visual acuity and fields	IC
For those on intravenous heparin, 4-hourly APTT	IC
For those on subcutaneous heparin, daily factor Xa	IC
For those who are unconscious and/or ventilated:	
Continuous EEG monitoring	IIC
Intracranial pressure monitoring	IIC
Repeat neuroimaging	IIC

hemorrhage occurs. This regimen is often followed by chronic anticoagulation with LMWH or Coumadin for 3 to 6 months. Anticoagulation should be carefully monitored, with activated partial thromboplastin time (APTT) for unfractionated heparin, anti-Xa for LMWH, or international normalized ratio for Coumadin, to achieve adequate levels for efficacy while preventing overdosage. However, anticoagulation may be terminated sooner than this if recanalization of the affected vessel(s) is demonstrated on follow-up neuroimaging with MR or CT venography. At some centers, there seems to be a reluctance to treat neonates with anticoagulation[12,13,78] due to perceived risks of worsening preexisting intracranial hemorrhage or causing hemorrhagic transformation of bland venous infarction, coupled with a lack of evidence demonstrating improved outcome in neonates treated with anticoagulation. However, treatment of neonates with LMWH appears to be safe, and should at least be considered.[79] Very few centers have reported on the use of antiplatelet agents such as acetylsalicylic acid (ASA)[7,12] or dipyridamole in the acute or chronic[1] settings.

There are currently no well-designed clinical trials in children to support acute or chronic antithrombotic therapy with anticoagulants or antiplatelet agents once the diagnosis of CSVT is made. The only randomized placebo-controlled trial of intravenous heparin in adults[80] was stopped early because there was clear evidence of benefit, particularly in terms of mortality. Subsequent to this, a randomized placebo-controlled trial of subcutaneous LMWH in adults[81] showed a trend for better outcome in the treated group, but the mortality was lower in this series and there were more patients with milder presentations in the placebo arm. Despite these limited data, a recent Cochrane review concluded that anticoagulation was safe, and there was some evidence for a clinically important benefit.[82]

Single-center and small multicenter series in children[7,57,74,83] have shown that intravenous and subcutaneous LMWH can be used safely in children, with close monitoring of heparin levels or anti-Xa levels when LMWH is employed (see **Table 8**). DeVeber and colleagues[84] initiated a prospective cohort study of anticoagulant therapy in 30 children with CSVT from 1992 to 1996, and reported a mortality rate of 3 out of 8 untreated compared with 0 of 22 treated children. One series suggested that cognitive outcome might be better in the anticoagulated group,[7] and pooled data from the European collaborative group found a reduced risk of recurrence in those who were anticoagulated.[4] In adult series, patients with hemorrhage were anticoagulated, and available evidence suggests that the benefit of anticoagulation on improved outcome outweighs the risk of new bleeding or extension of old hemorrhage. There is currently a consensus that in children beyond the neonatal period without hemorrhage, anticoagulation should be considered.[85–87]

There are no randomized data on thrombolysis,[1,3,88–90] thrombectomy,[91] or surgical decompression[92,93] in CSVT even in adults,[94] but each has been used with apparent success in isolated cases or small series of seriously ill patients, including children, usually in coma and with extensive thrombosis of superficial and deep venous structures.[79,88–90] A nonrandomized study comparing urokinase thrombolysis with heparin in adults suggested better functional outcome for the thrombolysed patients but higher risk of hemorrhage.[95] These patients have a high risk of secondary complications, including status epilepticus, hydrocephalus,[95] and raised intracranial pressure,[96,97] and may benefit from intensive care and monitoring of electroencephalograph and intracranial pressure as well as neuroimaging (see **Table 8**).

MORTALITY AND MORBIDITY

CSVT-specific mortality is less than 10%, but neurologic deficits are present at time of discharge or follow-up examination in 17% to 79% of survivors, and motor and cognitive sequelae may require long-term rehabilitative regimens.[1,7,28,98–100] Coma is a predictor of death in childhood CSVT.[7] Most published pediatric cohorts have followed affected children for relatively short periods, typically less than 2 years from time of diagnosis. Despite aggressive therapy with antithrombotic agents, antibiotics, and surgery in some cases, many children with CSVT suffer chronic neurologic symptoms, such as headache, visual impairment, and cranial nerve VI palsy related to increased intracranial pressure. Others display deficits related to venous infarction ranging from developmental delays and learning disabilities to hemiparesis and hemisensory loss. In the series by Sébire and colleagues of children who presented at more than 1 month of age,[7] older age, lack of parenchymal abnormality, anticoagulation, and lateral and/or sigmoid sinus involvement were independent predictors of good cognitive outcome, although the last predicted pseudotumor cerebri. More than 50% of neonates have a poor outcome, and mortality is high.[3,12]

FOLLOW-UP

All children with CSVT require close monitoring for neurologic and ophthalmologic symptoms and signs related to increased intracranial pressure and optic nerve compression. As visual impairment and failure may go undetected by parents, particularly in nonverbal children, ophthalmology follow-up is warranted in the first year after diagnosis. Persistent headache, nausea, or vomiting (particularly if nocturnal or early morning) mandate repeat neuroimaging to exclude hydrocephalus, CSVT propagation, and/or recurrence. Chronically elevated intracranial pressure may respond to treatment with steroids or acetazolamide, or may require lumboperitoneal shunting.[94,101,102] Occasionally patients with cryptogenic CSVT later manifest symptoms of an underlying disease (see **Fig. 1**), such as systemic lupus erythematosus or Behçet disease,[103] so patients should be encouraged to report back if they have any other medical concerns after diagnosis.

Follow-up neuroimaging with MR or CT venography should be undertaken in the acute phase and during the first year of follow-up to look for evidence of extension or persistence or recanalization of venous occlusion, or the development of venous stenosis. Some centers perform this at 3, 6, and 12 months after diagnosis. In the European study, complete and partial recanalization occurred in 46% and 42%, respectively.[4]

PREDICTION AND PREVENTION OF RECURRENCE

Between 10% and 20% of children who have a cerebral venous sinus thrombosis will experience a recurrent symptomatic venous event, at least half of which are systemic rather than cerebral (**Table 9**).[4,5,7,28] In a multicenter European study,[4] recurrent venous thrombosis only occurred in children whose first CSVT was diagnosed after age 2 years; the underlying medical condition had no effect. In Cox regression analyses, nonadministration of anticoagulant before relapse (hazard ratio [HR] 11.2, 95% confidence interval [CI] 3.4–37.0; $P<.0001$), persistent occlusion on repeat venous imaging (HR 4.1, 95% CI 1.1–14.8; $P = .032$), and heterozygosity for the G20210A mutation in factor II (HR 4.3, 95% CI 1.1–16.2; $P = .034$) were independently associated with recurrence. Among patients who had recurrent CSVT, 70% (15) occurred within 6 months after the initial episode.

There have been no trials of strategies to prevent recurrent cerebral or systemic venous thrombosis in children, but these cohort data suggest that anticoagulation should be considered for up to 6 months after the first episode. It would be difficult to recommend a higher risk strategy, such as prolonged oral anticoagulation, unless recurrence had already occurred, but there is a case for anticoagulation in acute settings where the risk of recurrence is likely to be high, for example, relapse of nephrotic syndrome or active inflammatory bowel disease.[4] There is also a little evidence that stopping the use of oral contraceptives reduces the risk, and there are several low-risk strategies, such as improving the quality of the diet, which can be recommended (see **Table 9**).

Table 9
Management of risk factors to prevent recurrence

	Level of Evidence
Improve diet, eg, 5 portions of fruit and/or vegetables per day	IC
Reduce cow's milk intake and increase solids in infants and toddlers	IC
Treat cause, eg, steroids for SLE, IBD	IC
Suggest alternative contraception	IB
Treat iron deficiency	IIC
Treat hyperhomocysteinemia/ frank vitamin deficiency, eg, folate, B_6, or B_{12}	IIC
Consider acute anticoagulation in high-risk settings	IIA
Consider prolonged oral anticoagulation after recurrence	IIC

SUMMARY

Cerebral sinovenous thrombosis is an underdiagnosed but important cause of stroke in childhood occurring most often in the neonatal period. Mortality and morbidity are significant. However, there are several unanswered questions regarding CSVT, particularly in relation to diagnosis in children presenting with hydrocephalus, or in coma or status epilepticus in the context of common conditions such as head injury, as well as the safety and efficacy of treatment in this age group. Hence the need for further high quality studies and where possible - well conducted randomized controlled trials.

REFERENCES

1. Mallick AA, Sharples PM, Calvert SE, et al. Cerebral venous sinus thrombosis: a case series including thrombolysis. Arch Dis Child 2009;94: 790–4.

2. Viera JP, Luis C, Monteiro JP, et al. Cerebral sinovenous thrombosis in children: clinical presentation and extension, localization and recanalization of thrombosis. Eur J Paediatr Neurol; 2010;14:80–5.
3. Wasay M, Dai AI, Ansari M, et al. Cerebral venous sinus thrombosis in children: a multicenter cohort from the United States. J Child Neurol 2008;23: 26–31.
4. Kenet G, Kirkham F, Niederstadt T, et al. Risk factors for recurrent venous thromboembolism in the European collaborative paediatric database on cerebral venous thrombosis: a multicentre cohort study. Lancet Neurol 2007;6:595–603.
5. Heller C, Heinecke A, Junker R, et al. Cerebral venous thrombosis in children: a multifactorial origin. Circulation 2003;108:1362–7.
6. Bonduel M, Sciuccati G, Hepner M, et al. Arterial ischemic stroke and cerebral venous thrombosis in children: a 12-year Argentinean registry. Acta Haematol 2006;115:180–5.
7. Sébire G, Tabarki B, Saunders DE, et al. Cerebral venous sinus thrombosis in children: risk factors, presentation, diagnosis and outcome. Brain 2005; 128:477–89.
8. Kenet G, Waldman D, Lubetsky A, et al. Paediatric cerebral sinus vein thrombosis: a multi-center, case-controlled study. Thromb Haemost 2004;92: 713–8.
9. Barnes C, Newall F, Furmedge J, et al. Cerebral sinus venous thrombosis in children. J Paediatr Child Health 2004;40:53–5.
10. Wu YW, Miller SP, Chin K, et al. Multiple risk factors in neonatal sinovenous thrombosis. Neurology 2002;59:438–40.
11. Huisman TA, Holzmann D, Martin E, et al. Cerebral venous thrombosis in childhood. Eur Radiol 2001; 11:1760–5.
12. deVeber G, Andrew M, Adams C, et al. Cerebral sinovenous thrombosis in children. N Engl J Med 2001;345:417–23.
13. Carvalho KS, Bodensteiner JB, Connolly PJ, et al. Cerebral venous thrombosis in children. J Child Neurol 2001;16:574–80.
14. Lynch JK, Nelson KB. Epidemiology of perinatal stroke. Curr Opin Pediatr 2001;13:499–505.
15. Schreiber SJ, Lurtzing F, Gotze R, et al. Extrajugular pathways of human cerebral venous blood drainage assessed by duplex ultrasound. J Appl Phys 2003;94:1802–5.
16. Al-Otibi M, Jea A, Kulkarni AV. Detection of important venous collaterals by computed tomography venogram in multisutural synostosis. Case report and review of the literature. J Neurosurg 2007; 107:508–10.
17. Valdueza JM, von MT, Hoffman O, et al. Postural dependency of the cerebral venous outflow. Lancet 2000;355:200–1.
18. Cowan F, Thoresen M. Changes in superior sagittal sinus blood velocities due to postural alterations and pressure on the head of the newborn infant. Pediatrics 1985;75:1038–47.
19. Dean LM, Taylor GA. The intracranial venous system in infants: normal and abnormal findings on duplex and color Doppler sonography. AJR Am J Roentgenol 1995;164:151–6.
20. Newton TH, Gooding CA. Compression of superior sagittal sinus by neonatal calvarial molding. Radiology 1975;115:635–40.
21. Tan MA, deVeber G, Miller E, et al. Alleviation of cerebral venous obstruction in supine lying neonates with use of a custom-designed pillow [abstract]. Ann Normandie 2008;64(Suppl 12):S131.
22. Ramenghi LA, Gill BJ, Tanner SF, et al. Cerebral venous thrombosis, intraventricular haemorrhage and white matter lesions in a preterm newborn with factor V (Leiden) mutation. Neuropediatrics 2002;33:97–9.
23. Wu YW, Hamrick SE, Miller SP, et al. Intraventricular hemorrhage in term neonates caused by sinovenous thrombosis. Ann Neurol 2003;54:123–6.
24. Kirton A, deVeber G, Pontigon AM, et al. Presumed perinatal ischemic stroke: vascular classification predicts outcomes. Ann Neurol 2008;63:436–43.
25. Maguire JL, deVeber G, Parkin PC. Association between iron-deficiency anemia and stroke in young children. Pediatrics 2007;120:1053–7.
26. Cottrill CM, Kaplan S. Cerebral vascular accidents in cyanotic congenital heart disease. Am J Dis Child 1973;125:484–7.
27. Barron TF, Gusnard DA, Zimmerman RA, et al. Cerebral venous thrombosis in neonates and children. Pediatr Neurol 1992;8:112–6.
28. deVeber G, Andrew M. The Canadian Paediatric Ischemic Stroke Study group. The epidemiology and outcome of sinovenous thrombosis in pediatric patients. N Engl J Med 2001;345:417–23.
29. Keane S, Gallagher A, Ackroyd S, et al. Cerebral venous thrombosis during diabetic ketoacidosis. Arch Dis Child 2002;86:204–5.
30. Fluss J, Geary D, deVeber G. Cerebral sinovenous thrombosis and idiopathic nephrotic syndrome in childhood: report of four new cases and review of the literature. Eur J Pediatr 2006; 165:709–16.
31. Belman AL, Roque CT, Ancona R, et al. Cerebral venous thrombosis in a child with iron deficiency anemia and thrombocytosis. Stroke 1990;21: 488–93.
32. Hartfield DS, Lowry NJ, Keene DL, et al. Iron deficiency: a cause of stroke in infants and children. Pediatr Neurol 1997;16:50–3.
33. Benedict SL, Bonkowsky JL, Thompson JA, et al. Cerebral sinovenous thrombosis in children:

another reason to treat iron deficiency anemia. J Child Neurol 2004;19:526–31.
34. Shiozawa Z, Ueda R, Mano T, et al. Superior sagittal sinus thrombosis associated with Evans' syndrome of haemolytic anaemia. J Neurol 1985; 232:280–2.
35. Incorpora G, Di GF, Romeo MA, et al. Focal neurological deficits in children with beta-thalassemia major. Neuropediatrics 1999;30:45–8.
36. Garcia JH. Thrombosis of cranial veins and sinuses: brain parenchymal effects. In: Einhaupl KM, Kempski O, Baethmann A, editors. Cerebral sinus thrombosis: experimental and clinical aspects. New York: Plenum Press; 1990. p. 27–37.
37. Oguz M, Aksungur EH, Soyupak SK, et al. Vein of Galen and sinus thrombosis with bilateral thalamic infarcts in sickle cell anaemia: CT follow-up and angiographic demonstration. Neuroradiology 1994; 36:155–6.
38. Di RC, Jourdan C, Yilmaz H, et al. [Cerebral deep vein thrombosis: three cases]. Rev Neurol (Paris) 1999;155:583–7 [in French].
39. van Mierlo TD, van den Berg HM, Nievelstein RA, et al. An unconscious girl with sickle-cell disease. Lancet 2003;361:136.
40. Sidani CA, Ballourah W, El Dassouki M, et al. Venous sinus thrombosis leading to stroke in a patient with sickle cell disease on hydroxyurea and high hemoglobin levels: treatme nt with thrombolysis. Am J Hematol 2008;83:818–20.
41. Kastenbauer S, Pfister HW. Pneumococcal meningitis in adults: spectrum of complications and prognostic factors in a series of 87 cases. Brain 2003;126:1015–25.
42. Narayanan JT, Murthy JM. Nonconvulsive status epilepticus in a neurological intensive care unit: profile in a developing country. Epilepsia 2007;48:900–6.
43. Norrell H, Wilson C, Howieson J, et al. Venous factors in infantile hydrocephalus. J Neurosurg 1969;31:561–9.
44. Tamimi A, bu-Elrub M, Shudifat A, et al. Superior sagittal sinus thrombosis associated with raised intracranial pressure in closed head injury with depressed skull fracture. Pediatr Neurosurg 2005; 41:237–40.
45. Yuen HW, Gan BK, Seow WT, et al. Dural sinus thrombosis after minor head injury in a child. Ann Acad Med Singap 2005;34:639–41.
46. Stiefel D, Eich G, Sacher P. Posttraumatic dural sinus thrombosis in children. Eur J Pediatr Surg 2000;10:41–4.
47. Matsushige T, Nakaoka M, Kiya K, et al. Cerebral sinovenous thrombosis after closed head injury. J Trauma 2009;66:1599–604.
48. Krishnan A, Karnad DR, Limaye U, et al. Cerebral venous and dural sinus thrombosis in severe falciparum malaria. J Infect 2004;48:86–90.
49. Prasad R, Singh R, Joshi B. Lateral sinus thrombosis in neurocysticercosis. Trop Doct 2005;35: 182–3.
50. Standridge S, de los Reyes E. Inflammatory bowel disease and cerebrovascular arterial and venous thromboembolic events in 4 pediatric patients: a case series and review of the literature. J Child Neurol 2008;23:59–66.
51. Uziel Y, Laxer RM, Blaser S, et al. Cerebral vein thrombosis in childhood systemic lupus erythematosus. J Pediatr 1995;126:722–7.
52. Yoshimura S, Ago T, Kitazono T, et al. Cerebral sinus thrombosis in a patient with Cushing's syndrome. J Neurol Neurosurg Psychiatr 2005;76:1182–3.
53. Siegert CE, Smelt AH, de Bruin TW. Superior sagittal sinus thrombosis and thyrotoxicosis. Possible association in two cases. Stroke 1995; 26:496–7.
54. McQueen A. "I think she's just crazy". Lancet 2005; 365:1513.
55. deVeber G, Monagle P, Chan A, et al. Prothrombotic disorders in infants and children with cerebral thromboembolism. Arch Neurol 1998;55:1539–43.
56. Bonduel M, Sciuccati G, Hepner M, et al. Factor V Leiden and prothrombin gene G20210A mutation in children with cerebral thromboembolism. Am J Hematol 2003;73:81–6.
57. Cakmak S, Derex L, Berruyer M, et al. Cerebral venous thrombosis: clinical outcome and systematic screening of prothrombotic factors. Neurology 2003;60:1175–8.
58. Johnson MC, Parkerson N, Ward S, et al. Pediatric sinovenous thrombosis. J Pediatr Hematol Oncol 2003;25:312–5.
59. Vorstman E, Keeling D, Leonard J, et al. Sagittal sinus thrombosis in a teenager: homocystinuria associated with reversible antithrombin deficiency. Dev Med Child Neurol 2002;44:498.
60. Hillier CE, Collins PW, Bowen DJ, et al. Inherited prothrombotic risk factors and cerebral venous thrombosis. QJM 1998;91:677–80.
61. Martinelli I, Battaglioli T, Pedotti P, et al. Hyperhomocysteinemia in cerebral vein thrombosis. Blood 2003;102:1363–6.
62. Cantu C, Alonso E, Jara A, et al. Hyperhomocysteinemia, low folate and vitamin B12 concentrations, and methylene tetrahydrofolate reductase mutation in cerebral venous thrombosis. Stroke 2004;35:1790–4.
63. Visentin A, Falco P, Pilu G, et al. Prenatal diagnosis of thrombosis of the dural sinuses with real-time and color Doppler ultrasound. Ultrasound Obstet Gynecol 2001;17:322–5.
64. Laurichesse DH, Winer N, Gallot D, et al. Prenatal diagnosis of thrombosis of the dural sinuses: report of six cases, review of the literature and suggested management. Ultrasound Obstet Gynecol 2008;32: 188–98.

65. Barbosa M, Mahadevan J, Weon YC, et al. Dural sinus malformations (DSM) with giant lakes, in neonates and infants. Review of 30 consecutive cases [abstract]. Intervent Neuroradiol 2003;9:407–24.
66. Marquardt G, Weidauer S, Lanfermann H, et al. Cerebral venous sinus thrombosis manifesting as bilateral subdural effusion. Acta Neurol Scand 2004;109:425–8.
67. Adaletli I, Sirikci A, Kara B, et al. Cerebral venous sinus thrombosis presenting with excessive subarachnoid hemorrhage in a 14-year-old boy. Emerg Radiol 2005;12:57–9.
68. Biousse V, Ameri A, Bousser MG. Isolated intracranial hypertension as the only sign of cerebral venous thrombosis. Neurology 1999;53:1537–42.
69. Cumurciuc R, Crassard I, Sarov M, et al. Headache as the only neurological sign of cerebral venous thrombosis: a series of 17 cases. J Neurol Neurosurg Psychiatr 2005;76:1084–7.
70. Baumgartner RW, Studer A, Arnold M, et al. Recanalisation of cerebral venous thrombosis. J Neurol Neurosurg Psychiatr 2003;74:459–61.
71. Teksam M, Moharir M, deVeber G, et al. Frequency and topographic distribution of brain lesions in pediatric cerebral venous thrombosis. AJNR Am J Neuroradiol 2008;29:1961–5.
72. Zubkov AY, McBane RD, Brown RD, et al. Brain lesions in cerebral venous sinus thrombosis. Stroke 2009;40:1509–11.
73. Kothare SV, Ebb DH, Rosenberger PB, et al. Acute confusion and mutism as a presentation of thalamic strokes secondary to deep cerebral venous thrombosis. J Child Neurol 1998;13:300–3.
74. Medlock MD, Olivero WC, Hanigan WC, et al. Children with cerebral venous thrombosis diagnosed with magnetic resonance imaging and magnetic resonance angiography. Neurosurgery 1992;31:870–6.
75. Selim M, Fink J, Linfante I, et al. Diagnosis of cerebral venous thrombosis with echo-planar T2*-weighted magnetic resonance imaging. Arch Neurol 2002;59:1021–6.
76. Goldenberg NA, Knapp-Clevenger R, Hays T, et al. Lemierre's and Lemierre's-like syndromes in children: survival and thromboembolic outcomes. Pediatrics 2005;116:e543–8.
77. Wong I, Kozak FK, Poskitt K, et al. Pediatric lateral sinus thrombosis: retrospective case series and literature review. J Otolaryngol 2005;34:79–85.
78. Fitzgerald KC, Williams LS, Garg BP, et al. Cerebral sinovenous thrombosis in the neonate. Arch Neurol 2006;63:405–9.
79. Kersbergen KC, de Vries LS, van Straaten HLM, et al. Anticoagulation therapy and imaging in neonates with a unilateral thalamic hemorrhage due to cerebral sinovenous thrombosis. Stroke 2009;40:2754–60.
80. Einhaupl KM, Villringer A, Meister W, et al. Heparin treatment in sinus venous thrombosis. Lancet 1991;338:597–600.
81. de Bruijn SF, Stam J. Randomized, placebo-controlled trial of anticoagulant treatment with low-molecular-weight heparin for cerebral sinus thrombosis. Stroke 1999;30:484–8.
82. Stam J, de Bruijn SF, deVeber G. Anticoagulation for cerebral sinus thrombosis. Cochrane Database Syst Rev 2002;4:CD002005.
83. Bousser MG, Ross-Russell R. Cerebral venous thrombosis. In: Major J, editor. 1st edition, In: Problems in neurology, vol. 1. London: WB Saunders; 1997.
84. deVeber G, Chan A, Monagle P, et al. Anticoagulation therapy in pediatric patients with sinovenous thrombosis: a cohort study. Arch Neurol 1998;55:1533–7.
85. Royal College of Physicians Paediatric Stroke Working Group. Stroke in Childhood: clinical guidelines for diagnosis, management and rehabilitation. Royal College of Physicians, London, November, 2004. Available at: http://www.rcplondon.ac.uk/pubs/books/childstroke/childstroke_guidelines.pdf. Accessed March 10, 2010.
86. Roach ES, Golomb MR, Adams R, et al. Management of stroke in infants and children: a scientific statement from a Special Writing Group of the American Heart Association Stroke Council and the Council on Cardiovascular Disease in the Young. Stroke 2008;39:2644–91.
87. Monagle P, Chalmers E, Chan A, et al. Antithrombotic therapy in neonates and children: American College of Chest Physicians evidence-based clinical practice guidelines (8th edition). Chest 2008;133:887S–968S.
88. Griesemer DA, Theodorou AA, Berg RA, et al. Local fibrinolysis in cerebral venous thrombosis. Pediatr Neurol 1994;10:78–80.
89. Soleau SW, Schmidt R, Stevens S, et al. Extensive experience with dural sinus thrombosis. Neurosurgery 2003;52:534–44.
90. Liebetrau M, Mayer TE, Bruning R, et al. Intra-arterial thrombolysis of complete deep cerebral venous thrombosis. Neurology 2004;63:2444–5.
91. Chahlavi A, Steinmetz MP, Masaryk TJ, et al. A transcranial approach for direct mechanical thrombectomy of dural sinus thrombosis. Report of two cases. J Neurosurg 2004;101:347–51.
92. Stefini R, Latronico N, Cornali C, et al. Emergent decompressive craniectomy in patients with fixed dilated pupils due to cerebral venous and dural sinus thrombosis: report of three cases. Neurosurgery 1999;45:626–9.
93. Keller E, Pangalu A, Fandino J, et al. Decompressive craniectomy in severe cerebral venous and

dural sinus thrombosis. Acta Neurochir Suppl 2005;94:177–83.
94. Ciccone A, Canhao P, Falcao F, et al. Thrombolysis for cerebral vein and dural sinus thrombosis. Cochrane Database Syst Rev 2004;1:CD003693.
95. Wasay M, Bakshi R, Kojan S, et al. Nonrandomized comparison of local urokinase thrombolysis versus systemic heparin anticoagulation for superior sagittal sinus thrombosis. Stroke 2001;32:2310–7.
96. Canhao P, Ferro JM, Lindgren AG, et al. Causes and predictors of death in cerebral venous thrombosis. Stroke 2005;36:1720–5.
97. Petzold A, Smith M. High intracranial pressure, brain herniation and death in cerebral venous thrombosis. Stroke 2006;37:331–2.
98. Hetherington R, Tuff L, Anderson P, et al. Short-term intellectual outcome after arterial ischemic stroke and sinovenous thrombosis in childhood and infancy. J Child Neurol 2005;20:553–9.
99. De Schryver EL, Blom I, Braun KP, et al. Long-term prognosis of cerebral venous sinus thrombosis in childhood. Dev Med Child Neurol 2004;46:514–9.
100. deVeber GA, MacGregor D, Curtis R, et al. Neurologic outcome in survivors of childhood arterial ischemic stroke and sinovenous thrombosis. J Child Neurol 2000;15:316–24.
101. Koitschev A, Simon C, Lowenheim H, et al. Delayed otogenic hydrocephalus after acute otitis media in pediatric patients: the changing presentation of a serious otologic complication. Acta Otolaryngol 2005;125:1230–5.
102. Standridge SM, O'Brien SH. Idiopathic intracranial hypertension in a pediatric population: a retrospective analysis of the initial imaging evaluation. J Child Neurol 2008;23:1308–11.
103. Panicker JN, Vinayan KP, Ahsan Moosa NV, et al. Juvenile Behcet's disease: highlighting neuropsychiatric manifestations and putative genetic mechanisms. Clin Neurol Neurosurg 2007;109:436–8.

Traumatic Intracranial and Extracranial Vascular Injuries in Children

Roukoz B. Chamoun, MD, Andrew Jea, MD*

KEYWORDS

• Trauma • Carotid artery • Vertebral artery • Dissection

TRAUMATIC INJURIES OF THE CAROTID ARTERY

Extracranial Carotid Injuries

The incidence of carotid artery dissection (CAD) in adults after blunt head and neck injury is estimated at 0.3 to 0.67%.[1–5] In children, this injury seems to be significantly less common (estimated at 0.03%).[6] However, because CAD can be clinically silent, its frequency may be underestimated. The traumatic event is usually that of hyperextension/rotation injury or a direct blow to the neck.

Extracranial CAD represents the most common location of traumatic vascular dissections in the head and neck area and is followed in frequency by the extracranial vertebral artery.[7] Arterial dissection has been associated with several conditions including fibromuscular dysplasia, Marfan syndrome, cystic medial necrosis, oral contraceptives, and drug abuse.[8] In connective tissue disease there is a structural defect leading to weakness in the arterial wall and predisposing to dissection either spontaneously or after a minor trauma. In other cases, environmental factors such as drug abuse can cause endothelial damage predisposing to this condition. On the other hand, traumatic dissection is also known to occur in otherwise healthy patients with no known risk factors.

CAD can be asymptomatic, especially in patients younger than 18 years of age. The dissection may remain in a subadventitial rather than subintimal plane, which may account for a delay in presentation[9]; a subadventitial dissection is believed to result in pseudoaneurysm with a potential for delayed presentation caused by emboli, whereas a subintimal one can lead to significant narrowing of the lumen with a more imminent clinical presentation (**Fig. 1**). A review of the literature showed that in most cases the diagnosis was suspected and then confirmed only after a focal neurologic deficit consistent with a stroke or transient ischemic attack (TIA) in the presence of a history of trauma.[10] Consequently, a high index of suspicion based on the mechanism of injury or physical signs and symptoms is of paramount importance to diagnose these lesions before the occurrence of severe neurologic deficit.

One mechanism of injury that deserves a special emphasis in children is soft palate traumatic injury. Pens and sticks are the most frequent traumatic agents and the mean age of occurrence is 4 years.[11] The proposed pathophysiology is related to an indirect compression of the internal carotid artery (ICA) against the skull base or against the upper cervical transverse process.[12] Although CAD is rare after such an injury, it is potentially associated with high mortality and morbidity. The initial symptoms are usually mild, such as minor and transient oral bleeding, small pharyngeal wound, and tenderness at the angle of the mandible. The neurologic symptoms typically appear after a silent period that can last from a few hours to several days.[13]

Division of Pediatric Neurosurgery, Department of Neurosurgery, Texas Children's Hospital, Baylor College of Medicine, CCC 1230.01, 12th Floor, Houston, TX 77030, USA
* Corresponding author.
E-mail address: ajea@bcm.edu

Neurosurg Clin N Am 21 (2010) 529–542
doi:10.1016/j.nec.2010.03.009
1042-3680/10/$ – see front matter

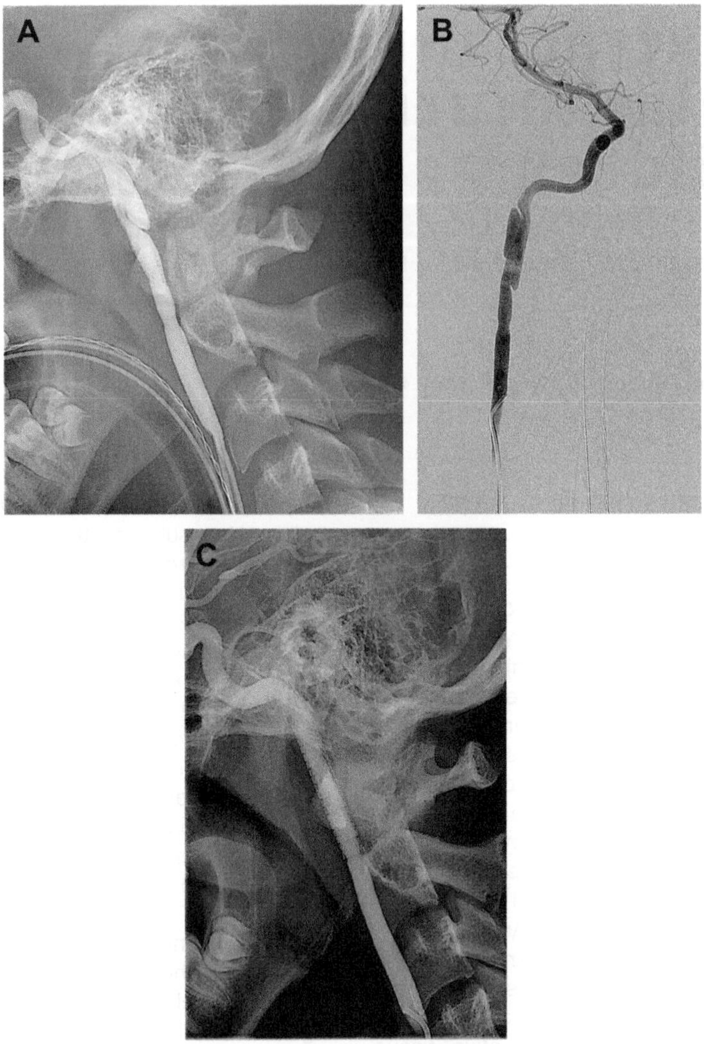

Fig. 1. 15-year-old boy with neck pain after football injury. (*A* and *B*) Lateral view of cerebral angiogram with (R) internal carotid injection shows a traumatic dissection with pseudoaneurysm of the extracranial ICA. (*C*) Lateral view of cerebral angiogram with (R) internal carotid injection at 6 months after endovascular treatment of the dissection using stent shows intimal healing and endothelialization.

Intracranial Carotid Injuries

Although intracranial location is rare among CAD in adults,[14,15] it seems to be common in children. In their review of the literature, Fullerton and colleagues[16] found that 60% of the reported cases of CAD were intracranial. A male predominance seems to be attributable to a higher incidence of trauma among young males. Similarly, Oka and colleagues[17] found that 25 of 45 patients who presented with intracranial carotid dissection were 18 years of age or younger. Although subarachnoid hemorrhage (SAH) is a real concern in these cases, strokes and TIAs remain the most common presenting feature.

Intracranial ICA dissection in children most commonly occurs spontaneously without any history of trauma. Among all reported cases of pediatric ICA dissection, the likelihood of intracranial dissection seems to be inversely proportional to the severity of trauma reported. Following severe trauma, 25% of the reported ICA dissections were intracranial, compared with 58% in the case of mild trauma, and 86% when no history of trauma is given.[16] This observation favors a traumatic cause in extracranial dissections and a spontaneous cause in the intracranial ones (possibly precipitated by a minor trauma). A predisposing risk factor (collagen vascular diseases, connective tissue disorders, use of oral contraceptives, smoking, hypertension, and migraine) was reported in several cases; however, in most cases the cause remains unknown. Overall, the mortality seems to be significantly higher in intracranial dissections compared with extracranial ones.[16]

Traumatic intracranial aneurysms are rare, comprising less than 1% of intracranial aneurysms in most large series.[18,19] Histologically, they can be true aneurysms (disruption of intima and media, with an intact adventia) or false aneurysms (disruption of all 3 layers with formation of a contained hematoma). False aneurysms are considered the most common, although the relative incidence of these histologic types is unknown.[20] Traumatic intracranial aneurysms in children are best categorized by mechanism of injury and location (**Table 1**).[21] Traumatic aneurysms can be caused by penetrating or nonpenetrating trauma. Aneurysms secondary to nonpenetrating trauma can be divided further into skull base and peripheral lesions. Peripheral traumatic aneurysms can again be divided into aneurysms of the distal anterior cerebral artery (ACA) secondary to trauma against the falcine edge (**Fig. 2**), distal posterior cerebral artery secondary to trauma against the tentorial edge, and distal cortical artery aneurysms frequently associated with an overlying skull fracture (**Fig. 3**). At the base of the skull, traumatic aneurysms most commonly involve the petrous and cavernous carotid artery and are almost invariably associated with a skull base fracture.[22,23] Injury to the ICA at the skull base can cause immediate rupture, leading to a carotid-cavernous fistula or to massive epistaxis.[24] Maurer and colleagues[25] stated that the triad of unilateral blindness, basal skull fracture, and recurrent severe epistaxis is diagnostic of ICA injury at the skull base.

Traumatic carotid-cavernous fistula (TCCF) is another rare entity that can occur after head injury. The estimated incidence ranges between 0.1 and 1%.[26,27] In a recent study, a skull base fracture was documented in 67% of the cases, and among 312 patients with a fracture at the skull base, TCCF was found in 3.4%.[28] TCCF most commonly results from a direct connection between the carotid artery and the cavernous sinus, leading to high-flow fistula. These lesions are unlikely to regress spontaneously and require prompt diagnosis and management. Clinically, these patients most commonly present with exophthalmos, bruit, chemosis, decreased vision, and limited ocular movements.

Table 1
Classification of traumatic intracranial aneurysms

Penetrating trauma
Nonpenetrating trauma
Skull base
Peripheral
Distal ACA: parafalcine
Distal cortical artery

TRAUMATIC INJURIES OF THE VERTEBRAL ARTERY

Extracranial Vertebral Injuries

Traumatic extracranial vertebral artery injuries may include dissections, pseudoaneurysms, or arteriovenous fistulas. Trauma remains the most common cause of dissection of the extracranial vertebral artery.[16] Other causes include mainly vasculopathy and connective tissue disease. In some cases the dissection can be spontaneous, with no history of trauma or predisposing factors identified. In accordance with the adult literature, the most common segment involved is at the mobile C1-C2 level.[29,30] The predilection for injury of this segment of vertebral artery has been observed in traumatic as well as in spontaneous cases. In most reported cases, vertebral dissections are preceded by a mild head or neck trauma.[31,32] Typically, there is a history of neck hyperextension with torsion.[33] When the dissection involves a segment below C2, an alternative mechanism must be sought because rotation between adjacent lower cervical vertebrae is minimal (**Fig. 4**). Typically, more severe trauma with cervical spine fractures is found in these cases.

Arteriovenous fistulas involving the vertebral artery are rare lesions, defined by the presence of an abnormal shunt between the extracranial vertebral artery or 1 of its muscular or radicular branches and the adjacent perivertebral venous plexus.[34,35] Approximately one-third of arteriovenous fistulas are asymptomatic,[36] discovered incidentally after auscultation of a neck bruit. However, these lesions can have ischemic symptoms of vertigo, diplopia, and cephalgia secondary to arterial steal. The presence of myelopathy or cervical neuralgia is rare but can result after arterial blood reflux into spinal pial veins, causing venous hypertension (Foix-Alajouanine syndrome) or after root compression by engorged epidural veins.[37] The main goal of treatment is closure of the arteriovenous fistula or pseudoaneurysm with preservation of the parent artery, frequently attained through an endovascular approach.[36]

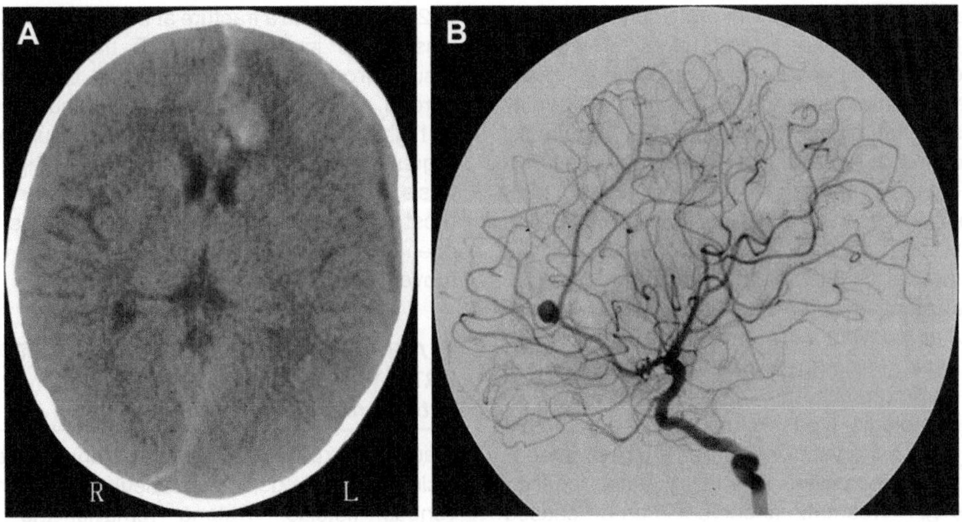

Fig. 2. A 7-year-old boy after a motor vehicle accident. (*A*) Axial CT scan of the brain without contrast shows evidence of interhemispheric subarachnoid and intraparenchymal hemorrhage. (*B*) Lateral view of cerebral angiogram with (L) internal carotid injection illustrates a traumatic distal ACA aneurysm.

The natural history of extracranial vertebral artery dissection in children remains poorly understood. Late complications in children include pseudoaneurysm formation, thrombosis, and recurrent stroke.[38] Stroke can result either from thrombosis leading to critical narrowing of the vessel or from emboli. The dynamic processes involved with vascular injury and healing may span years and result in variable outcomes. Because of the unpredictable evolution of these vascular changes, long-term clinical and radiologic follow-up are warranted.

Intracranial Vertebral Injuries

Intracranial dissection constitutes around 11% of reported vertebral artery injuries in children.[39] Unlike intracranial carotid dissections, trauma remains the most common cause in intracranial vertebral dissections.[16,40] Intracranial vertebral

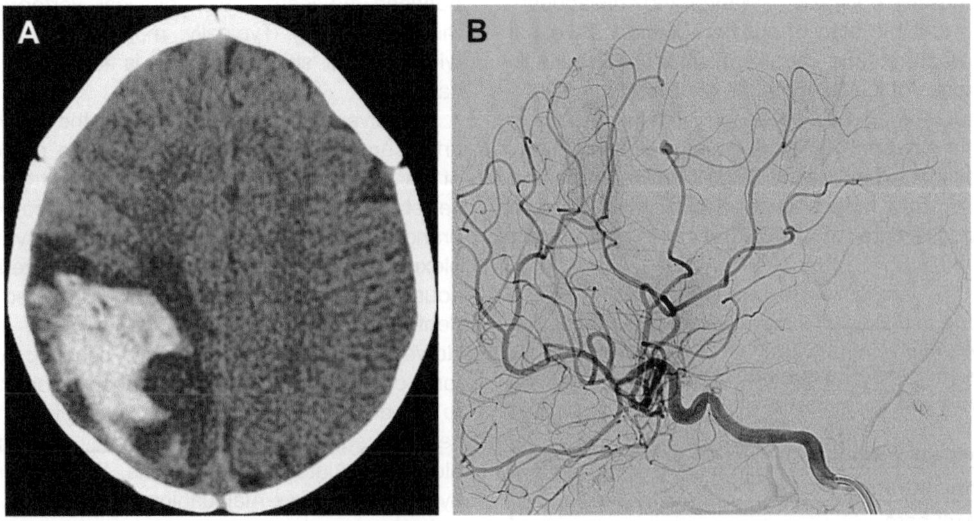

Fig. 3. A 3-month-old baby in a suspected case of nonaccidental trauma. (*A*) Axial CT of the brain without contrast shows large (R) intraparenchymal hemorrhage. (*B*) Lateral view of cerebral angiogram with (R) internal carotid injection illustrates a traumatic aneurysm of a distal cortical branch of the middle cerebral artery. Although distal cortical aneurysms are frequently associated with skull fractures, no fracture was identified in this case.

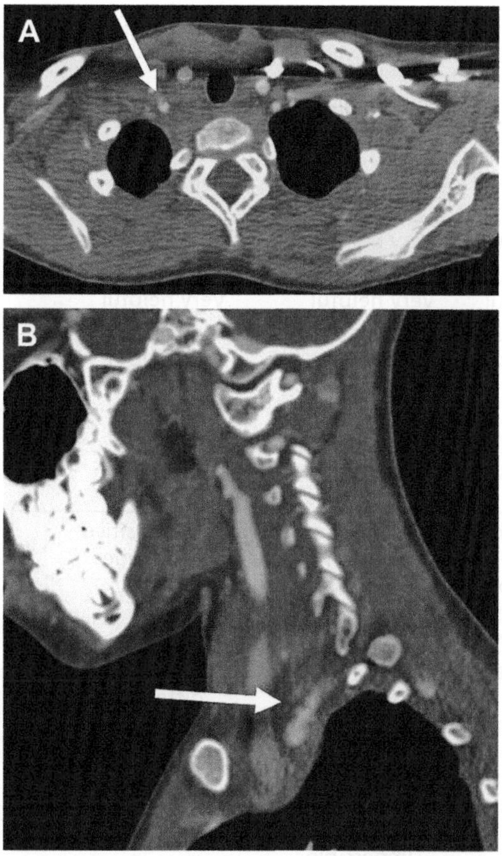

Fig. 4. A 9-year-old boy after whiplash injury from a motor vehicle accident. (*A*) Axial and (*B*) sagittal CTA shows a dissection and intimal flap (*arrow*) of the proximal part of the right extracranial vertebral artery.

artery dissections also differ from extracranial dissections, which are usually associated with strokes, as mentioned earlier.[41] Their prognosis is worse than extracranial dissections. Intracranial vertebral artery dissections are more susceptible to rupture than the extracranial segment, because the intracranial vertebral artery has thinner adventitia, and few elastic fibers in the media.[42] SAH is commonly reported in these cases with a high risk of rebleed (in up to 30%–70% of cases in some series), resulting in high mortality and morbidity.[43] Rare cases of nonaccidental trauma resulting in intracranial vertebral artery injury have been reported.[44] The presence of retinal hemorrhage in these cases should be interpreted with caution as it can be simply the consequence of SAH (Terson syndrome).

Patients with vertebral artery dissections usually have a lucid interval after trauma until they present with symptoms.[45,46] Ipsilateral headache, neck pain, dizziness, and neurologic deficits are the most common symptoms of vertebral artery dissections.[47] Patients who develop neurologic deficit may have speech deficits, dysphagia, and vision defects.

DIAGNOSTIC MODALITIES

Cerebral angiography remains the gold standard diagnostic modality (**Table 2**). It is currently the most accurate modality and provides fine detail of vascular anatomy and intimal injury near bony structures such as the skull base or the transverse foramen for the vertebral artery.[48] One of the major advantages of angiography is the ability to detect collateral circulation, which is critical when dealing with a dissected or occluded vessel. Furthermore, three-dimensional reconstructed images enable circumferential spatial evaluation of the vessel and estimation of flow compromise. However, because of its invasive nature and associated risk of iatrogenic injuries, it is advisable to reserve formal angiography for confirmation of findings detected on a screening diagnostic examination.

Magnetic resonance angiography (MRA) offers a high-resolution noninvasive approach for diagnosis and follow-up of traumatic vascular injuries. It is helpful in visualization of the arterial wall and detection of intramural hematoma.[49] However, the accuracy of MRA is limited in detecting small intimal injuries (<25% luminal stenosis) and early pseudoaneurysm formation.[50] MRA is less suited for acute unstable trauma patient, and because of logistical difficulties with access for critically ill patients. In a prospective comparative study by Biffl and colleagues[51] of trauma patients, the sensitivity and specificity of MRA for the diagnosis of cerebrovascular injuries were 75% and 67%, respectively. In a similar study by Miller and colleagues[52] the sensitivity of MRA was 50% in carotid injuries and 47% in vertebral injuries. However, the sensitivity of MR imaging/MRA is highest 2 days after dissections. The resolution of MRA now approaches that of conventional angiography. MR imaging can show not only vessel occlusion, but its effect on the brain. It is also noninvasive and should become the investigation of choice for patients in whom blunt cervical vascular trauma is clinically suspected.[53]

Because computed tomography (CT) is noninvasive and widely available, CT angiography (CTA) has been used for the screening and diagnosis of traumatic vascular injuries. Early studies using old generation scanners have been disappointing, suggesting a high rate of false-negative and false-positive results.[51,52,54] The main disadvantage of CTA is related to bony artifact limiting its ability to identify injuries in some areas such as carotid canal or transverse foramina. However, current generation 16-detector scanners are

Table 2
Diagnostic modalities in case of carotid and vertebral artery injury

	Doppler Ultrasound	CTA	MR Imaging/MRA	Angiography
Information				
Flow interruption	Very helpful	Very helpful	Very helpful	Sometimes helpful
Thrombus versus spasm	Very helpful	Very helpful	Very helpful	Very helpful
Thrombus extension	Useless	Very helpful	Very helpful	Very helpful
Permeability of circle of Willis	Sometimes helpful (transcranial Doppler)	Very helpful	Very helpful	Very helpful
Cerebral ischemia	Useless	Sometimes helpful	Very helpful	Useless
Advantages	Noninvasive, easy to obtain, and readily available	Rapid, high spatial resolution, usually easy to obtain	Noninvasive; no adverse effect with contrast	Most sensitive technique
Disadvantages	No visualization of intracranial vessels. Limited use for the vertebral	Risks resulting from intravenous injection of iodinated contrast; irradiation; sedation required in patients <2 years old	Sedation usually required in patients less than 5 years old; not easy to obtain; impossible in case of metallic foreign body	Invasive; may not differentiate between dissection and vasospasm; irradiation

Data from Pierrot S, Bernardeschi D, Morrisseau-Durand MP, et al. Dissection of the internal carotid artery following trauma of the soft palate in children. Ann Otol Rhinol Laryngol 2006;115:323–9.

capable of rendering high-resolution images along with high-speed data acquisition. In a recent large study, the accuracy of new generation CTA in diagnosing and excluding blunt carotid or vertebral artery injuries was evaluated by comparing it with angiography. Dissections as well as pseudoaneurysms were included in this study. The overall sensitivity, specificity, and positive and negative predictive values of CTA were 74%, 86%, 65%, and 90%, respectively; no significant difference was found between carotid and vertebral artery injuries.[55]

Doppler ultrasonography is able to provide high-resolution real-time images of the carotid artery bifurcation and proximal ICA. It has proved reliable in evaluating the presence and severity of atherosclerotic disease. Ultrasonography is also a noninvasive and widely available test. However, its role in the diagnosis of traumatic vascular injuries is hampered by several limitations. For obvious reasons related to surrounding bony structures, this modality is unable to assess intracranial injuries or high cervical vascular lesions close to the skull base. Furthermore, most of the extracranial vertebral artery cannot be assessed for the same reason. Small series reporting the use of Doppler ultrasonography have been published.[56–58] The diagnostic accuracy for identification of a vascular injury was found to be around 86% for the cervical carotid[59] and 79% for vertebral artery.[60] This modality is suboptimal for the screening and diagnosis of traumatic vascular injuries, but may have a role in the follow-up of known traumatic cervical lesions of carotid and vertebral vessels.

MANAGEMENT OPTIONS

Choosing a treatment option represents a significant challenge for the clinician in traumatic cerebrovascular injuries in children because of the lack of high-quality clinical data comparing 1 modality with another, and the absence of a clear consensus. As a result, decisions are largely based on individualized, single-center experience supported by data from case reports and small case series. The individual application of these modalities may also be extrapolated from adult experience, but the unique features of children need to be recalled (eg, the safety profile of full anticoagulation in active toddlers).

In general, penetrating trauma is more likely to require surgical repair for control of bleeding than is the case with blunt injury, although endovascular occlusion may be used. Blunt trauma is most often managed by medical therapy or endovascular approaches.[61]

Extracranial Carotid Artery Injury

Medical therapy is based on the premise that most neurologic events are related to thrombus within the lumen and are potentially preventable with anticoagulation or antiplatelet drugs (**Fig. 5**).[62–64] Imaging studies suggest that more than 90% of infarcts caused by dissection are thrombotic rather than hemodynamic in origin.[62,63] Transcranial Doppler studies show a high frequency of intracranial microemboli.[64]

Antithrombotic therapy has been advocated since the 1970s.[65] However, there were no randomized trials to assess the effects of antithrombotic therapy or surgical treatment. As no reliable data from randomized trials were available, it is not possible to draw any definite conclusions.[66,67] Reported nonrandomized studies have, likewise, not shown evidence of a significant difference between anticoagulant and antiplatelet agents.

Based on some open-label studies and anecdotal experience, several investigators favor anticoagulation with heparin followed by coumadin therapy as a reasonable approach in symptomatic CADs.[68,69] Treatment with coumadin for 6 months

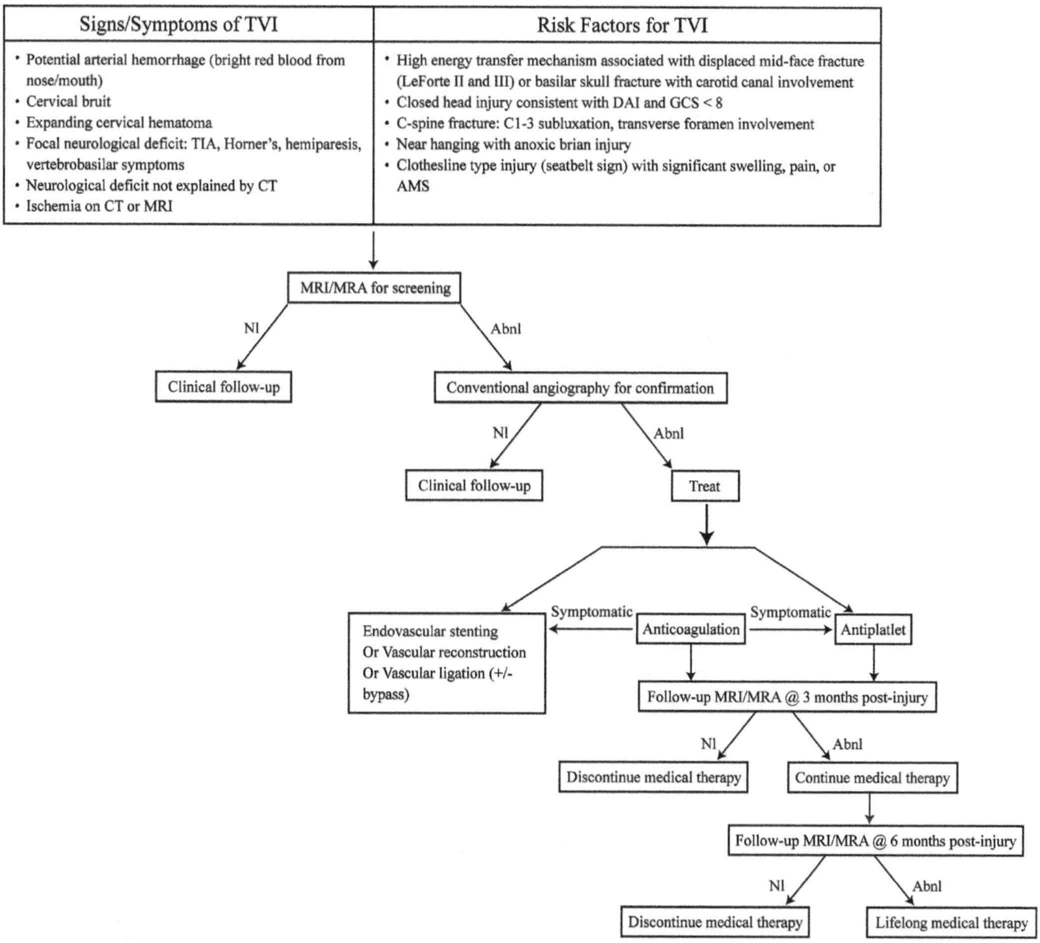

Fig. 5. An approach to the diagnosis and treatment of extracranial carotid and vertebral artery injuries. AMS, altered mental status; TVI, traumatic vascular injuries.

to 1 year has traditionally been advocated with a target international normalized ratio of 2 to 3.[63,70] In a study of the treatment of a blunt carotid artery injury, anticoagulation was suggested to be the treatment of choice when dissection or pseudoaneurym was diagnosed.[71] There are no data from controlled studies on the safety of heparin, although several consecutive series showed no significant side effects.[72,73]

Caution should be exercised when anticoagulant agents are used in patients who have concurrent intracranial dissections, because of the risk of SAH and a worsening of deficits after early anticoagulation.[74] The fear that anticoagulation or tissue-plasminogen activator therapy will extend the dissection seems to be unfounded.[14,75]

Antiplatelet agents have been used in the management of dissection, but there is less information about their efficacy.[76] If anticoagulation is contraindicated, many investigators recommend antiplatelet therapy.[63]

In studies comparing antiplatelet and anticoagulation treatment, there were no statistically significant differences in primary outcome measures. In a 1-year follow-up study, patients who were treated with aspirin had higher event rates (TIAs, stroke, or death) compared with patients treated with anticoagulants (12.4% compared with 8.3%)[66]; however, this was statistically not significant. Therefore, it cannot be concluded that antiplatelet therapy is less effective than anticoagulation therapy in preventing stroke occurrences and recurrence in patients with extracranial CAD.[67]

Antithrombotic therapy is recommended as initial medical treatment in extracranial carotid dissection. Antiplatelet therapy with its safer pharmacologic profile for children in terms of administration, maintenance, and complications may be favored over anticoagulation (see **Fig. 5**).[10]

Surgical intervention for carotid dissection is reserved for patients with recurrent TIAs or progressive neurologic deficits secondary to hypoperfusion or embolic phenomenon despite maximal medical therapy. Eligibility for surgery is determined by the patient's clinical status as well as the duration of the occlusion as suggested by imaging criteria. In general, patients are excluded who have severe fixed deficits after a completed stroke or TIA for an extended period with a chronic occlusion. Those patients with recent onset of multiple TIAs, transient monocular blindness, and acute occlusion may benefit from endarterectomy and thrombectomy or carotid ligation.[77]

One review indicated that the presence of a large or expanding pseudoaneurysm is also an indication for surgical intervention.[78] Chronic carotid dissections have also been treated with surgical reconstruction to prevent further ischemic or thromboembolic complications, if medical treatment with 6-month anticoagulation fails or if carotid aneurysms and/or high-grade stenosis persist.[79]

In most cases, endovascular treatment has supplanted open surgery as the initial treatment of choice once medical therapy fails in adults.[80,81] Endovascular stenting for carotid atherosclerotic disease was not in use before 1989; studies published before 1989 may not have reflected endovascular stenting as an available treatment option for carotid dissection. The decreased tortuosity of pediatric vessels makes stent placement feasible in the extracranial carotid artery.[82] Nonetheless, the long-term results and effects of carotid stenting in children are unknown (eg, poststenting restenosis), and the treatment of stent-related complications can be complex.[83]

Extracranial Vertebral Artery Injury

The natural history of vertebral artery dissection is unknown (see **Fig. 5**). It can heal spontaneously, develop occlusion, or form a pseudoaneurysm. Like extracranial carotid dissection, treatment of extracranial vertebral artery dissection is controversial; it is not clear whether patients must be heparinized, be treated with antiplatelets, or treated at all. Hasan and colleagues[39] in their review of 68 children found that the most common treatment of extracranial vertebral artery dissection was antiplatelet therapy. These investigators found that asymptomatic recovery occurred in 12 of 15 (80%) children who received antiplatelet therapy compared with 4 of 15 (27%) patients who received anticoagulation therapy with or without antiplatelet therapy. Once thrombus occurs, it is also controversial whether anticoagulation or antiplatelet therapy should be the treatment of choice. Beletsky and colleagues[66] showed that the recurrence rate for embolization is decreased significantly in patients on anticoagulation compared with those on antiplatelets (8.3% vs 12.4%). The difference in outcome at 1 year was not significantly different, however. It is therefore prudent to consider prophylactic treatment with antithrombotic therapy (unless contraindicated) because the consequence of brainstem ischemia is so poor.

Attempts at primary repair of an injured extracranial vertebral artery are rarely successful. Because of its location deep within the posterior triangle of the neck, the vertebral artery is difficult to approach surgically. Osteotomy of the middle portion of the transverse process may be required. Furthermore, craniotomy may be necessary for exposure of the distal portion.[84]

Open surgical ligation or endovascular occlusion (via balloon occlusion or coil embolization) of an injured artery with progressive dissection, pseudoaneurysm, arteriovenous fistula, or thromboembolic events despite antithrombotic therapy is frequently the procedure of choice. Only 10% of cerebral blood flow is from the vertebrobasilar system. A hypoplastic left vertebral artery occurs in 3.1% of individuals; on the right, 1.8% are hypoplastic. Thus, the risk of neurologic deficit from unilateral ligation is small.[85] Controversy persists in the literature as to whether proximal ligation alone is adequate; some believe that proximal and distal ligation must be done to avert distal thrombus propagation. Most agree that the risk of this complication is reduced by prophylactic heparinization in the acute phase for any patient who has undergone vertebral artery ligation.[86]

The surgical and endovascular procedures described earlier involve the occlusion of the arterial lumen, which is the main disadvantage of these methods. For the patients whose contralateral vertebral artery is hypoplastic, it is often impossible to perform an arterial occlusion because of lack of an adequate intracranial collateral circulation and consequent ischemia.[87] In these cases, the use of a stent graft placed by endovascular means may halt progressive dissection, seal a pseudoaneurysm, or occlude an arteriovenous fistula, yet preserving the parent artery.[88]

In the very young pediatric population, the femoral artery can accommodate only a 4-French catheter system. Placement of a stent, which typically requires larger guide catheters, may not be an option in this population. Moreover, stent placement is associated with a risk of thrombosis that increases significantly with decreasing arterial diameter; for this reason, stents are rarely, if ever, placed when the patient is younger than 1 year of age.[40]

Intracranial Carotid Artery Injury

Dissecting aneurysm

The goal of treatment is to exclude an intracranial dissecting aneurysm from the circulation by surgical or endovascular methods. In 1975, Fleischer and colleagues[89] reported 41% mortality in patients treated conservatively compared with 18% mortality in surgically treated patients. Other investigators also described poor outcome in conservatively treated pediatric patients.[21] Given its poor natural history, aggressive surgical management with clipping, resection, or trapping of intracranial dissecting aneurysms of the carotid artery and its branches seems the most appropriate treatment.[21,90–94]

Endovascular techniques such as trapping, in which detachable balloons or embolization with detachable coils are used, have also been performed in the treatment of traumatic aneurysms.[21,95] The advantages of surgical clipping include the ability to isolate the aneurysm with the opportunity to reconstruct the parent artery, and allowing the opportunity to evacuate the associated intracranial hematoma.[20] On the other hand, endovascular therapy avoids prolonged anesthesia, eliminates retraction of an inflamed and irritated brain, and allows diagnostic angiography to be performed throughout the case.[96]

Carotid-cavernous fistula

Rupture of a large or giant aneurysm of the intracavernous carotid artery can result in sudden and massive epistaxis, requiring emergent packing of the nose as a life-saving measure. Parkinson first proposed a direct surgical repair of intracavernous aneurysms with preservation of the carotid artery by a transcavernous approach, but the morbidity was high from multiple cranial nerve dysfunction, and it subsequently fell out of favor.[97]

Contemporary management of carotid-cavernous fistula is nearly always accomplished by endovascular techniques.[98–100] An endovascular approach to these lesions is attractive in that the procedure can usually be performed using local anesthesia in older children and adolescents. Test occlusion and antiaggregant medication for at least 3 months are recommended to avoid secondary thromboembolic complications.[101] Balloon test occlusion, however, is often not technically feasible in children. Few data are available in children regarding the correlation of collateral artery caliber and the tolerance to cerebral circulation occlusion.[40]

Occlusion

Management of traumatic intracranial carotid artery occlusion is problematic, with death or severe neurologic deficit resulting in up to 85% of patients.[101] Steroids, revascularization, and anticoagulation have all been tried with limited success. Control of intracranial pressure (ICP) is essential in patients in whom distal ischemia and infarction can be expected to incite cerebral swelling, but maintenance of blood pressure and even hypervolemia are most effective in limiting the neurologic deficit and extent of infarction from thrombotic vascular occlusion.[101]

Vasospasm

Although rarely symptomatic in children, treatment of traumatic vasospasm when it does become symptomatic remains problematic. Blood pressure support with the goal of normotension, establishment of normovolemia, and surveillance with transcranial Doppler ultrasound may be reasonable first steps in treating symptomatic traumatic vasospasm. The standard prophylactic course of artificially maintained hypertension, hypervolemia, and hemodilution used in vasospasm following aneurysm rupture and SAH may be counterproductive in patients whose injury is often complicated by cerebral edema, increased ICP, and tenuous tissue perfusion. Calcium channel blockade with calcium antagonists may be a more benign regimen, and good results have been reported in vasospasm associated with aneurysm rupture.[102] However, calcium channel blockers have been shown to interfere with autoregulation, to undermine the integrity of the blood-brain barrier, and to increase the sodium content of cerebral edema fluid. Their indiscriminant use in the context of increased ICP from trauma or radiographic signs of brain swelling is, therefore, dangerous and not recommended until further information is available for children.[103]

Angioplasty has been proposed by Higashida and colleagues[104] for management of cerebral vasospasm secondary to aneurysmal bleeding. However, this technique has not been used in posttraumatic vasospasm in children, and its safety and efficacy in this background remain to be proved.[104] Endovascular infusion of vasodilatory medications such as papaverine, or of calcium channel blockers such as verapamil, is also used in the treatment of vasospasm in adults. The safety and efficacy of this treatment in children is unknown.

Intracranial Vertebral Artery Injury

Traumatic dissections isolated to the intracranial vertebral artery approaching the vertebrobasilar junction are rare. At the level of the pontomedullary sulcus, the vertebrobasilar junction is tethered by thick trabeculae, the medial pontomedullary membrane, separating the premedullary and prepontine cisterns. The tethered vertebrobasilar junction may therefore represent another intracranial site prone to motion-induced arterial injury.

For intracranial dissections presenting with ischemia, spontaneous healing is regularly observed, and therefore anticoagulation or antiplatelet therapy with close follow-up suffice in most cases. On the other hand, dissecting aneurysms presenting with SAH portend a high risk of rehemorrhage (30%–70% in adults and unknown in children[88,105]).

The most definitive treatment of arterial dissection involves excluding the aneurysm and the injured segment of the parent vessel from the circulation, using either surgical or endovascular trapping procedures. When only the aneurysm sac is obliterated, the associated injured parent vessel segment remains vulnerable to rerupture, particularly in the acute phase. Combined occlusion of the aneurysm and the parent vessel is not feasible in every case, and the treatment plan must be formulated case by case.[40]

Introduction of a microcatheter and placement of coils into the friable aneurysm sac may be associated with a high risk of intraprocedural perforation. In addition, packing coils against the pseudoaneurysm wall, composed largely of fibrin, thrombus, and collagen, may be associated with a high risk of delayed recanalization.[40]

SUMMARY

Traumatic vascular injuries are uncommon in children. The clinical experience with this entity is limited and there is a lack of clear recommendations regarding diagnosis and treatment practices. Because of the rarity of this condition in children, it is unlikely that recommendations based on high-level evidence will be available soon. With these limitations in mind, several points can be concluded:

1. These injuries are frequently missed, and a high index of suspicion needs to be maintained for diagnosis before the occurrence of severe neurologic deficits
2. The natural history of these injuries is unique and stratified on the type of vessel injured (carotid vs vertebral) and location of injury (extracranial vs intracranial)
3. Noninvasive screening with MRA or CTA for cases of high suspicion, reserving catheter angiography for definitive diagnosis
4. Use of antiplatelet therapy rather than anticoagulation in children as first-line medical therapy in asymptomatic extracranial vascular injury without pseudoaneurysm formation, because of lack of evidence in favor of the latter, and the safer pharmacologic profile of the former
5. Endovascular treatment seems safe and efficacious and preferred to open surgery in failed medical treatment of extracranial vascular injuries
6. Surgical and/or endovascular approaches represent primary treatment rather than medical therapy for intracranial vascular injuries.

REFERENCES

1. de Virgilio C, Mercado PD, Arnell T, et al. Noniatrogenic pediatric vascular trauma: a ten-year experience at a level I trauma center. Am Surg 1997;63:781–4.

2. Meagher DP Jr, Defore WW, Mattox KL, et al. Vascular trauma in infants and children. J Trauma 1979;19:532–6.
3. Klinkner DB, Arca MJ, Lewis BD, et al. Pediatric vascular injuries: patterns of injury, morbidity, and mortality. J Pediatr Surg 2007;42:178–82 [discussion: 182–3].
4. Fabian TC, Patton JH Jr, Croce MA, et al. Blunt carotid injury. Importance of early diagnosis and anticoagulant therapy. Ann Surg 1996;223:513–22 [discussion: 522–5].
5. Laitt RD, Lewis TT, Bradshaw JR. Blunt carotid arterial trauma. Clin Radiol 1996;51:117–22.
6. Lew SM, Frumiento C, Wald SL. Pediatric blunt carotid injury: a review of the National Pediatric Trauma Registry. Pediatr Neurosurg 1999;30:239–44.
7. Guillon B, Levy C, Bousser MG. Internal carotid artery dissection: an update. J Neurol Sci 1998; 153:146–58.
8. Klufas RA, Hsu L, Barnes PD, et al. Dissection of the carotid and vertebral arteries: imaging with MR angiography. AJR Am J Roentgenol 1995; 164:673–7.
9. Pozzati E, Giuliani G, Poppi M, et al. Blunt traumatic carotid dissection with delayed symptoms. Stroke 1989;20:412–6.
10. Chamoun RB, Mawad ME, Whitehead WE, et al. Extracranial traumatic carotid artery dissections in children: a review of current diagnosis and treatment options. J Neurosurg Pediatr 2008;2:101–8.
11. Hellmann JR, Shott SR, Gootee MJ. Impalement injuries of the palate in children: review of 131 cases. Int J Pediatr Otorhinolaryngol 1993;26:157–63.
12. Pitner SE. Carotid thrombosis due to intraoral trauma. An unusual complication of a common childhood accident. N Engl J Med 1966;274:764–7.
13. Pierrot S, Bernardeschi D, Morrisseau-Durand MP, et al. Dissection of the internal carotid artery following trauma of the soft palate in children. Ann Otol Rhinol Laryngol 2006;115:323–9.
14. Mokri B, Sundt TM Jr, Houser OW, et al. Spontaneous dissection of the cervical internal carotid artery. Ann Neurol 1986;19:126–38.
15. Treiman GS, Treiman RL, Foran RF, et al. Spontaneous dissection of the internal carotid artery: a nineteen-year clinical experience. J Vasc Surg 1996;24:597–605 [discussion: 605–7].
16. Fullerton HJ, Johnston SC, Smith WS. Arterial dissection and stroke in children. Neurology 2001;57:1155–60.
17. Oka F, Shimizu H, Matsumoto Y, et al. Ischemic stroke due to dissection of intracranial internal carotid artery: implications for early surgical treatment. Surg Neurol 2008;69:578–84 [discussion: 584–5].
18. Benoit BG, Wortzman G. Traumatic cerebral aneurysms. Clinical features and natural history. J Neurol Neurosurg Psychiatry 1973;36:127–38.
19. Laun A. Traumatic aneurysms. Berlin: Springer-Verlag; 1979.
20. Larson PS, Reisner A, Morassutti DJ, et al. Traumatic intracranial aneurysms. Neurosurg Focus 2000;8:e4.
21. Buckingham MJ, Crone KR, Ball WS, et al. Traumatic intracranial aneurysms in childhood: two cases and a review of the literature. Neurosurgery 1988;22:398–408.
22. Pozzati E, Gaist G, Servadei F. Traumatic aneurysms of the supraclinoid internal carotid artery. J Neurosurg 1982;57:418–22.
23. Yonas H, Dujovny M. "True" traumatic aneurysm of the intracranial internal carotid artery: case report. Neurosurgery 1980;7:499–502.
24. Hahn YS, Welling B, Reichman OH, et al. Traumatic intracavernous aneurysm in children: massive epistaxis without ophthalmic signs. Childs Nerv Syst 1990;6:360–4.
25. Maurer JJ, Mills M, German WJ. Triad of unilateral blindness, orbital fractures and massive epistaxis after head injury. J Neurosurg 1961;18:837–40.
26. Takenoshita Y, Hasuo K, Matsushima T, et al. Carotid-cavernous sinus fistula accompanying facial trauma. Report of a case with a review of the literature. J Craniomaxillofac Surg 1990;18:41–5.
27. Zachariades N, Papavassiliou D. Traumatic carotid-cavernous sinus fistula. J Craniomaxillofac Surg 1988;16:385–8.
28. Liang W, Xiaofeng Y, Weiguo L, et al. Traumatic carotid cavernous fistula accompanying basilar skull fracture: a study on the incidence of traumatic carotid cavernous fistula in the patients with basilar skull fracture and the prognostic analysis about traumatic carotid cavernous fistula. J Trauma 2007;63:1014–20 [discussion: 1020].
29. Greselle JF, Zenteno M, Kien P, et al. Spontaneous dissection of the vertebro-basilar system. A study of 18 cases (15 patients). J Neuroradiol 1987;14: 115–23.
30. Saver J, Easton J. Dissections and trauma of cervicocerebral arteries. Philadelphia: WB Saunders; 1998.
31. Hope EE, Bodensteiner JB, Barnes P. Cerebral infarction related to neck position in an adolescent. Pediatrics 1983;72:335–7.
32. Khurana DS, Bonnemann CG, Dooling EC, et al. Vertebral artery dissection: issues in diagnosis and management. Pediatr Neurol 1996;14:255–8.
33. Garg BP, Ottinger CJ, Smith RR, et al. Strokes in children due to vertebral artery trauma. Neurology 1993;43:2555–8.
34. Halbach VV, Higashida RT, Hieshima GB. Treatment of vertebral arteriovenous fistulas. AJR Am J Roentgenol 1988;150:405–12.
35. Nagashima C, Iwasaki T, Kawanuma S, et al. Traumatic arteriovenous fistula of the vertebral artery

with spinal cord symptoms. Case report. J Neurosurg 1977;46:681–7.
36. Beaujeux RL, Reizine DC, Casasco A, et al. Endovascular treatment of vertebral arteriovenous fistula. Radiology 1992;183:361–7.
37. Herrera DA, Vargas SA, Dublin AB. Endovascular treatment of traumatic injuries of the vertebral artery. AJNR Am J Neuroradiol 2008;29:1585–9.
38. Tan MA, Armstrong D, MacGregor DL, et al. Late complications of vertebral artery dissection in children: pseudoaneurysm, thrombosis, and recurrent stroke. J Child Neurol 2009;24:354–60.
39. Hasan I, Wapnick S, Tenner MS, et al. Vertebral artery dissection in children: a comprehensive review. Pediatr Neurosurg 2002;37:168–77.
40. Wang H, Orbach DB. Traumatic dissecting aneurysm at the vertebrobasilar junction in a 3-month-old infant: evaluation and treatment strategies. Case report. J Neurosurg Pediatr 2008;1:415–9.
41. Malek AM, Halbach VV, Phatouros CC, et al. Endovascular treatment of a ruptured intracranial dissecting vertebral aneurysm in a kickboxer. J Trauma 2000;48:143–5.
42. Shin JH, Suh DC, Choi CG, et al. Vertebral artery dissection: spectrum of imaging findings with emphasis on angiography and correlation with clinical presentation. Radiographics 2000;20:1687–96.
43. Peluso JP, van Rooij WJ, Sluzewski M, et al. Endovascular treatment of symptomatic intradural vertebral dissecting aneurysms. AJNR Am J Neuroradiol 2008;29:102–6.
44. Nguyen PH, Burrowes DM, Ali S, et al. Intracranial vertebral artery dissection with subarachnoid hemorrhage following child abuse. Pediatr Radiol 2007;37:600–2.
45. McCrory P. Vertebral artery dissection causing stroke in sport. J Clin Neurosci 2000;7:298–300.
46. Parbhoo AH, Govender S, Corr P. Vertebral artery injury in cervical spine trauma. Injury 2001;32:565–8.
47. Nadgir RN, Loevner LA, Ahmed T, et al. Simultaneous bilateral internal carotid and vertebral artery dissection following chiropractic manipulation: case report and review of the literature. Neuroradiology 2003;45:311–4.
48. Hoit DA, Schirmer CM, Weller SJ, et al. Angiographic detection of carotid and vertebral arterial injury in the high-energy blunt trauma patient. J Spinal Disord Tech 2008;21:259–66.
49. Oelerich M, Stogbauer F, Kurlemann G, et al. Craniocervical artery dissection: MR imaging and MR angiographic findings. Eur Radiol 1999;9:1385–91.
50. Biffl WL, Moore EE, Offner PJ, et al. Blunt carotid and vertebral arterial injuries. World J Surg 2001;25:1036–43.
51. Biffl WL, Ray CE Jr, Moore EE, et al. Noninvasive diagnosis of blunt cerebrovascular injuries: a preliminary report. J Trauma 2002;53:850–6.
52. Miller PR, Fabian TC, Croce MA, et al. Prospective screening for blunt cerebrovascular injuries: analysis of diagnostic modalities and outcomes. Ann Surg 2002;236:386–93 [discussion: 393–5].
53. Bok AP, Peter JC. Carotid and vertebral artery occlusion after blunt cervical injury: the role of MR angiography in early diagnosis. J Trauma 1996;40:968–72.
54. Schneidereit NP, Simons R, Nicolaou S, et al. Utility of screening for blunt vascular neck injuries with computed tomographic angiography. J Trauma 2006;60:209–15 [discussion: 215–6].
55. Malhotra AK, Camacho M, Ivatury RR, et al. Computed tomographic angiography for the diagnosis of blunt carotid/vertebral artery injury: a note of caution. Ann Surg 2007;246:632–42 [discussion: 642–3].
56. Davis JW, Holbrook TL, Hoyt DB, et al. Blunt carotid artery dissection: incidence, associated injuries, screening, and treatment. J Trauma 1990;30:1514–7.
57. Fry WR, Dort JA, Smith RS, et al. Duplex scanning replaces arteriography and operative exploration in the diagnosis of potential cervical vascular injury. Am J Surg 1994;168:693–5 [discussion: 695–6].
58. Martin RF, Eldrup-Jorgensen J, Clark DE, et al. Blunt trauma to the carotid arteries. J Vasc Surg 1991;14:789–93 [discussion: 793–5].
59. Cogbill TH, Moore EE, Meissner M, et al. The spectrum of blunt injury to the carotid artery: a multicenter perspective. J Trauma 1994;37:473–9.
60. Sturzenegger M, Mattle HP, Rivoir A, et al. Ultrasound findings in spontaneous extracranial vertebral artery dissection. Stroke 1993;24:1910–21.
61. Partington MD. Traumatic vascular injuries. In: Albright AL, Adelson PD, Pollack IF, editors. Principles and practice of pediatric neurosurgery. 2nd edition. New York: Thieme; 2008. p. 828–32.
62. Lucas C, Moulin T, Deplanque D, et al. Stroke patterns of internal carotid artery dissection in 40 patients. Stroke 1998;29:2646–8.
63. Schievink WI. Spontaneous dissection of the carotid and vertebral arteries. N Engl J Med 2001;344:898–906.
64. Srinivasan J, Newell DW, Sturzenegger M, et al. Transcranial Doppler in the evaluation of internal carotid artery dissection. Stroke 1996;27:1226–30.
65. Fisher CM, Ojemann RG, Roberson GH. Spontaneous dissection of cervico-cerebral arteries. Can J Neurol Sci 1978;5:9–19.
66. Beletsky V, Nadareishvili Z, Lynch J, et al. Cervical arterial dissection: time for a therapeutic trial? Stroke 2003;34:2856–60.
67. Lyrer P, Engelter S. Antithrombotic drugs for carotid artery dissection. Cochrane Database Syst Rev 2003;3:CD000255.

68. Selim M, Caplan LR. Carotid artery dissection. Curr Treat Options Cardiovasc Med 2004;6:249–53.
69. Stapf C, Elkind MS, Mohr JP. Carotid artery dissection. Annu Rev Med 2000;51:329–47.
70. Leys D, Lucas C, Gobert M, et al. Cervical artery dissections. Eur Neurol 1997;37:3–12.
71. Singh RR, Barry MC, Ireland A, et al. Current diagnosis and management of blunt internal carotid artery injury. Eur J Vasc Endovasc Surg 2004;27: 577–84.
72. Desfontaines P, Despland PA. Dissection of the internal carotid artery: aetiology, symptomatology, clinical and neurosonological follow-up, and treatment in 60 consecutive cases. Acta Neurol Belg 1995;95:226–34.
73. Sturzenegger M, Mattle HP, Rivoir A, et al. Ultrasound findings in carotid artery dissection: analysis of 43 patients. Neurology 1995;45:691–8.
74. Gomez CR, May AK, Terry JB, et al. Endovascular therapy of traumatic injuries of the extracranial cerebral arteries. Crit Care Clin 1999;15: 789–809.
75. Derex L, Nighoghossian N, Turjman F, et al. Intravenous tPA in acute ischemic stroke related to internal carotid artery dissection. Neurology 2000; 54:2159–61.
76. Shintani S, Shiigai T, Tsuruoka S, et al. TIAs in a spontaneously dissecting aneurysm of the internal carotid artery–a case report. Angiology 1992;43:621–4.
77. Heros R. Acute carotid occlusion. Toronto: BC Decker; 1989.
78. Adkins AL, Zelenock GB, Bendick PJ, et al. Duplex ultrasound recognition of spontaneous carotid dissection–a case report and review of the literature. Vasc Endovascular Surg 2004;38: 455–60.
79. Muller BT, Luther B, Hort W, et al. Surgical treatment of 50 carotid dissections: indications and results. J Vasc Surg 2000;31:980–8.
80. Liu AY, Paulsen RD, Marcellus ML, et al. Long-term outcomes after carotid stent placement treatment of carotid artery dissection. Neurosurgery 1999; 45:1368–73 [discussion: 1373–4].
81. Malek AM, Higashida RT, Phatouros CC, et al. Endovascular management of extracranial carotid artery dissection achieved using stent angioplasty. AJNR Am J Neuroradiol 2000;21:1280–92.
82. Wolfe SQ, Mueller-Kronast N, Aziz-Sultan MA, et al. Extracranial carotid artery pseudoaneurysm presenting with embolic stroke in a pediatric patient. Case report. J Neurosurg Pediatr 2008;1:240–3.
83. Schievink WI, Thompson RC, Lavine SD, et al. Superficial temporal artery to middle cerebral artery bypass and external carotid reconstruction for carotid restenosis after angioplasty and stent placement. Mayo Clin Proc 2000;75:1087–90.
84. Mas JL, Bousser MG, Hasboun D, et al. Extracranial vertebral artery dissections: a review of 13 cases. Stroke 1987;18:1037–47.
85. Golueke P, Sclafani S, Phillips T, et al. Vertebral artery injury–diagnosis and management. J Trauma 1987;27:856–65.
86. Blickenstaff KL, Weaver FA, Yellin AE, et al. Trends in the management of traumatic vertebral artery injuries. Am J Surg 1989;158:101–5 [discussion: 105–6].
87. Chiaradio JC, Guzman L, Padilla L, et al. Intravascular graft stent treatment of a ruptured fusiform dissecting aneurysm of the intracranial vertebral artery: technical case report. Neurosurgery 2002; 50:213–6 [discussion: 216–7].
88. Aoki N, Sakai T. Rebleeding from intracranial dissecting aneurysm in the vertebral artery. Stroke 1990;21:1628–31.
89. Fleischer AS, Patton JM, Tindall GT. Cerebral aneurysms of traumatic origin. Surg Neurol 1975;4:233–9.
90. Amirjamshidi A, Rahmat H, Abbassioun K. Traumatic aneurysms and arteriovenous fistulas of intracranial vessels associated with penetrating head injuries occurring during war: principles and pitfalls in diagnosis and management. A survey of 31 cases and review of the literature. J Neurosurg 1996;84:769–80.
91. Dario A, Dorizzi A, Scamoni C, et al. Iatrogenic intracranial aneurysm. Case report and review of the literature. J Neurosurg Sci 1997;41:195–202.
92. Holmes B, Harbaugh RE. Traumatic intracranial aneurysms: a contemporary review. J Trauma 1993;35:855–60.
93. Loevner LA, Ting TY, Hurst RW, et al. Spontaneous thrombosis of a basilar artery traumatic aneurysm in a child. AJNR Am J Neuroradiol 1998;19:386–8.
94. Yazbak PA, McComb JG, Raffel C. Pediatric traumatic intracranial aneurysms. Pediatr Neurosurg 1995;22:15–9.
95. Han MH, Sung MW, Chang KH, et al. Traumatic pseudoaneurysm of the intracavernous ICA presenting with massive epistaxis: imaging diagnosis and endovascular treatment. Laryngoscope 1994; 104:370–7.
96. Martin NA. The combination of endovascular and surgical techniques for the treatment of intracranial aneurysms. Neurosurg Clin N Am 1998;9:897.
97. Parkinson D. Carotid cavernous fistula: direct repair with preservation of the carotid artery. Technical note. J Neurosurg 1973;38:99–106.
98. Corradino G, Gellad FE, Salcman M. Traumatic carotid-cavernous fistula. South Med J 1988;81:660–3.
99. Lewis AI, Tomsick TA, Tew JM Jr, et al. Long-term results in direct carotid-cavernous fistulas after treatment with detachable balloons. J Neurosurg 1996;84:400–4.

100. Wilms G, Demaerel P, Lagae L, et al. Direct caroticocavernous fistula and traumatic dissection of the ipsilateral internal carotid artery: endovascular treatment. Neuroradiology 2000;42:62–5.
101. Giannotta S, Gruen P. Vascular complications of head trauma. Chicago: American Association of Neurological Surgeons; 1992.
102. Kostron H, Rumpl E, Stampfl G, et al. Treatment of cerebral vasospasm following severe head injury with the calcium influx blocker nimodipine. Neurochirurgia (Stuttg) 1985;28(Suppl 1):103–9.
103. Compton JS, Lee T, Jones NR, et al. A double blind placebo controlled trial of the calcium entry blocking drug, nicardipine, in the treatment of vasospasm following severe head injury. Br J Neurosurg 1990;4:9–15.
104. Higashida RT, Halbach VV, Dormandy B, et al. New microballoon device for transluminal angioplasty of intracranial arterial vasospasm. AJNR Am J Neuroradiol 1990;11:233–8.
105. Yamaura A, Watanabe Y, Saeki N. Dissecting aneurysms of the intracranial vertebral artery. J Neurosurg 1990;72:183–8.

Moyamoya: Epidemiology, Presentation, and Diagnosis

Edward R. Smith, MD*, R. Michael Scott, MD

KEYWORDS

- Moyamoya • Epidemiology • Stroke
- Natural history • Diagnosis

DEFINITION AND HISTORY

Moyamoya syndrome is an increasingly recognized arteriopathy associated with cerebral ischemia and has been associated with approximately 6% of childhood strokes.[1–3] It is characterized by chronic progressive stenosis at the apices of the intracranial internal carotid arteries (ICA), including the proximal anterior cerebral arteries and middle cerebral arteries. Occurring in tandem with reduction in flow in the major vessels of the anterior circulation of the brain, there is compensatory development of collateral vasculature by small vessels near the carotid apices, on the cortical surface, leptomeninges, and branches of the external carotid artery supplying the dura and skull base.

These collateral vessels, when visualized on angiography, have been likened to the appearance of a puff of smoke, which translates to moyamoya in Japanese. First described in 1957 as "hypoplasia of the bilateral internal carotid arteries,"[4] the descriptive title of moyamoya was applied more than a decade later by Suzuki and Takaku in 1969 (**Fig. 1**).[5] The use of the term moyamoya has subsequently been adopted by the International Classification of Diseases as the specific name for this disorder.[6]

NOMENCLATURE (DISEASE VS SYNDROME)

Patients with the characteristic moyamoya vasculopathy who also have well-recognized associated conditions (see later discussion) are categorized as having moyamoya syndrome, whereas those patients with no known associated risk factors are said to have moyamoya disease. By definition, the pathognomic arteriographic findings are bilateral in moyamoya disease (although severity can vary between sides).[5] Patients with unilateral findings have moyamoya syndrome, even if they have no other associated risk factors.[6] However, up to nearly 40% of patients who initially present with unilateral findings later progress to develop disease on the unaffected side.[7,8] When used alone, without the distinguishing modifier of disease or syndrome, the term moyamoya refers solely to the distinctive findings on cerebral arteriography, independent of cause.

It is important to recognize that the angiographic changes in patients with moyamoya represent a final common pathway shared by a diverse collection of genetic and acquired conditions.[1] Investigations into the pathogenesis of moyamoya suggest that the clinical presentation of affected patients may be the result of disparate underlying genetic and environmental cues. The heterogeneity of pathophysiologic processes underlying the radiographic findings that define moyamoya predicts distinct moyamoya populations, with individual clinical presentations and responses to therapeutic interventions.

EPIDEMIOLOGY

First described in Japan and originally considered a disease that predominantly affected individuals

Department of Neurosurgery, Children's Hospital Boston, Harvard Medical School, 300 Longwood Avenue, Boston, MA 02115, USA
* Corresponding author.
E-mail address: edward.smith@childrens.harvard.edu

Neurosurg Clin N Am 21 (2010) 543–551
doi:10.1016/j.nec.2010.03.007

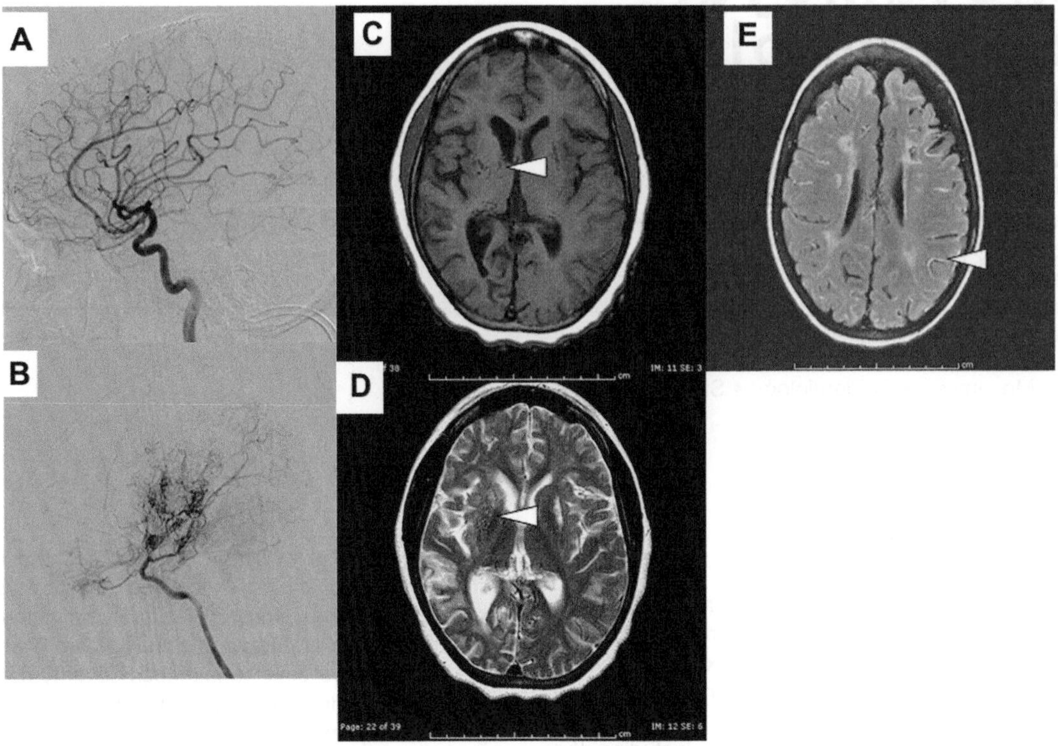

Fig. 1. Radiographic findings in moyamoya. Representative angiograms illustrating a normal study compared with moyamoya. (*A*) Normal lateral projection angiogram with injection of the internal carotid artery (ICA). (*B*) Suzuki grade III to IV with significant ICA narrowing and characteristic puff-of-smoke collaterals; note diminished cortical perfusion compared with (*A*). (*C–E*) Typical MRI images of moyamoya. (*C*) T1- and (*D*) T2-weighted studies reveal cortical atrophy, old infarcts, and flow void signals resulting from basal collaterals (*white arrowheads*). (*E*) FLAIR images demonstrating ivy sign consistent with bilateral ischemia (*white arrowhead*).

of Asian heritage, moyamoya syndrome has now been observed throughout the world and affects individuals of many ethnic backgrounds, with increasing detection of this disease in American and European populations.[9,10] There are 2 peak age groups: children at 5 years of age and adults in their mid-40s.[11–14] There is a gender predominance with females affected nearly twice as often as males.[11,12,15] Moyamoya is the most common pediatric cerebrovascular disease in Japan with a prevalence of approximately 3/100,000.[3,11,12] A recent European study cited an incidence about 1/10th of that in Japan.[16] Studies in the United States suggest an incidence of 0.086/100,000 persons (about 1 in a million).[17] Studies of individual ethnic groups suggest that moyamoya is more common in Americans of Asian or African American descent compared with whites or Hispanics. Ethnicity-specific incidence rate ratios compared with whites were 4.6 for Asian Americans, 2.2 for African Americans, and 0.5 for Hispanics.[17]

Although the cause and pathogenesis of moyamoya disease are poorly understood, genetic factors play a major role. The familial incidence of affected first-degree relatives in Japan is 10%, with a rate of 6% reported in a recent series in the United States.[15,18] Associations with loci on chromosomes 3, 6, 8, and 17 (MYMY1, MYMY2, MYMY3) as well as specific human leukocyte antigen haplotypes have been described.[19–24] However, despite evidence supporting a genetic basis of moyamoya, important caveats remain. Reports exist of identical twins with only 1 affected sibling.[15,25] These data support the premise that environmental factors precipitate the syndrome's clinical emergence in susceptible patients. Ultimately, the pathogenesis of moyamoya will likely involve genetic and environmental factors.

PRESENTATION

Patients with moyamoya present with signs and symptoms resulting from changes in flow to the ICAs. These signs and symptoms can be categorized into 2 groups: (1) ischemic injury, producing transient ischemic attacks (TIAs), seizures, and strokes[1,15,26–28]; (2) deleterious consequences of compensatory mechanisms responding to this ischemia including hemorrhage from fragile collateral vessels, flow-related aneurysms, or headache from dilated transdural collaterals.[1,13–15,29–31] Individual variation in degrees of arterial involvement, rates of progression, regions of ischemic cortex, and response to the reduction in blood supply helps to explain the wide range of presentations seen in practice.

In the United States, most adults and children present with ischemic symptoms, although the rate of hemorrhage is approximately 7 times greater in adults (20% vs 2.8%).[15,31] Some degree of geographic variability exists; reports from Asian populations indicate adults have much higher rates of hemorrhage as a presenting symptom (42%) compared with US populations (20%).[13–15,29–31] In contrast, it is extremely rare for children to present with hemorrhage (2.8%); they predominantly present with TIAs or ischemic strokes (68%) as shown in the largest current report of pediatric moyamoya patients (**Table 1**).[15] The much higher rate of completed strokes found in children may be related to less developed verbal skills in this age group as young children may not be able to clearly communicate TIA symptoms, thus delaying diagnosis and subsequent treatment and increasing the risk of progressive disease culminating in a stroke.[32]

Headache is a frequent presenting symptom in moyamoya, particularly in children. A recent review has speculated that dilatation of meningeal and leptomeningeal collateral vessels may stimulate dural nociceptors.[33] Typically, headache is migrainelike in quality, refractory to medical therapies, and may persist in up to 63% of patients even after successful surgical revascularization.[33] Headache may improve in patients within 1 year after surgical treatment of moyamoya, possibly concordant with regression of basal collateral vessels. Unfortunately, headache can cause persisting disability even after successful treatment of the syndrome.

Associated Conditions

There are numerous published links between moyamoya and a wide variety of other disorders. The clinical associations identified in a recently reported series are summarized in **Table 2**.[1,15] These include prior radiotherapy to the head or neck for optic gliomas, craniopharyngiomas, and pituitary tumors; genetic disorders such as Down syndrome, neurofibromatosis type 1 (NF1) (with or without hypothalamic-optic pathway tumors), large facial hemangiomas, sickle cell anemia, and other hemoglobinopathies; autoimmune disorders such as Graves disease; congenital cardiac disease; renal artery stenosis; meningeal infections including tuberculous meningitis; and a host of unique syndromes such as Williams, Alagille, and so forth.[1,15,34–36]

Two of these conditions merit particular attention. First, the association between moyamoya and radiotherapy to the head or neck has been well described, but to date the dose of radiation capable of causing this effect is unknown and the time between treatment and disease onset is highly variable, ranging from months to decades. Second, patients with sickle cell disease may represent a population with a markedly underreported prevalence of moyamoya, especially amongst individuals who suffer repeated strokes in the setting of failed transfusion therapy.[1,37] The prevalence of these 2 groups, especially the large number of individuals with sickle cell disease in the United States, suggest that careful observation of these patients for signs or symptoms of cerebral ischemia may be warranted.

Table 1
Symptoms at presentation in 143 patients

	Number of Patients With Symptom	% of Patients With Symptom
Stroke	97	67.8
TIAs (including drop attacks)	62	43.4
Seizures	9	6.3
Headache	9	6.3
Choreiform movements	6	4.2
Incidental	6	4.2
Intraventricular or intracerebral bleed	4	2.8

Symptom totals are greater than patient numbers, because some patients had multiple symptoms at presentation.

Table 2
Associated conditions, risk factors, or syndromes

Syndrome	Number
No associated conditions (idiopathic)	66
Neurofibromatosis type 1 (NF1)	16
Asian	16
Cranial therapeutic radiation	15
Hypothalamic-optic system glioma	8
Craniopharyngioma	4
Medulloblastoma, with Gorlin syndrome	1
Acute lymphocytic leukemia, intrathecal chemotherapy	2
Down syndrome	10
Congenital cardiac anomaly, previously operated	7
Renal artery stenosis	4
Hemoglobinopathy (2 sickle cell, 1 Bryn Mawr)	3
Other hematologic (1 spherocytosis, 1 ITP)	2
Giant cervicofacial hemangiomas	3
Shunted hydrocephalus	3
Idiopathic hypertension requiring medication	3
Hyperthyroidism (1 with Graves syndrome)	2

Other syndromes, 1 patient each: Reyes (remote), Williams, Alagille, cloacal extrophy, renal artery fibromuscular dysplasia, and congenital cytomegalic inclusion virus infection (remote). Two patients had unclassified syndromic presentations. There were 4 African Americans, 2 of whom had sickle cell disease.

NATURAL HISTORY AND PROGNOSIS

The prognosis of moyamoya syndrome is difficult to predict because the natural history of this disorder is not well known. The progression of disease can be slow with rare intermittent events, or can be fulminant with rapid neurologic decline.[15,38] However, regardless of the course, it seems clear that moyamoya syndrome, in terms of arteriopathy and clinical symptoms, inevitably progresses in untreated patients.[5,39] A 2005 study revealed that the rate of disease progression is high even in asymptomatic patients and that medical therapy alone does not halt disease progression.[40] It has been estimated that up to 66% of patients with moyamoya have symptomatic progression in a 5-year period with poor outcomes if left untreated.[41–43] This number contrasts strikingly to an estimated rate of only 2.6% of symptomatic progression following surgical treatment in a recent meta-analysis of 1156 patients.[44]

The single greatest predictor of overall outcome for patients with moyamoya is the neurologic status at time of treatment.[15,45]

Other factors that influence outcome include the speed and degree of arterial narrowing, the patient's ability to develop functional collateral vessels, the age at diagnosis, and the extent of infarction as demonstrated radiographically at the time of initial presentation.[46] Because neurologic status at the time of treatment is of paramount importance to outcome, early diagnosis is imperative and needs to be coupled with the timely delivery of therapy. If surgical revascularization is performed before disabling infarction in moyamoya syndrome, even if severe angiographic changes are present, the prognosis tends to be excellent.[15]

DIAGNOSIS

The diagnosis of moyamoya is made based on characteristic radiographic findings involving narrowing of the terminal segments of the ICA, often with the associated development of collateral vessels. Consideration of moyamoya syndrome should be given to any patient, particularly those in the pediatric age group who present with clinical findings suggestive of stroke or TIA. An important aspect of the diagnostic evaluation hinges on accurate recognition of the condition, which can be greatly increased with rapid referral to centers experienced in the care of these patients. Any child with unexplained symptoms suggestive of cerebral ischemia should be considered as possibly at-risk for moyamoya. Although the differential diagnosis for these symptoms is broad, the presence of moyamoya can be readily confirmed radiographically. Radiographic evaluation of a patient suspected of having moyamoya usually proceeds through several studies.

The workup of a patient in whom the diagnosis of moyamoya syndrome is suspected typically begins with a either a magnetic resonance imaging (MRI) study or computerized tomography (CT) of the brain. On CT, small areas of hypodensity suggestive of stroke are commonly observed in cortical watershed zones, basal ganglia, deep white matter, or periventricular regions.[47,48] Although rare in children, hemorrhage from moyamoya vessels can be readily diagnosed on head CT with the most common sites of hemorrhage being the basal ganglia, ventricular system, medial temporal lobes, and thalamus.

Patients with these findings on CT are often subsequently evaluated with MRI/magnetic resonance angiography (MRA). Acute infarcts are well seen using diffusion-weighted imaging (DWI), chronic infarcts are better delineated with T1 and T2 imaging and cortical ischemia may be inferred from fluid attenuated inversion recovery (FLAIR) sequences, which demonstrate linear high signal following a sulcal pattern, felt to represent slow flow in poorly perfused cortical circulation (the so-called ivy sign).[49,50] Most suggestive of moyamoya on MRI is the finding of diminished flow voids in the internal carotid and middle and anterior cerebral arteries coupled with prominent collateral flow voids in the basal ganglia and thalamus. These imaging findings are virtually diagnostic of moyamoya syndrome (see **Fig. 1**).[48,51–55]

Because of the excellent diagnostic yield and noninvasive nature of MRI, it has been proposed that MRA be used as the primary diagnostic imaging modality for moyamoya syndrome instead of conventional cerebral angiography.[51,56–60] Although MRA can detect stenosis of the major intracranial vessels, visualization of basal moyamoya collateral vessels and smaller vessel occlusions is frequently subject to artifact. Therefore, to confirm the diagnosis of moyamoya syndrome and to visualize the anatomy of the vessels involved and the patterns of flow through the hemispheres, conventional cerebral angiography is typically required.

Definitive diagnosis is based on a distinct arteriographic appearance characterized by bilateral stenosis of the distal intracranial ICA extending to the proximal anterior (ACA) and middle (MCA) arteries (see **Fig. 1**). Disease severity is frequently classified into 1 of 6 progressive stages originally defined by Suzuki and Takaku[5] (**Table 3**). Development of an extensive collateral network at the base of the brain along with the classic puff of smoke appearance on angiography is seen during the intermediate stages of the Suzuki grading system.

Table 3
Suzuki stages of moyamoya disease

Stage	Appearance
1	Bilateral ICA stenosis
2	Collateral vessels begin to form
3	Prominence of collateral vessels
4	Severe stenosis/complete occlusion of circle of Willis, moyamoya vessels narrow, extracranial collaterals begin to form
5	Prominence of extracranial collaterals
6	Complete carotid occlusion

Angiography should consist of a full 6-vessel series, including selective injection of the external carotid systems (both internal carotid arteries, external carotid arteries, and vertebral arteries). External carotid imaging is essential to identify preexisting collateral vessels so that surgery, if performed, will not disrupt them. Aneurysms or AVMs, known to be associated with some cases of moyamoya, can also be best detected by conventional angiography. In a study of 190 angiograms of pediatric patients, the risk of complications from performing angiography in children with moyamoya syndrome has been demonstrated to be no higher than the risk of performing angiography in nonmoyamoya populations being evaluated for cerebrovascular disease, with a rate of serious complications of less than 1%.[61]

Periprocedural hydration for these patients is useful along with aggressive measures to control pain and anxiety. Crying can lower P_{CO_2} with resultant cerebral vasoconstriction and a subsequent increased risk of stroke. Class III data support the use of these measures, with studies demonstrating decreased frequency of TIAs and strokes when patients are treated with these techniques.[62] In addition, the risk of angiography is increased in patients with sickle cell disease because of the contrast load on the kidneys. It is recommended that these patients undergo preangiography exchange transfusion and preprocedural hydration when feasible.

Cerebral blood flow studies, using techniques such as transcranial Doppler ultrasonography (TCD), xenon-enhanced CT, positron emission tomography (PET), and single photon emission computed tomography (SPECT) with acetazolamide challenge, can also be helpful in the diagnostic evaluation of patients with moyamoya syndrome as well as assisting in treatment decisions. For example, transcranial Doppler examination provides a noninvasive way to follow changes in blood flow patterns with time in larger cerebral vessels; xenon CT, PET, and SPECT can be used to detect regional perfusion instability before treatment and to determine the extent of improvement of functional perfusion after therapy.[63–70]

There is compelling class I data to support the use of TCD as an initial screening study for stroke in the sickle cell population. In a recent randomized trial, the stroke prevention trial in sickle cell anemia (STOP) evaluated more than 2000 children with sickle cell disease and validated the use of TCD as a screening study for stroke in this patient group.[71] Use of the information gained from these TCD studies resulted in a more than 90% decreased risk of strokes through the use of transfusions.[71] Although this trial was not primarily focused on moyamoya disease, the anticipated widespread use of TCDs will likely increase the number of MRI/MRA studies in this population, with a corresponding increase in the number of diagnosed cases of sickle cell–related moyamoya.

Another diagnostic evaluation that has been used in the workup of patients with moyamoya syndrome includes electroencephalography (EEG). Specific alterations of EEG recordings are usually observed only in pediatric patients and include posterior or centrotemporal slowing, a hyperventilation-induced diffuse pattern of monophasic slow waves (ie, buildup), and a characteristic re-buildup phenomenon.[72] The re-buildup phenomenon looks identical to the buildup slow waves seen in nonmoyamoya patients, but differs from buildup in timing of presentation; buildup occurs during hyperventilation and re-buildup occurs after the hyperventilation is completed and indicates diminished cerebral perfusion reserve.

Although each of these studies has the potential to add information in the diagnosis and management of moyamoya, not all are routinely used in the United States. MRI/MRA and conventional angiography are the standard diagnostic tools used for most patients with moyamoya. Following surgical treatment, an angiogram and/or MRI/MRA are often obtained 1 year after operation and, depending on the age of the patient, subsequent yearly MRI. The role of SPECT and PET scans in the evaluation and management of moyamoya syndrome has been increasing in the past decade.[69,70] Further studies are needed to optimize screening and follow-up imaging protocols for patients with moyamoya.

SCREENING

Although there are neither broad-based initiatives nor any class I data supporting screening protocols for moyamoya syndrome, particular note should be made of the association of moyamoya with NF1, Down syndrome, and sickle cell disease. These diseases are relatively common in pediatric practice and class III data support the premise of prospective noninvasive screening for moyamoya syndrome in these selected populations.[36,73–75] Recent literature reviewing the treatment of patients with sickle cell disease and moyamoya may provide additional evidence favoring screening of patients with sickle cell disease who fail transfusion therapy for moyamoya.[37]

There is less compelling evidence to suggest some usefulness to screening first-degree relatives of patients with moyamoya. The familial incidence of affected first-degree relatives in Japan is 7% to 12% and a similar rate of approximately 6% was found in the Children's Hospital Boston series.[15,76–78] Despite these relatively small percentages, the compelling association between neurologic status at presentation and long-term outcome after treatment may support a more aggressive posture toward screening in this population.[15]

TREATMENT

Once the diagnosis of moyamoya is made, rapid referral of the patient to a center experienced with moyamoya should be made to develop a plan for treatment. Current therapies are designed to prevent strokes by improving blood flow to the affected cerebral hemisphere, not to reverse the primary disease process for which there is no known treatment. Improvement in cerebral blood flow can protect against future strokes, effect a concurrent reduction in collaterals, and reduce symptom frequency.

Most of the data available supports the use of surgical revascularization as a first-line therapy for the treatment of moyamoya syndrome, particularly for patients with recurrent or progressive symptoms.[1,44,79] Many different operative techniques have been described; all with the main goal of preventing further ischemic injury by increasing collateral blood flow to hypoperfused areas of cortex, commonly using the external carotid circulation as a donor supply.[15,38] Abundant type III data including 2 relatively large studies with long-term follow-up have demonstrated a good safety profile for surgical treatment of moyamoya (4% risk of stroke within 30 days of surgery per hemisphere) with a 96% probability of remaining stroke-free in a 5-year follow-up period.[15,41] These type III data suggest that surgical therapy for moyamoya is an effective durable treatment of the disease. Recent guidelines published by the American Heart Association support the use of surgery to treat moyamoya.[79]

SUMMARY

Moyamoya is an increasingly recognized entity associated with cerebral ischemia. Diagnosis is made from clinical and radiographic findings, including a characteristic stenosis of the internal

carotid arteries in conjunction with abundant collateral vessel development. Surgical revascularization is recommended for definitive treatment of children with moyamoya syndrome.

REFERENCES

1. Scott RM, Smith ER. Moyamoya disease and moyamoya syndrome. N Engl J Med 2009; 360(12):1226–37.
2. Soriano SG, Sethna NF, Scott RM. Anesthetic management of children with moyamoya syndrome. Anesth Analg 1993;77(5):1066–70.
3. Nagaraja D, Verma A, Taly AB, et al. Cerebrovascular disease in children. Acta Neurol Scand 1994; 90(5):251–5.
4. Takeuchi K, Shimizu K. Hypoplasia of the bilateral internal carotid arteries. Brain Nerve 1957;9:37–43.
5. Suzuki J, Takaku A. Cerebrovascular "moyamoya" disease: disease showing abnormal net-like vessels in base of brain. Arch Neurol 1969;20(3):288–99.
6. Fukui M. Guidelines for the diagnosis and treatment of spontaneous occlusion of the circle of Willis ('moyamoya' disease). Research Committee on Spontaneous Occlusion of the Circle of Willis (Moyamoya Disease) of the Ministry of Health and Welfare, Japan. Clin Neurol Neurosurg 1997;99(Suppl 2): S238–40.
7. Kelly ME, Bell-Stephens TE, Marks MP, et al. Progression of unilateral moyamoya disease: a clinical series. Cerebrovasc Dis 2006;22(2–3):109–15.
8. Smith ER, Scott RM. Progression of disease in unilateral moyamoya syndrome. Neurosurg Focus 2008; 24(2):E17.
9. Caldarelli M, Di Rocco C, Gaglini P. Surgical treatment of moyamoya disease in pediatric age. J Neurosurg Sci 2001;45(2):83–91.
10. Suzuki J, Kodama N. Moyamoya disease–a review. Stroke 1983;14(1):104–9.
11. Baba T, Houkin K, Kuroda S. Novel epidemiological features of moyamoya disease. J Neurol Neurosurg Psychiatry 2007;79(8):900–4.
12. Wakai K, Tamakoshi A, Ikezaki K, et al. Epidemiological features of moyamoya disease in Japan: findings from a nationwide survey. Clin Neurol Neurosurg 1997;99(Suppl 2):S1–5.
13. Han DH, Nam DH, Oh CW. Moyamoya disease in adults: characteristics of clinical presentation and outcome after encephalo-duro-arterio-synangiosis. Clin Neurol Neurosurg 1997;99(Suppl 2):S151–5.
14. Han DH, Kwon OK, Byun BJ, et al. A co-operative study: clinical characteristics of 334 Korean patients with moyamoya disease treated at neurosurgical institutes (1976–1994). The Korean Society for Cerebrovascular Disease. Acta Neurochir (Wien) 2000; 142(11):1263–73 [discussion: 1273–4].
15. Scott RM, Smith JL, Robertson RL, et al. Long-term outcome in children with moyamoya syndrome after cranial revascularization by pial synangiosis. J Neurosurg 2004;100(2 Suppl Pediatrics):142–9.
16. Yonekawa Y, Ogata N, Kaku Y, et al. Moyamoya disease in Europe, past and present status. Clin Neurol Neurosurg 1997;99(Suppl 2):S58–60.
17. Uchino K, Johnston SC, Becker KJ, et al. Moyamoya disease in Washington State and California. Neurology 2005;65(6):956–8.
18. Fukui M, Kono S, Sueishi K, et al. Moyamoya disease. Neuropathology 2000;20(Suppl):S61–4.
19. Ikeda H, Sasaki T, Yoshimoto T, et al. Mapping of a familial moyamoya disease gene to chromosome 3p24.2-p26. Am J Hum Genet 1999;64(2):533–7.
20. Nanba R, Tada M, Kuroda S, et al. Sequence analysis and bioinformatics analysis of chromosome 17q25 in familial moyamoya disease. Childs Nerv Syst 2005;21(1):62–8.
21. Inoue TK, Ikezaki K, Sasazuki T, et al. Linkage analysis of moyamoya disease on chromosome 6. J Child Neurol 2000;15:179–82.
22. Inoue TK, Ikezaki K, Sasazuki T, et al. Analysis of class II genes of human leukocyte antigen in patients with moyamoya disease. Clin Neurol Neurosurg 1997;99(Suppl 2):S234–7.
23. Han H, Pyo CW, Yoo DS, et al. Associations of Moyamoya patients with HLA class I and class II alleles in the Korean population. J Korean Med Sci 2003; 18(6):876–80.
24. Sakurai K, Horiuchi Y, Ikeda H, et al. A novel susceptibility locus for moyamoya disease on chromosome 8q23. J Hum Genet 2004;49(5):278–81.
25. Tanghetti B, Capra R, Giunta F, et al. Moyamoya syndrome in only one of two identical twins. Case report. J Neurosurg 1983;59(6):1092–4.
26. Karasawa J, Touho H, Ohnishi H, et al. Cerebral revascularization using omental transplantation for childhood moyamoya disease. J Neurosurg 1993;79(2):192–6.
27. Lubman DI, Pantelis C, Desmond P, et al. Moyamoya disease in a patient with schizophrenia. J Int Neuropsychol Soc 2003;9(5):806–10.
28. Miyamoto S, Kikuchi H, Karasawa J, et al. Study of the posterior circulation in moyamoya disease. Part 2: visual disturbances and surgical treatment. J Neurosurg 1986;65(4):454–60.
29. Yilmaz EY, Pritz MB, Bruno A, et al. Moyamoya: Indiana University Medical Center experience. Arch Neurol 2001;58(8):1274–8.
30. Ikezaki K, Han DH, Kawano T, et al. A clinical comparison of definite moyamoya disease between South Korea and Japan. Stroke 1997;28(12):2513–7.
31. Hallemeier CL, Rich KM, Grubb RL Jr, et al. Clinical features and outcome in North American adults with moyamoya phenomenon. Stroke 2006;37(6):1490–6.
32. Nishimoto A, Ueta K, Onbe H. Cooperative study on moyamoya disease in Japan. Abstracts of the 10th

meeting on surgery for stroke. Tokyo: Nyuuron-sha; 1981. p. 53–8.
33. Seol HJ, Wang KC, Kim SK, et al. Headache in pediatric moyamoya disease: review of 204 consecutive cases. J Neurosurg 2005;103(Suppl 5):439–42.
34. Hankinson TC, Bohman LE, Heyer G, et al. Surgical treatment of moyamoya syndrome in patients with sickle cell anemia: outcome following encephaloduroarteriosynangiosis. J Neurosurg Pediatr 2008;1(3): 211–6.
35. Ullrich NJ, Robertson R, Kinnamon DD, et al. Moyamoya following cranial irradiation for primary brain tumors in children. Neurology 2007;68(12):932–8.
36. Jea A, Smith ER, Robertson R, et al. Moyamoya syndrome associated with Down syndrome: outcome after surgical revascularization. Pediatrics 2005;116(5):e694–701.
37. Smith ER, McClain CD, Heeney M, et al. Pial synangiosis in patients with moyamoya syndrome and sickle cell anemia: perioperative management and surgical outcome. Neurosurg Focus 2009;26(4):E10.
38. Ohaegbulam C, Magge S, Scott RM. Moyamoya syndrome. In: McLone D, editor. Pediatric neurosurgery. Philadelphia: WB Saunders; 2001. p. 1077–92.
39. Imaizumi T, Hayashi K, Saito K, et al. Long-term outcomes of pediatric moyamoya disease monitored to adulthood. Pediatr Neurol 1998;18(4):321–5.
40. Kuroda S, Ishikawa T, Houkin K, et al. Incidence and clinical features of disease progression in adult moyamoya disease. Stroke 2005;36(10):2148–53.
41. Choi JU, Kim DS, Kim EY, et al. Natural history of moyamoya disease: comparison of activity of daily living in surgery and non surgery groups. Clin Neurol Neurosurg 1997;99(Suppl 2):S11–8.
42. Kurokawa T, Chen YJ, Tomita S, et al. Cerebrovascular occlusive disease with and without the moyamoya vascular network in children. Neuropediatrics 1985;16(1):29–32.
43. Ezura M, Takahashi A, Yoshimoto T. Successful treatment of an arteriovenous malformation by chemical embolization with estrogen followed by conventional radiotherapy. Neurosurgery 1992;31(6):1105–7.
44. Fung LW, Thompson D, Ganesan V. Revascularisation surgery for paediatric moyamoya: a review of the literature. Childs Nerv Syst 2005;21(5):358–64.
45. Fukuyama Y, Umezu R. Clinical and cerebral angiographic evolutions of idiopathic progressive occlusive disease of the circle of Willis ("moyamoya" disease) in children. Brain Dev 1985;7(1):21–37.
46. Maki Y, Enomoto T. Moyamoya disease. Childs Nerv Syst 1988;4(4):204–12.
47. Shin IS, Cheng R, Pordell GR. Striking CT scan findings in a case of unilateral moyamoya disease–a case report. Angiology 1991;42(8):665–71.
48. Fujita K, Shirakuni T, Kojima N, et al. Magnetic resonance imaging in moyamoya disease. No Shinkei Geka 1986;14(Suppl 3):324–30.
49. Chabbert V, Ranjeva JP, Sevely A, et al. Diffusion- and magnetisation transfer-weighted MRI in childhood moya-moya. Neuroradiology 1998;40(4):267–71.
50. Fujiwara H, Momoshima S, Kuribayashi S. Leptomeningeal high signal intensity (ivy sign) on fluid-attenuated inversion-recovery (FLAIR) MR images in moyamoya disease. Eur J Radiol 2005;55(2):224–30.
51. Yamada I, Matsushima Y, Suzuki S. Moyamoya disease: diagnosis with three-dimensional time-of-flight MR angiography. Radiology 1992;184(3):773–8.
52. Sunaga Y, Fujinaga T, Ohtsuka T. MRI findings of moyamoya disease in children. No To Hattatsu 1992;24(4):375–9.
53. Brady AP, Stack JP, Ennis JT. Moyamoya disease–imaging with magnetic resonance. Clin Radiol 1990;42(2):138–41.
54. Rolak LA. Magnetic resonance imaging in moyamoya disease. Arch Neurol 1989;46(1):14.
55. Bruno A, Yuh WT, Biller J, et al. Magnetic resonance imaging in young adults with cerebral infarction due to moyamoya. Arch Neurol 1988;45(3):303–6.
56. Yamada I, Suzuki S, Matsushima Y. Moyamoya disease: diagnostic accuracy of MRI. Neuroradiology 1995;37(5):356–61.
57. Yamada I, Suzuki S, Matsushima Y. Moyamoya disease: comparison of assessment with MR angiography and MR imaging versus conventional angiography. Radiology 1995;196(1):211–8.
58. Katz DA, Marks MP, Napel SA, et al. Circle of Willis: evaluation with spiral CT angiography, MR angiography, and conventional angiography. Radiology 1995;195(2):445–9.
59. Takanashi JI, Sugita K, Niimi H. Evaluation of magnetic resonance angiography with selective maximum intensity projection in patients with childhood moyamoya disease. Eur J Paediatr Neurol 1998;2(2):83–9.
60. Chang KH, Yi JG, Han MH, et al. MR imaging findings of moyamoya disease. J Korean Med Sci 1990;5(2):85–90.
61. Robertson RL, Chavali RV, Robson CD, et al. Neurologic complications of cerebral angiography in childhood moyamoya syndrome. Pediatr Radiol 1998;28(11):824–9.
62. Nomura S, Kashiwagi S, Uetsuka S, et al. Perioperative management protocols for children with moyamoya disease. Childs Nerv Syst 2001;17(4-5):270–4.
63. Takase K, Kashihara M, Hashimoto T. Transcranial Doppler ultrasonography in patients with moyamoya disease. Clin Neurol Neurosurg 1997;99(Suppl 2): S101–5.
64. Morgenstern C, Griewing B, Muller-Esch G, et al. Transcranial power-mode duplex ultrasound in two patients with moyamoya syndrome. J Neuroimaging 1997;7(3):190–2.
65. Takeuchi S, Tanaka R, Ishii R, et al. Cerebral hemodynamics in patients with moyamoya disease. A

study of regional cerebral blood flow by the 133Xe inhalation method. Surg Neurol 1985;23(5):468–74.
66. Nambu K, Suzuki R, Hirakawa K. Cerebral blood flow: measurement with xenon-enhanced dynamic helical CT. Radiology 1995;195(1):53–7.
67. Liu HM, Peng SS, Li YW. The preoperative and postoperative cerebral blood flow and vasoreactivity in childhood moyamoya disease. Keio J Med 2000; 49(Suppl 1):A86–9.
68. Shirane R, Yoshida Y, Takahashi T, et al. Assessment of encephalo-galeo-myo-synangiosis with dural pedicle insertion in childhood moyamoya disease: characteristics of cerebral blood flow and oxygen metabolism. Clin Neurol Neurosurg 1997;99(Suppl 2):S79–85.
69. Khan N, Yonekawa Y. Moyamoya angiopathy in Europe. Acta Neurochir Suppl 2005;94:149–52.
70. Ikezaki K, Matsushima T, Kuwabara Y, et al. Cerebral circulation and oxygen metabolism in childhood moyamoya disease: a perioperative positron emission tomography study. J Neurosurg 1994;81(6):843–50.
71. Gebreyohanns M, Adams RJ. Sickle cell disease: primary stroke prevention. CNS Spectr 2004;9(6):445–9.
72. Kodama N, Aoki Y, Hiraga H, et al. Electroencephalographic findings in children with moyamoya disease. Arch Neurol 1979;36(1):16–9.
73. Kirkham FJ, DeBaun MR. Stroke in children with sickle cell disease. Curr Treat Options Neurol 2004;6(5):357–75.
74. Roach ES. Etiology of stroke in children. Semin Pediatr Neurol 2000;7(4):244–60.
75. Rosser TL, Vezina G, Packer RJ. Cerebrovascular abnormalities in a population of children with neurofibromatosis type 1. Neurology 2005;64(3):553–5.
76. Kitahara T, Ariga N, Yamaura A, et al. Familial occurrence of moya-moya disease: report of three Japanese families. J Neurol Neurosurg Psychiatry 1979; 42(3):208–14.
77. Sogaard I, Jorgensen J. Familial occurrence of bilateral intracranial occlusion of the internal carotid arteries (Moya Moya). Acta Neurochir (Wien) 1975; 31(3–4):245–52.
78. Hamada JI, Yoshioka S, Nakahara T, et al. Clinical features of moyamoya disease in sibling relations under 15 years of age. Acta Neurochir (Wien) 1998;140(5):455–8.
79. Roach ES, Golomb MR, Adams R, et al. Management of stroke in infants and children: a scientific statement from a Special Writing Group of the American Heart Association Stroke Council and the Council on Cardiovascular Disease in the Young. Stroke 2008;39(9):2644–91.

Indirect Revascularization Techniques for Treating Moyamoya Disease

Neil N. Patel, DO, MBA[a,*], Francesco T. Mangano, DO[a],
Paul Klimo Jr, MD, MPH, Maj, USAF[b]

KEYWORDS

- Indirect revascularization techniques
- Moyamoya disease • Omental transplantation
- Multiple burr holes • EMS • EDAS • Pial synangiosis
- Combined

Moyamoya disease (MD), originally described by Takeuchi in the 1950s, is a disease that results in cerebral ischemia from progressive bilateral stenosis of the internal carotid arteries. Children with MD typically present with symptoms of ischemia, while adult patients tend to present with intracranial hemorrhage. Definitive diagnosis originally required cerebral angiography, which demonstrated the stenotic arteries and the classic puff of smoke, the description given to the slowly filling basal perforator angiogenesis. As noninvasive vasculature imaging modalities such as magnetic resonance (MRA) and computed tomography angiography (CTA) have dramatically improved over the last 10 years, this technology has assumed a greater role in both pre- and post-treatment.

MD is a surgical disease and as such, there are a multitude of different techniques. Medical management most often is used to complement surgery but not replace it. The evolution of surgical procedures has been described by Reis and colleagues.[1] None of the surgical procedures described to treat MD are curative, but rather preventative in nature. The true underlying etiology of moyamoya still is not fully understood. The article by Smith and Scott in this volume of *Neurosurgery Clinics of North America* discussed the epidemiology, presentation, diagnosis and prognosis of moyamoya disease.

Surgical revascularization techniques for moyamoya are divided into direct, indirect and combined approaches. In general, indirect techniques require less time and have a decreased overall risk than direct revascularization approaches.[2–4] Direct techniques can be difficult to perform because of the small diameter of donor or recipient vessels, and an increased risk of middle cerebral artery (MCA) cerebrovascular accident, or intracerebral hemorrhage.[5] Direct revascularization techniques, however, appear to provide improved results over a shorter time frame[6] and may lead to more robust revascularization as suggested by the literature review conducted by Fung and colleagues.[7]

This article reviews numerous indirect revascularization procedures, focusing more on the technical aspects, as there have been numerous more outcome-focused articles published recently. A PubMed and Medline review of the English literature for moyamoya was conducted.

[a] Division of Pediatric Neurosurgery, Cincinnati Children's Hospital Medical Center, 3333 Burnet Avenue, MLC 2019, Cincinnati, OH 45229, USA
[b] Neurosurgery, 88th Medical Group, SGOS/SGCXN, 4881 Sugar Maple Dr Wright-Patterson Air Force Base, OH 45433, USA
* Corresponding author.
E-mail address: npatel777@aol.com

Neurosurg Clin N Am 21 (2010) 553–563
doi:10.1016/j.nec.2010.03.008

This yielded 26 articles specifically focused on indirect revascularization techniques. The procedures reviewed include

- Cervical sympathectomy (CS)
- Omental transplantation (OT)
- Multiple burr holes (MBH)
- Encephalo-myo-synangiosis (EMS)
- Encephalo-arterio-synangiosis (EAS)
- Encephalo-duro-synangiosis (EDS)
- Encephalo-myo-arterio-synangiosis (EMAS)
- Encephalo-duro-arterio-synangiosis (EDAS)
- Encephalo-duro-arterio-myo-synangiosis (EDAMS)
- Encephalo-duro-galeo (periosteal)-synangiosis (EDGS)
- Multiple combined indirect procedures (MCI)
- Indirect combined with direct procedures (I+D).

CERVICAL CAROTID SYMPATHECTOMY AND SUPERIOR CERVICAL GANGLIONECTOMY

CS and ganglionectomy were the first surgical procedures used in the treatment of moyamoya by Suzuki and Takaku in 1969.[8] Previous research had demonstrated loss of adrenergic axons within the walls of arteries and arterioles in dogs after a superior cervical ganglionectomy. The authors theorized that this would promote dilation of cerebral arteries and thus improve the collateral circulation. They performed this procedure in 10 children. Even though clinical symptoms initially improved, the progression of moyamoya was not halted both clinically and angiographically. Although the procedure now can be performed using a thoracoscopic approach, it has fallen out of favor because of the development of alternate revascularization techniques with better results and less surgical morbidity.

OMENTRAL TRANSPLANTATION

OT first was described in a case report by Karasawa in 1978.[9] The patient presented with bilateral motor ischemic events and blindness. The procedure consisted of a fronto-parieto-occipital skin incision, preserving the superficial temporal artery, and associated superficial temporal vein. The anteroinferior border of the craniotomy was used for insertion of the omentum. Via a midline laparotomy, a large 13 cm × 13 cm segment of omentum containing perforating vessels of the gastroepiploic artery and vein was isolated. An end-to-end anastomosis between the superficial temporal artery and vein to the gastroepiploic artery and vein, respectively, was performed. Durotomy and arachnoid incision permitted spreading of the transplanted omentum to the cortical surface. The patient improved clinically over the next 2 years without any new cerebrovascular events. Havlik and colleagues[10] described a procedure whereby a pedicled graft of omentum was tunneled subcutaneously to the cerebral cortex in a patient who failed a direct (superficial temporal artery [STA]-MCA) bypass. The rate for patency of the omental graft has been reported to be as high as 70% over a 2-year period.[11]

Touho and colleagues[12] performed OT in five children who failed prior EMS, EDAS, or STA-MCA direct bypass surgeries. All patients experienced resolution of their neurologic deficits after several months. Similar results also were achieved by Karasawa and colleagues.[13] His study involved 30 children, of whom 19 patients underwent omental transplant using the anterior cerebral artery distribution, and 13 patients underwent omental transplant using posterior cerebral artery distribution. All these patients except two in the posterior artery distribution group demonstrated neurologic improvement and increase in collateral vessels on follow-up angiography.[5]

MULTIPLE BURR HOLES

MBH were developed as a treatment for MD after the discovery of neovascularization around burr holes performed for ventriculostomies. Endo and colleagues[14] first reported this in 1984 in a pediatric patient who required bifrontal ventriculostomies. Using this observation as a starting point, Endo performed the first multiple burr hole procedure for MD in 1986. Angiographically adequate neovascularization at 12 months follow-up was noted with no ischemic events.[14]

More recently this procedure was reported on 15 patients and 24 hemispheres by Sainte-Rose and colleagues.[15] The patient is placed supine with head flexed to expose the entire calvarium if bilateral procedures are necessary. The incision is bi-coronal in a zigzag form for cosmesis. The exposure allows access to the frontal, parietal, temporal, and partial occipital regions bilaterally. If a unilateral procedure is indicated, the head is rotated to the contralateral side, and a T-shaped incision is fashioned.

The galea is dissected carefully, in a meticulous fashion to preserve vascularity of the scalp. The periosteum should remain intact, to preserve the vessels that will form future collateral networks. The reason that complete subperiosteal dissection is not preferred is mainly to prevent postoperative collection of cerebrospinal fluid (CSF), and also to minimize blood loss. Many triangular incisions are made in the periosteum and lifted as small flaps to expose the skull (**Fig. 1**). These openings are placed roughly 3 cm apart, covering the appropriately targeted vascular territories, and 3 cm from the midline to avoid bleeding resulting from injury to the superior sagittal sinus or the associated draining veins. Burr holes then are made at each exposed area (**Fig. 2**). The dura is opened through each burr hole using the microscope to avoid middle meningeal arterial branches. The arachnoid and pia are carefully opened while preventing any bleeding. Hemostasis is obtained by using cottonoid patties and gentle saline irrigation, as cautery is to be avoided to preserve any potential anastomotic vessels. The periosteal flap that elevated was previously is now placed in contact with the exposed parenchyma through each burr hole. The galea is carefully repositioned, with a two-layered skin/galea closure. A compressive dressing is applied for 4 days to facilitate hemostasis and limit facial swelling. Postoperative skull radiographs and a CT scan are obtained to exclude complications and assess placement of burr holes as a baseline, for comparison to follow-up angiograms and to assess for hemorrhage and CSF collections. None of their patients suffered ischemic events postoperatively, and angiography revealed excellent revascularization of the hemisphere by the external carotid system. Subcutaneous CSF collections occurred in 5 of the 18 procedures, but were treated successfully by tapping and wrapping the head; one patient also required a temporary lumbar drain.

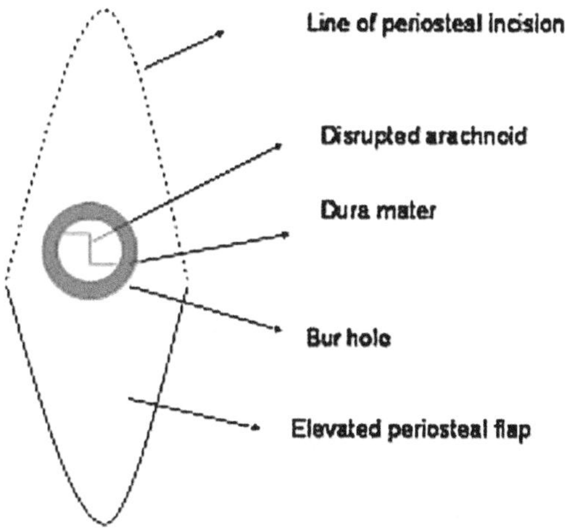

Fig. 1. Multiple burr hole technique (MBH). Schematic diagram depicting the location of the periosteal incision, elevation of the flap, and opening of the dura. (*Reprinted from* Sainte-Rose C, Oliveira R, Puget S, et al. Multiple bur hole surgery for the treatment of moyamoya disease in children. J Neurosurg 2006;105(6):439; with permission.)

The most significant benefit of this technique is the ability to use it anywhere on the cranium. It can be, and often is, combined with other procedures, direct or indirect, and it is technically simpler than other approaches. Another potential benefit as discussed by Baaj and colleagues[5] is that certain patients can undergo this procedure under local anesthesia, thus avoiding the risks of general anesthesia.

ENCEPHALOMYOSYNANGIOSIS

Encephalomyosynangiosis (EMS) first was described by Karasawa and colleagues[16] in 1975 and represented the first indirect revascularization technique for the treatment of MD. It was developed after reports in 1950 from Henschen, who demonstrated revascularization from muscle flaps after cerebral injuries.[17] EMS requires opening the dura and arachnoid layer of the cerebral cortex, then placing a vascularized section of temporalis muscle directly over it (**Fig. 3**). The muscle then is sutured or tacked up to the superior aspect of the durotomy, to prevent mobility of the muscle, and resultant mass effect. The dural flap is sutured back in place over the muscle, allowing a portion of the temporalis to enter the inferior aspect of the durotomy. A small craniectomy at the site where the temporalis enters the calvarium may be necessary to prevent ischemic compression of the muscle. Over time, collateral angiogenesis will develop between the vascular-rich muscle and the ischemic underlying cerebral tissue. One must be careful to allow the inflow vessels of the transplant to be patent and perfusing through the temporalis muscle by not applying too much pressure on it with the head wrap.[5] Touho and colleagues[18] have described a gracilis muscle transplantation technique, unilaterally and bilaterally, to revascularize frontal and occipital regions with good results.

Takeuchi and colleagues[19] performed EMS on 13 patients and 24 total hemispheres. Seventy-five percent of these patients achieved revascularization in more than one third of the MCA distribution. In addition, seven of these patients presented with transient ischemic attacks (TIAs) preoperatively, and four of seven had complete resolution of the TIAs, the remainder having significant decreases in the frequency of TIAs postoperatively. Similar good results were reported by Caldarelli and colleagues.[20] Disadvantages of EMS include the need for a larger craniotomy, and reported postoperative complications include seizures, mass effect from the muscle, and associated increase in intracranial pressure. A case report by Touho[21] described calcification of the graft with significant

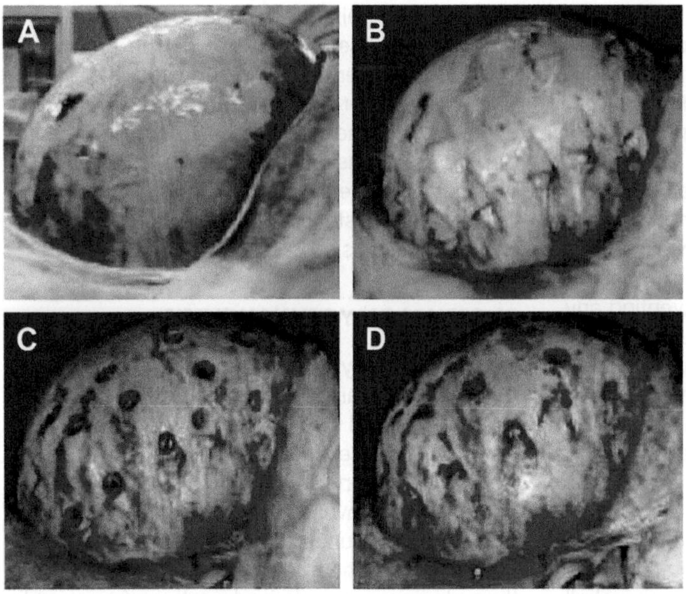

Fig. 2. MBH technique. After the scalp is reflected (*A*), multiple triangular incisions in the periosteum are made (*B*). The burr holes then are made in the exposed skull, approximately 3 cm apart (*C*). The dura is opened, followed by the arachnoid and pia. The triangular flap of periosteum then is placed into the burr hole, making direct contact with the exposed cortex (*D*). (*Reprinted from* Sainte-Rose C, Oliveira R, Puget S, et al. Multiple bur hole surgery for the treatment of moyamoya disease in children. J Neurosurg 2006;105(6):438; with permission.)

mass effect and ischemia 6 years after EMS. This complication resulted in removal of the graft. The use of EMS now is incorporated more often into a combination of procedures and used less frequently as a single operation.

ENCEPHALOARTERIOSYNANGIOSIS

Encephaloarteriosynangiosis (EAS) is mainly an intermediate procedure most often used as part of an EDAS or EDAMS. It, however, has been described as a single procedure in the past when a direct anastomosis between the STA and the MCA cannot be achieved due to MCA insufficiency, especially in posthemorrhagic presentation of moyamoya disease.[22] Because it is commonly used as part of the EDAS or EDAMS, the results on its isolated use are not readily available. The technique involves first carefully dissecting the STA. It then is retracted softly while a temporal craniotomy and durotomy are performed. The STA then simply is placed in contact with the brain. Using this technique, Touho[23] recently reported complete resolution of TIAs in 19 of 21 operative sides, with the remaining two sides having marked decrease in TIA frequency. Houkin and colleagues[24] found that neovascularization from the superficial temporal artery in EAS often was insufficient and that the deep temporal artery (temporalis muscle) and middle meningeal artery (dura) were better sources. Thus EAS, like EMS, often is used in combination with other procedures both direct and indirect.

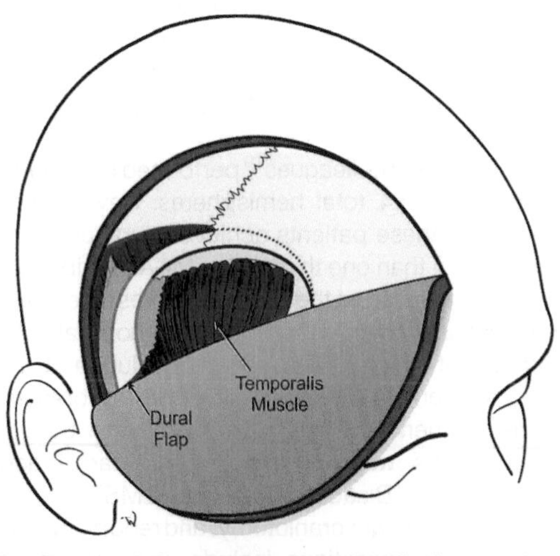

Fig. 3. Encephalomyosynangiosis (EMS). The temporalis muscle is freed from its fascia and placed directly on the exposed surface of the brain. The dura is reflected posteriorly.

ENCEPHALODUROSYNANGIOSIS

Encephalodurosynangiosis (EDS) is also an intermediate procedure that is used as part of the EDAS or the EDAMS. EDS involves the direct placement of dura with its blood supply (usually the middle meningeal artery) on the pial surface. The same principle can be applied in a more localized fashion by a burr hole with a dural incision as described with the MBH technique. EDS is used most commonly to generate collaterals to ischemic anterior cerebral artery (ACA) territories.[25] This procedure, like the EMS and the EAS mentioned previously, can be used in combination with other procedures both direct and indirect. As an isolated procedure, EDS has not been studied in depth, and results of its isolated use are not available.

ENCEPHALOMYOARTERIOSYNANGIOSIS

Encephalomyoarteriosynangiosis (EMAS) is also basically a sum of its parts. Matsushima and colleagues[26] explained the procedure in detail. They described it in variants of a frontal EMAS. In the frontal EMAS, the anterior superficial temporal artery is exposed using a cut-down technique, and then divided distally to make a muscle flap attached to it. The skin incision is extended to create a horseshoe skin flap with the epicenter in the anteroinferior skull, at the origin of the STA. A craniotomy then is performed and the dura resected. The temporalis muscle flap with the STA branch attached is sutured to the dural edge to make contact with the frontal cortical surface.[22] This technique can be applied to posterior and middle cerebral circulation as well using the posterior branch of the superficial temporal artery and the posterior auricular or the occipital artery as needed. In Matsushima's study, 10 patients and 16 hemispheres were studied. The results of this technique yielded vascular collateral formation in 88% of the procedures as evidenced by angiogram at 25 months after surgery.[22] EMAS was used as a combined technique in this study and therefore clinical outcomes were not directly correlated to revascularization from EMAS alone.

ENCEPHALODUROARTERIORSYNANGIOSIS

Encephalo-duro-arterio-synangiosis (EDAS) is probably the most commonly performed indirect procedure for moyamoya. This being the case, there are many variants and adjuncts put onto the technique by individual surgeons for additional support for revascularization. This includes most commonly the following combinations

EDAS + pial synangiosis
EDAS + dural inversion
EDAS + split dura technique.

The origin of this procedure dates back to 1979.[27] At that time, the best current surgical therapy used was STA-MCA bypass with associated high frequency of neurologic decline and seizures in pediatric patients. The first patient was a 9-year-old boy with moyamoya disease. Over the course of 4 years, the authors reported 75% success rates and decreased complication rates compared with direct STA-MCA bypass.[26,28]

The procedure can be completed in many different ways, but the basics remain the same. The procedure is best described in detail by Kashiwagi and colleagues.[29] The patient is in supine position, with head turned to the side facing anesthesia and away from the surgeon and held on a head rest. The anterior and posterior branches of the STA are palpated and marked with a Doppler ultrasound probe. The skin incision is made along the course of the parietal (posterior) branch of the STA, starting at a point 2 cm above the zygoma in front of the tragus and extending vertically and posteriorly to a point 10 cm above the zygoma, then curving anteriorly to a point 2 cm lateral to the midline at the level of the hairline. The STA is dissected at its proximal portion and separated from the inner surface of the skin.

A plane between the subcutaneous fat and the STA is dissected, and the skin incision is performed above this plane so as not to encroach upon the STA. The galea is incised parallel to the STA to provide a cuff of tissue over the exposed length of the vessel. The STA then is dissected carefully away and isolated from the fascia below, including the point at which the artery crosses the skin incision. The skin incision then is extended to the frontal region just behind the hairline. The skin flap is turned over a moist sponge used to prevent ischemic compression. The temporalis muscle is separated from the bone with a periosteal elevator and retracted posteriorly with the STA. Three burr holes are made. The first one, inferior temporal, is under the proximal portion of the STA, and the second one, superior temporal, under the distal portion of the STA. The third one, anterior frontal, is located 2 cm lateral to the midline, just in front of the coronal suture. The craniotomy is performed by connecting these burr holes, taking care not to injure the dural vasculature. A Penfield dissector is helpful in dissecting dural attachments from the inner aspect of the skull. A linear durotomy is made along the course of the STA, and the galeal cuffs on the STA strip are sutured to the edges of the dural incision to hold the STA in place over the cortex using interrupted silk or nylon sutures to complete the EDAS (**Fig. 4**). Isono and colleagues[30] performed EDAS on 16 hemispheres in 10 patients and found that it produced more robust neovascularization than EMS or EDAMS. Fujita and colleagues[31] found more revascularization from the external carotid artery in sides treated with EDAS than with sides treated with EMS.

In an EDAS with pial synangiosis, the dura is not opened in a linear fashion, but is opened into at least six flaps to increase the surface area of dura exposed to the pial surface while sparing any of the dural vessels, specifically the middle meningeal artery (MMA) and its branches (**Fig. 5**A).[32] This is thought to increase the

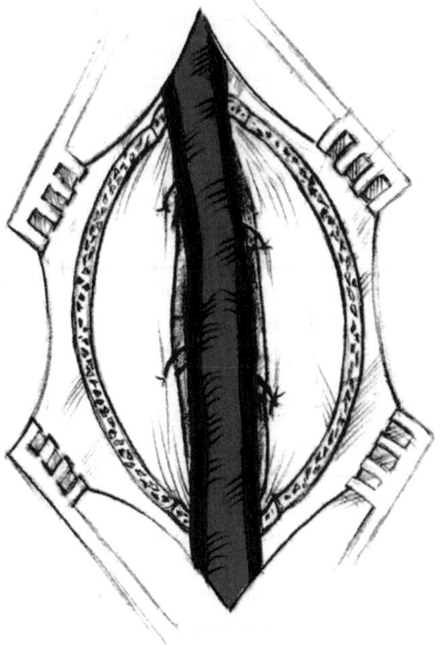

Fig. 4. Encephaloduroarteriosynangiosis (EDAS). The dissected superficial temporal artery is attached to the edges of the dura with interrupted silk or nylon sutures.

formation of collateral vessels from the dural vascular supply. The arachnoid is opened widely over the surface of the brain exposed by the durotomy. Then, the donor STA is sutured directly to the pial surface using four to six interrupted 10–0 nylon sutures placed through the donor vessel adventitia and the underlying pia (see **Fig. 5**B). A large piece of gel foam is used to cover the durotomy defect, and the bone flap is placed softly over it to avoid compression of the donor artery. This procedure aims at opening the arachnoid, which is believed to be a barrier to the ingrowth of new blood vessels onto the brain parenchyma.[20]

In 2004, Scott and colleagues[33] reported their extensive experience with pial synangiosis over a 17-year period at the Children's Hospital Boston. There were 143 patients (89 females and 54 males), with stroke being the presentation in 67.8%, and 43.4% experiencing one or more TIAs preoperatively. Average follow-up was 5.1 years. Within the first 30 days following 271 craniotomies for pial synangiosis, there were 11 episodes of stroke and three severe TIAs. In 126 patients followed for more than 1 year, four suffered a late-onset stroke; one suffered a severe reversible TIA, and two experienced persistent TIAs. In 46 patients followed for more than 5 years in whom the major initial presentation was stroke alone, only two late-onset strokes have occurred.

In an EDAS with dural inversion described by Dauser and colleagues[34] the craniotomy is completed after the posterior branch of the STA is dissected and protected. This craniotomy is completed so that the posterior branch of the MMA is visualized in the center of the craniotomy, so planned from the preoperative angiogram. The dura then is cut on either side of the MMA branch, thereby creating two rectangular dural flaps, each of which is situated around the artery itself. Care must be taken not to compromise flow through the vessel. The dural flaps then are inverted so that one passes over the artery and the other beneath it (**Fig. 6**). This maneuver allows the outer, richly vascularized layer of the dura to have direct contact with the surface of the cortex while maintaining both inflow and outflow through the middle meningeal artery supplying the inverted dura. The flaps are held into position loosely with absorbable suture, taking care not to twist and stenose the

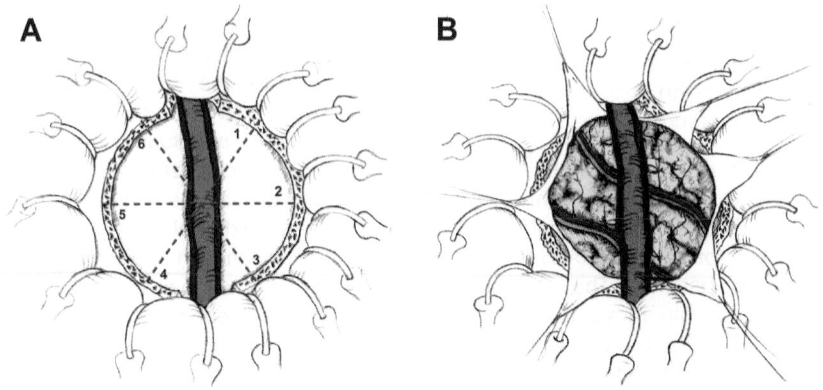

Fig. 5. Pial synangiosis. Rather than a linear opening as performed in EDAS, the dura is opened in 6 leaflets, thus maximizing the potential in growth of blood vessels from the cut edges of the dura (*A*). With the dural leaflets under fish hook-type retractors and the arachnoid widely opened, the STA is secured to the pia (*B*).

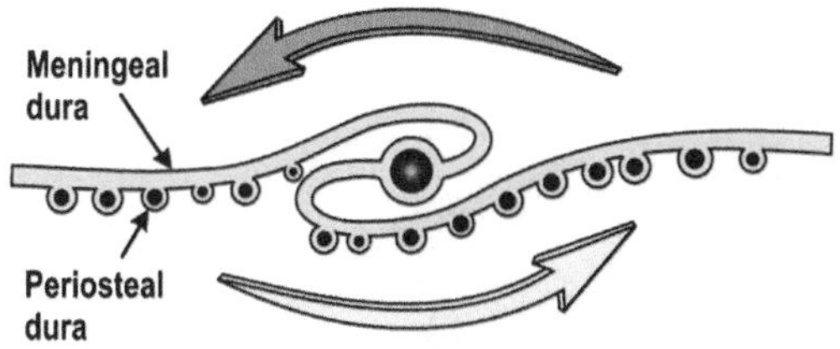

Fig. 6. Dural inversion technique. This cross-sectional schematic diagram shows how the dural flaps on either side of the middle meningeal artery are inverted, thus placing the vascular rich outer surface (periosteal dura) in direct contact with the cortex.

MMA branch. The superficial temporal artery then is sutured to the dura along the posterior margin of the exposed area under the dural flap, allowing this vessel to be in contact with the surface of the brain, as is done in the a standard EDAS procedure.

In an EDAS with the split-dural technique described by Kashiwagi and colleagues,[35] a similar approach is taken. After the STA is sutured to the linear durotomy avoiding the MMA, the course of the dural arteries, especially that of the anterior and posterior branches of the MMA, is inspected thoroughly. An H-shaped linear incision is made carefully through the outer layer of the dura adjacent to the MMA and the STA, not encroaching upon either vessel. This is done usually between the parietal STA and the posterior branch of MMA, and just anterior to the anterior branch of the MMA. The outer layer of the dura is separated, or split, from the inner layer and turned over. The inner layer is incised along the same H-shaped configuration as the initial incision and then folded over into the subdural space so that this split surface is attached to the cortical surface. This in-folding of the inner layer also exposes a window of cortical surface. The outer layer is closed with interrupted silk sutures, so that the internal surface of the outer layer is attached to the cortical surface. Bleeding from the dural incision or separation is controlled with oxycellulose and cottonoid patties but with minimal use of bipolar coagulation so as not to lose the blood supply to the dura. The results for this technique demonstrate 85% disappearance in TIAs by 1 year, and complete loss of TIAs by 1.5 years. Muto and Oi recently described a similar dural splitting-type technique called intradural arteriosynangiosis in which the supratemporal artery is anastomosed to the inner layer of the dura mater and surrounded by the outer layer as a sandwich with a blunt procedure of dural layer separation.[36]

The EDAS has been a widely used and successful technique that allows for the use of multiple variations. For this reason, as well as its relative ease and safety, it is the prime indirect revascularization technique used for pediatric moyamoya disease.

ENCEPHALODUROARTERIOMYOSYNANGIOSIS

EDAMS is an extended technique from the EDAS and the EMS that uses the temporalis muscle's deep temporal artery (DTA), the STA, and the MMA to act as adjuncts to facilitate neovascularization (**Fig. 7**). The EDAMS technique is one of the most powerful indirect techniques available to create neovascularization but requires all three donor areas to be adequate in size.

It was proposed and developed in 1984 by Kinugasa and colleagues[37] to combine aspects of all the indirect revascularization techniques. The procedure is summarized best by the technique described by Kim.[38] A skin incision is made along the parietal STA branch and the distal frontal branch of the STA in question mark shape in the fronto-parieto-temporal (FPT) region. After reflecting the skin flap anteriorly, both branches of the STA with attached strip of galea of 10 to 15 mm are carefully dissected from the pericranium and the fascia below. The underlying temporalis fascia and muscle and frontal pericranium are incised in a T-shape and elevated from the skull so that the temporalis has a posterior and an anterior cuff. A wide craniotomy is made in the fronto-parietal-temporal region while protecting the middle meningeal artery and other dural vessels as well as the dissected STA branches. The dura is opened in both the frontal and temporo–parietal regions alongside the MMA, creating two flaps with the MMA free-floating in the center. The stripped frontal STA branch is placed on the surface of the frontal region, and only the proximal and the distal portions of its galea are roughly sutured with one or two stitches to the opened dural margin. The parietal branch of the STA, however, is anastomosed near the largest cortical branch of the MCA on the temporo–parietal region. This posterior opened dural edge is multiply incised and folded inward into the subdural space to lay on the exposed brain surface. The split temporalis muscles are placed on the intact arachnoid membrane of the frontal and temporo–parietal cortex, respectively and sutured to the adjacent dura to facilitate CSF permeation. After rongeuring the lower parts of the squamous temporal bone as well as the bone flap itself to prevent compression of the temporalis muscle pedicle, the bone flap is replaced and secured to the cranium and the scalp is closed. The results for the EDAMS technique have demonstrated on average 85% revascularization rate over 2 years.[25]

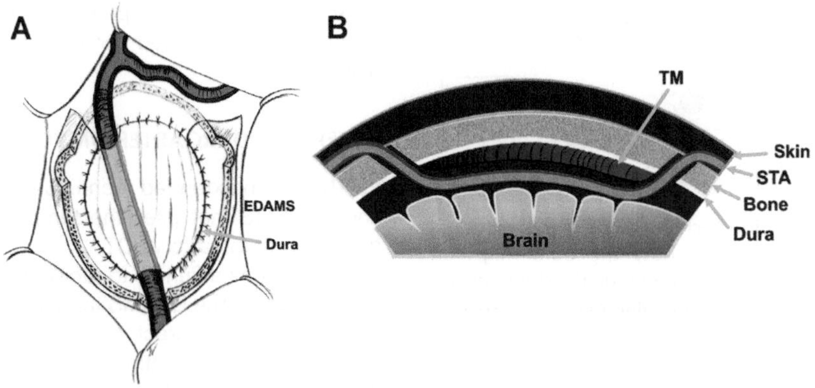

Fig. 7. Encephaloduroarteriomyosynangiosis (EDAMS). This technique takes advantage of all local vascularized structures. The parietal branch of the STA is placed between the parenchyma and the temporalis muscle; suturing of the dura mater to the temporalis muscle has been done (*A, B*).

In 2006, Ozgur developed a slightly modified version.[39] This version involves complete excision of the remaining dural flaps. In addition, Ozgur also recommend incising the pia–arachnoid surface and adding several small incisions overlying and parallel to the sulci, while avoiding vascular structures. After the arachnoid incision, the parenchyma is punctured, and then irrigated to eliminate any micro/macro hemorrhages. The temporalis muscle can be put back sparingly (or just the posterior cuff placed) if the muscle is too bulky to avoid causing mass effect and other complications associated with EMS.

ENCEPHALODUROGALEOSYNANGIOSIS

Encephalodurogaleo (periosteal)-synangiosis (EDGS) has been an adjunct that has been used alongside an EDAS or an EDAMS. It incorporates multiple incisions and has been shown to be beneficial mainly for ACA territory ischemia. Kawamoto and colleagues,[40] who coined the term galeoduroencephalosynangiosis (GDES), first described it in 2000, but this term later was switched to the reverse anatomic name (EDGS) to correlate with the remainder of indirect techniques. This technique has been described using two different methods. In a unilateral case of moyamoya disease, a small elliptical incision is fashioned just off midline with the apex toward the midline. Two incisions can be made in a curvilinear fashion just paramedian from two burr holes.[41] After a burr hole is made, the galea is dissected off the curvilinear skin flap, and a durotomy is performed. The galea is placed over the medial cortex and into the interhemispheric fissure. The galea then is tacked to the dura, and the skin is closed. Another method described by Kim and colleagues[42] that can be used for bilateral procedures begins with a horizontal S-shaped incision, 2 cm anterior to and parallel with the coronal suture crossing over the midline (**Fig. 8**A). Although the authors use the term galea, it is actually the periosteum that then is incised in a zigzag pattern, creating two rectangular flaps. A 4 $\times$ 8 cm craniotomy, crossing the superior sagittal sinus, is made. The dura then is incised separately on both hemispheres, and if preferred, the arachnoid membrane also may be incised for added benefit. The apex of the galeal/periosteal flaps is inserted as deeply as possible into the interhemispheric fissure and sutured to the dura (see **Fig. 8**B). Revascularization (20-month angiogram) rate for this technique was reported at 83% in a total of 159 patients.

COMBINED INDIRECT PROCEDURES

Multiple combined indirect procedures use many of the previously mentioned techniques to obtain the widest and safest coverage and allow revascularization of oligemic cerebrum. These techniques have included many different combinations, some of which were mentioned in the previous sections, but the more commonly described are EDAS plus bifrontal EGDS,[42] bilateral or unilateral concomitant EDAS,[43] EDAS plus EMS plus EMAS,[44] EDAS plus EMS only,[26,45,46] parietal EMAS with a frontotemporal EDAMS,[47] MBH with EMS, and EDAS and pial synangiosis.[3] The results for these procedures vary depending on specific technique combinations and the authors.

COMBINED INDIRECT AND DIRECT PROCEDURES

Indirect combined with direct procedures are performed more commonly in adults with moyamoya disease mainly because of the difficulty in

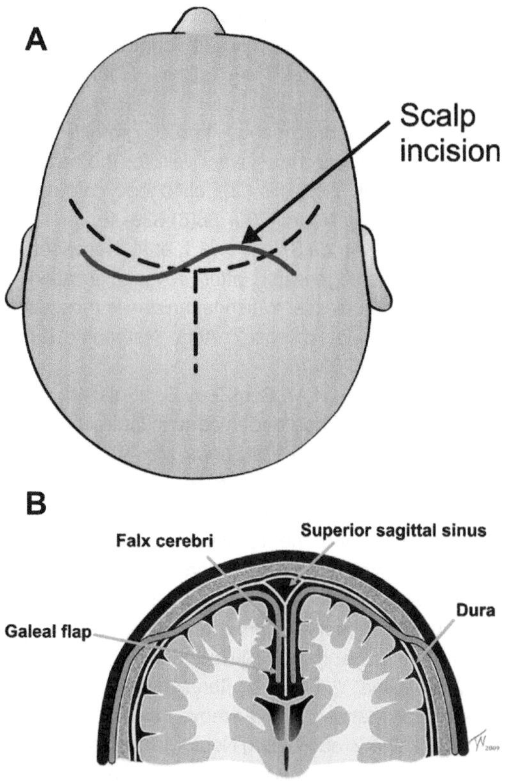

Fig. 8. Encephalodurogaleo (periosteal)-synangiosis (EDGS). An S-shaped scalp incision is made centered in the midline to access the interhemispheric space bilaterally (*A*). The periosteal (or what Kim and colleagues[51] call the galea) flaps then are advanced as far as possible into the interhemispheric space (*B*).

obtaining adequate vessel caliber for pediatric patients for direct anastomosis, as well as frequent complications in pediatric patients as opposed to adults. In the most recent review of direct versus indirect bypass, Starke and colleagues[4] state that there is evidence that both the direct and indirect bypass techniques are effective means of revascularization and reduce the incidence of ischemic events in patients with moyamoya disease. In their experience, they feel that the best collateral formation resulted from EDAMS procedures given the wider coverage to both MCA and ACA distributions. They recommended these procedures primarily for pediatric patients and combined direct and indirect bypass in adult patients. Veeravugu and colleagues[43] reviewed outcomes of many indirect and direct procedures and concluded that for children, there is as of yet no compelling evidence to support one technique over another. The authors did find that indirect procedures alone were less efficacious in elderly patients possibly because of an age-associated reduction in angiogenic capability.

Of the indirect/direct procedure combinations available, the most common is the STA-MCA anastomosis with an EMS using the same craniotomy.[2,48] Other combinations have included STA-MCA anastomosis with EDAS, MMA-MCA anastomosis with EDAS, occipital artery–PCA anastomosis with EGDS,[49] STA-MCA anastomosis with EDAMS.[50] The results of these techniques are variable. Specific techniques using direct anastomoses will be discussed in a separate article by Steinberg elsewhere in this issue.

SUMMARY

Revascularization surgery for moyamoya disease in pediatric patients is recommended to prevent ischemia or hemorrhage. For this reason, it is crucial to minimize the perioperative risks. This is accomplished most commonly with indirect techniques. To date, there have been no controlled trials to determine the efficacy of surgical revascularization and to establish specific benefit/risk ratios. Also, no standard surgical approaches for the treatment of moyamoya disease have been established as evidenced by the multitude of techniques that have been described over the last 50 years. Therefore the decision ultimately is based on the surgeon's experience and favor of technique.

Based on the literature review completed, not one of the articles individually discusses all the techniques identified and illustrated in this article. The procedures detailed in this article represent most of the indirect techniques being performed (or that have been performed) for moyamoya disease.

REFERENCES

1. Reis CV, Safavi-Abbasi S, Zabramski JM, et al. The history of neurosurgical procedures for moyamoya disease. Neurosurg Focus 2006;20(6):E7.
2. Matsushima T, Inoue T, Ikezaki K, et al. Multiple combined indirect procedure for the surgical treatment of children with moyamoya disease. A comparison with single indirect anastomosis and direct anastomosis. Neurosurg Focus 1998;5(5):e4.
3. Smith JL. Understanding and treating moyamoya disease in children. Neurosurg Focus 2009;26(4):E4.
4. Starke RM, Komotar RJ, Connolly ES. Optimal surgical treatment for moyamoya disease in adults: direct versus indirect bypass. Neurosurg Focus 2009;26(4):E8.
5. Baaj AA, Agazzi S, Sayed ZA, et al. Surgical management of moyamoya disease: a review. Neurosurg Focus 2009;26(4):E7.

6. Golby AJ, Marks MP, Thompson RC, et al. Direct and combined revascularization in pediatric moyamoya disease. Neurosurgery 1999;45(1):50–8 [discussion: 58–60].
7. Fung LW, Thompson D, Ganesan V. Revascularisation surgery for paediatric moyamoya: a review of the literature. Childs Nerv Syst 2005;21(5):358–64.
8. Suzuki J, Takaku A. Cerebrovascular moyamoya disease. Disease showing abnormal net-like vessels in base of brain. Arch Neurol 1969;20(3):288–99.
9. Karasawa J, Kikuchi H, Kawamura J, et al. Intracranial transplantation of the omentum for cerebrovascular moyamoya disease: a two-year follow-up study. Surg Neurol 1980;14(6):444–9.
10. Havlik RJ, Fried I, Chyatte D, et al. Encephalo-omental synangiosis in the management of moyamoya disease. Surgery 1992;111(2):156–62.
11. Gerber M, Spetzler RF. Burr holes for moyamoya disease. Barrow Quarterly 2002;18:22–4.
12. Touho H, Karasawa J, Tenjin H, et al. Omental transplantation using a superficial temporal artery previously used for encephaloduroarteriosynangiosis. Surg Neurol 1996;45(6):550–8 [discussion 558–9].
13. Karasawa J, Touho H, Ohnishi H, et al. Cerebral revascularization using omental transplantation for childhood moyamoya disease. J Neurosurg 1993; 79(2):192–6.
14. Endo M, Kawano N, Miyaska Y, et al. Cranial burr hole for revascularization in moyamoya disease. J Neurosurg 1989;71(2):180–5.
15. Sainte-Rose C, Oliveira R, Puget S, et al. Multiple burr hole surgery for the treatment of moyamoya disease in children. J Neurosurg 2006;105(6):437–43.
16. Karasawa J, Kikuchi H, Furuse S, et al. A surgical treatment of moyamoya disease encephalo-myo synangiosis. Neurol Med Chir (Tokyo) 1977;17:29–37.
17. Henschen C. Surgical revascularization of cerebral injury of circulatory origin by means of stratification of pedunculated muscle flaps. Langenbecks Arch Klin Chir Ver Dtsch Z Chir 1950;264:392–401.
18. Touho H, Karasawa J, Ohnishi H. Cerebral revascularization using gracilis muscle transplantation for childhood moyamoya disease. Surg Neurol 1995; 43(2):191–7 [discussion: 197–8].
19. Takeuchi S, Tsuchida T, Kobayashi K, et al. Treatment of moyamoya disease by temporal muscle graft encephalo-myo-synangiosis. Childs Brain 1983;10(1):1–15.
20. Caldarelli M, Di Rocco C, Gaglini P. Surgical treatment of moyamoya disease in pediatric age. J Neurosurg Sci 2001;45(2):83–91.
21. Touho H. Cerebral ischemia due to compression of the brain by ossified and hypertrophied muscle used for encephalomyosynangiosis in childhood moyamoya disease. Surg Neurol 2009;72:725–7.
22. Matsushima T, Inoue T, Katsuta T, et al. An indirect revascularization method in the surgical treatment of moyamoya disease–various kinds of indirect procedures and a multiple combined indirect procedure. Neurol Med Chir (Tokyo) 1998; 38(Suppl):297–302.
23. Touho H. Subcutaneous tissue graft including a scalp artery and a relevant vein for the treatment of cerebral ischemia in childhood moyamoya disease. Surg Neurol 2007;68(6):639–45.
24. Houkin K, Kuroda S, Ishikawa T, et al. Neovascularization (angiogenesis) after revascularization in moyamoya disease. Which technique is most useful for moyamoya disease? Acta Neurochir (Wien) 2000;142(3):269–76.
25. Nissim O, Bakon M, Ben Zeev B, et al. Moyamoya disease—diagnosis and treatment: indirect cerebral revascularization at the Sheba Medical Center. Isr Med Assoc J 2005;7(10):661–6.
26. Matsushima T, Inoue TK, Suzuki SO, et al. Surgical techniques and the results of a fronto-temporo-parietal combined indirect bypass procedure for children with moyamoya disease: a comparison with the results of encephalo-duro-arterio-synangiosis alone. Clin Neurol Neurosurg 1997;99(Suppl 2):S123–7.
27. Matsushima Y, Fukai N, Tanaka K, et al. A new surgical treatment of moyamoya disease in children: a preliminary report. Surg Neurol 1981;15(4):313–20.
28. Matsushima Y, Suzuki R, Ohno K, et al. Angiographic revascularization of the brain after encephaloduroarteriosynangiosis: a case report. Neurosurgery 1987; 21(6):928–34.
29. Kashiwagi S, Kato S, Yasuhara S, et al. Use of a split dura for revascularization of ischemic hemispheres in moyamoya disease. J Neurosurg 1996;85(3): 380–3.
30. Isono M, Ishii K, Kamida T, et al. Long-term outcomes of pediatric moyamoya disease treated by encephalo-duro-arterio-synangiosis. Pediatr Neurosurg 2002; 36(1):14–21.
31. Fujita K, Tamaki N, Matsumoto S. Surgical treatment of moyamoya disease in children: which is more effective procedure, EDAS or EMS? Childs Nerv Syst 1986;2(3):134–8.
32. Hannon KE. Pial synangiosis for treatment of moyamoya syndrome in children. AORN J 1996;64(4): 540–54 [quiz 557–60].
33. Scott RM, Smith JL, Robertson RL, et al. Long-term outcome in children with moyamoya syndrome after cranial revascularization by pial synangiosis. J Neurosurg 2004;100(Suppl 2):142–9.
34. Dauser RC, Tuite GF, McCluggage CW. Dural inversion procedure for moyamoya disease. Technical note. J Neurosurg 1997;86(4):719–23.
35. Kashiwagi S, Kato S, Yamashita K, et al. Revascularization with split duro-encephalo-synangiosis in the pediatric moyamoya disease–surgical result and clinical outcome. Clin Neurol Neurosurg 1997; 99(Suppl 2):S115–7.

36. Muto J, Oi S. Intradural arteriosynangiosis in pediatric moyamoya disease: modified technique of encephalo-duro-arterio-synangiosis with reduced operative damage to already growing revascularization. Childs Nerv Syst 2009;25(5):607–12.
37. Kinugasa K, Mandai S, Kamata I, et al. Surgical treatment of moyamoya disease: operative technique for encephalo-duro-arterio-myo-synangiosis, its follow-up, clinical results, and angiograms. Neurosurgery 1993;32(4):527–31.
38. Kim DS, Kye DK, Cho KS, et al. Combined direct and indirect reconstructive vascular surgery on the fronto-parieto-occipital region in moyamoya disease. Clin Neurol Neurosurg 1997;99(Suppl 2):S137–41.
39. Ozgur BM, Aryan HE, Levy ML. Indirect revascularisation for paediatric moyamoya disease: the EDAMS technique. J Clin Neurosci 2006;13(1):105–8.
40. Kawamoto H, Kiya K, Mizoue T, et al. A modified burr hole method galeoduroencephalosynangiosis in a young child with moyamoya disease. A preliminary report and surgical technique. Pediatr Neurosurg 2000;32(5):272–5.
41. Kawamoto H, Inagawa T, Ikawa F, et al. A modified burr hole method in galeoduroencephalosynangiosis for an adult patient with probable moyamoya disease—case report and review of the literature. Neurosurg Rev 2001;24(2–3):147–50.
42. Kim SK, Wang KC, Kim IO, et al. Combined encephaloduroarteriosynangiosis and bifrontal encephalogaleo (periosteal)synangiosis in pediatric moyamoya disease. Neurosurgery 2002;50(1):88–96.
43. Veeravagu A, Guzman R, Patil CG, et al. Moyamoya disease in pediatric patients: outcomes of neurosurgical interventions. Neurosurg Focus 2008; 24(2):E16.
44. Miyamoto S, Kikuchi H, Karasawa J, et al. Pitfalls in the surgical treatment of moyamoya disease. Operative techniques for refractory cases. J Neurosurg 1988;68(4):537–43.
45. Ishii K, Fujiki M, Kobayashi H. Invited article: surgical management of Moyamoya disease. Turk Neurosurg 2008;18(2):107–13.
46. Matsushima T, Inoue T, Suzuki SO, et al. Surgical treatment of moyamoya disease in pediatric patients–comparison between the results of indirect and direct revascularization procedures. Neurosurgery 1992;31(3):401–5.
47. Takahashi A, Kamiyama H, Houkin K, et al. Surgical treatment of childhood moyamoya disease–comparison of reconstructive surgery centered on the frontal region and the parietal region. Neurol Med Chir (Tokyo) 1995;35(4):231–7.
48. Shrestha P, Sakamoto S, Ohba S, et al. Multiple concurrent anastomotic procedures in the management of moyamoya disease: a case report with review of literature. Hiroshima J Med Sci 2008;57(1):47–51.
49. Hayashi T, Shirane R, Tominaga T. Additional surgery for postoperative ischemic symptoms in patients with moyamoya disease: the effectiveness of occipital artery–posterior cerebral artery bypass with an indirect procedure: technical case report. Neurosurgery 2009;64(1):E195–6 [discussion E196].
50. Houkin K, Kuroda S, Nakayama N. Cerebral revascularization for moyamoya disease in children. Neurosurg Clin N Am 2001;12(3):575–84, ix.
51. Kim CY, Wang KC, Kim SK, et al. Encephaloduroarteriosynangiosis with bifrontal encephalogaleo (periosteal)synangiosis in the pediatric moyamoya disease: the surgical technique and its outcomes. Childs Nerv Syst 2003;19:316–24.

Direct Bypass Techniques for the Treatment of Pediatric Moyamoya Disease

Raphael Guzman, MD[a], Gary K. Steinberg, MD, PhD[b,*]

KEYWORDS

• Moyamoya disease • Pediatric • Direct bypass

INDICATIONS

Moyamoya disease (MMD) has been recognized as a devastating condition in adults and in pediatric patients. Large pediatric epidemiologic studies have shown that MMD is a significant contributor to childhood stroke. Independent studies in the American, Asian, and European literature found a pediatric stroke incidence between 2.1 and 13/100,000/y,[1–3] with MMD accounting for 6% of the ischemic strokes.[1,3] With an untreated morbidity estimated to be greater than 70%,[4] and with a 5-year risk of recurrent ipsilateral stroke of 65% in medically treated symptomatic hemispheres,[5] surgical intervention has become the standard of treatment of patients with MMD.[6–8] In children, the most common presentation is cerebral ischemia. In a study by Scott and colleagues of 143 pediatric patients diagnosed with MMD in North America, nearly all patients presented with either symptoms of stroke or transient ischemic attack (TIA).[9] Similarly, in large populations of Asian patients, approximately 40% of those less than 10 years of age presented with a TIA and nearly 30% presented with cerebral infarction,[10] although some presented with headaches and seizures. Similar findings were made in European studies.[4,11] In our series including 272 adult and 96 pediatric patients with MMD, we found stroke and TIA to be the most common presenting symptoms in the pediatric patients followed by headache, seizures, and rarely intracerebral hemorrhage (**Fig. 1**).[12]

The diagnostic guidelines for identifying patients with MMD differ in centers around the world. The Research Committee on MMD of the Ministry of Health and Welfare of Japan has identified 4 criteria necessary for the diagnosis of MMD: (1) stenosis or occlusion of the terminal portion of the internal carotid artery (ICA); (2) a coexisting abnormal vascular network in the base of the brain or basal ganglia; (3) bilaterality; and (4) no other identifiable cause.[13,14] These guidelines have been modified case by case at various institutions around the United States. Although classically bilateral, unilateral MMD can occur. Patients with the characteristic moyamoya vasculopathy who also have well-recognized associated conditions are categorized as having moyamoya syndrome, whereas patients with no known associated risk factors have MMD. In our series 21% of the children had unilateral disease. We have previously reported that 71% of patients with equivocal or mild stenotic changes in the initially unaffected side eventually progressed to bilateral MMD at a mean follow-up time of 12.7 months.[15]

In light of the findings describing a natural history with a devastating disease course,

Funding sources: Huber Family Moyamoya Fund, William Randolph Hearst Foundation, Bernard and Ronni Lacroute, Russell and Elizabeth Siegelman.
[a] Division of Pediatric Neurosurgery, Lucile Packard Children's Hospital, Stanford University School of Medicine, 300 Pasteur Drive, R211, Stanford, CA 94305-5327, USA
[b] Department of Neurosurgery, Stanford University School of Medicine, Stanford, CA, USA
* Corresponding author.
E-mail address: raphaelg@stanford.edu

Neurosurg Clin N Am 21 (2010) 565–573
doi:10.1016/j.nec.2010.03.013

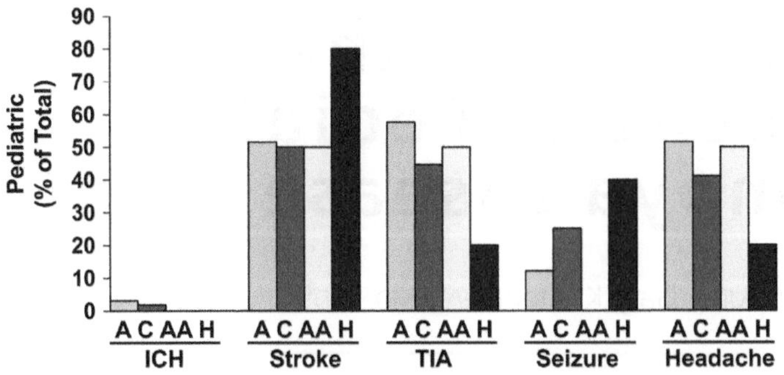

Fig. 1. Presenting symptoms in 96 pediatric patients consisting of intracerebral hemorrhage (ICH), stroke, TIA, seizures and headaches. Comparison between Asian (A), White (C), African American (AA), and Hispanic (H) patients did not reveal any statistically significant differences. Note that the high incidence of stroke in Hispanic pediatric patients is based on a small n. (*Data from* Guzman R, Lee M, Achrol A, et al. Clinical outcome after 450 revascularization procedures for moyamoya disease. J Neurosurg 2009;11(5):927–35.)

a poor response to medical therapy, and a good response to surgery, we strongly advocate surgical treatment of symptomatic pediatric patients with MMD. There is ongoing debate about the treatment of asymptomatic or incidentally discovered MMD. Because there are only limited data on the natural history of MMD in children, decision-making is complex. However, substantial evidence suggests inevitable disease progression and therefore close follow-up would be recommended. In our experience, careful history taking and physical examination often uncover signs and symptoms suggestive of cerebral hypoperfusion, such as recurrent TIAs. To avoid devastating strokes, early treatment is advocated.

PATIENT SELECTION

All patients undergo a detailed clinical assessment as part of the evaluation as a potential surgical candidate. In particular subgroups of patients with syndromes known to be associated with moyamoya, such as neurofibromatosis, Down syndrome, and primordial dwarfism, identifying comorbidities is essential. At our institution, we found a higher risk of postsurgical morbidities in patients with moyamoya syndrome compared with the rest of our cohort (odds ratio 4.16, $P = .09$[12]). Diagnosis of MMD is made based on angiography according to published guidelines.[13] All patients are evaluated with magnetic resonance (MR) imaging including diffusion-weighted imaging (DWI) and fluid attenuated inversed recovery imaging to assess the overall stroke burden. Acute strokes, as identified by diffusion-weighted MR imaging, have to be recognized, because they may put patients at a greater risk for perioperative strokes. The preoperative 6-vessel (including both external carotid arteries [ECAs], both ICAs, and 1 or both vertebral arteries) catheter angiography is important to determine the severity of the disease[16] and to evaluate the presence of the superficial temporal artery (STA) (**Fig. 2**). All patients undergo a cerebral blood flow analysis using MR imaging and single-photon emission computed tomography (SPECT) studies with and without acetazolamide (Diamox) challenge.

Surgical interventions for MMD have been divided into direct and indirect bypass techniques. The principal difference between the 2 strategies lies in the method of cerebral reperfusion. Whereas direct methods are believed to provide immediate flow increase in the affected areas of the brain, indirect methods aim to stimulate the development of a new vascular network over time. The arteriopathy of moyamoya affects the ICA and spares the ECA. Surgical treatment of moyamoya typically uses the ECA as a source of new blood flow to the ischemic hemisphere. Two general methods of revascularization are used: direct and indirect. In direct revascularization, a branch of the ECA (usually the STA) is directly anastomosed to a cortical artery. Indirect techniques involve the placement of vascularized tissue supplied by the ECA such as dura, temporalis muscle, or the STA itself in direct contact with the brain, leading to an ingrowth of new blood vessels to the underlying cortex. The direct bypass techniques that have been proposed include STA to middle cerebral artery (MCA), occipital artery to MCA, and middle meningeal artery[17] to MCA anastomoses. The indirect techniques include encephalomyosynangiosis (EMS), encephaloduroarteriosynangiosis (EDAS),[9,18,19]

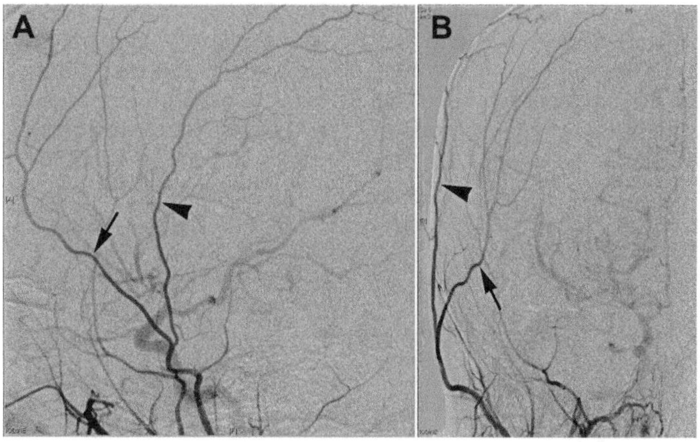

Fig. 2. Angiogram with injection of the ECA on the right side in the lateral (*A*) and anteroposterior view (*B*). Example of the STA splitting into a frontal (*arrow*) and parietal (*arrowhead*) branch.

encephaloduroarteriomyosynangiosis (EDAMS), encephalomyoarteriosynangiosis, multiple cranial bur holes,[4] and omental transposition.

There has not been a controlled randomized trial comparing direct and indirect revascularization techniques. Therefore, there are currently no data to support either direct or indirect revascularization techniques in the pediatric population with MMD.[20] Some investigators advocate that indirect techniques do not result in an immediate revascularization and may carry an increased risk for postoperative stroke.[18,21] Thus, it has been suggested to combine direct and indirect techniques to take advantage of immediate revascularization with the security of more diffuse neovascularization.

We advocate the use of direct bypass techniques when possible. In our pediatric series of 96 patients 67% received a direct bypass. The strongest predictor of the feasibility of a direct bypass was the age at surgery.[12] The mean age of pediatric patients undergoing indirect surgery was 6.5 years, whereas it was 11.2 years in children undergoing direct surgery ($P<.05$) (**Fig. 3**). The youngest child to receive a direct bypass was 4.3 years old.[12] The presence of the STA has to be confirmed on cerebral angiogram. However, we found that a small STA on angiogram does not necessarily preclude a direct bypass approach. Generally we consider a direct bypass possible if the STA and the MCA are 0.6 mm or greater.

At our institution, it is our practice to operate on the most symptomatic side first. If both hemispheres are symptomatic, we revascularize the right side first. In bilateral MMD, the second side is usually revascularized 1 week after the first surgery if tolerated by the patient.

OVERVIEW OF TECHNIQUE

All surgeries are performed under mild hypothermia with a target core temperature of 33°C. Cooling is achieved either with surface cooling using a cooling blanket or through placement of an intravenous catheter (Innercool Therapies, San Diego, CA, USA) into the inferior vena cava as described earlier.[17] The Innercool method is applicable only in older children and adults. Patients are monitored intraoperatively with somatosensory evoked potentials and electroencephalography (EEG). The patients are positioned supine with a shoulder role on the side ipsilateral to the surgery and fixed in a Mayfield 3-pin head

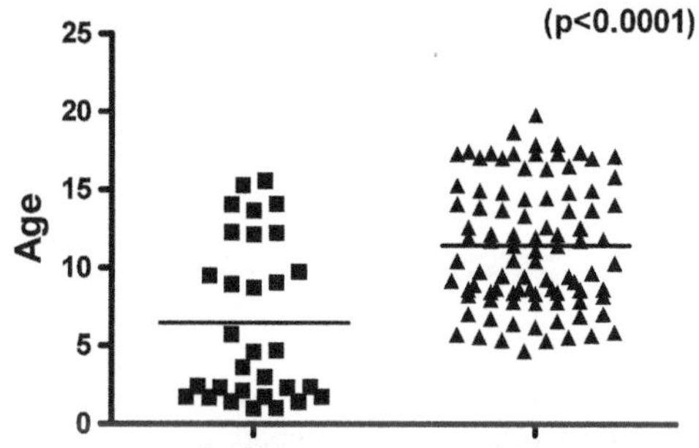

Fig. 3. Mean age at surgery of 96 patients undergoing either indirect or direct revascularization surgery. Patients undergoing an indirect bypass were significantly younger than patients undergoing a direct bypass ($P<.0001$).

clamp. Starting in front of the tragus within the hairline the STA is mapped for 7 to 8 cm. The size of the frontal and parietal branch of the STA is determined on the ECA angiography and the decision is made whether the frontal or parietal branch is to be used based on artery diameter. The STA is prepared under the surgical microscope, leaving an approximately 8-mm tissue cuff around the vessel (**Figs. 4–6**). A 4 × 4-cm craniotomy is performed over the sylvian fissure and the size of the M4 branches of the MCA evaluated at high magnification. The largest M4

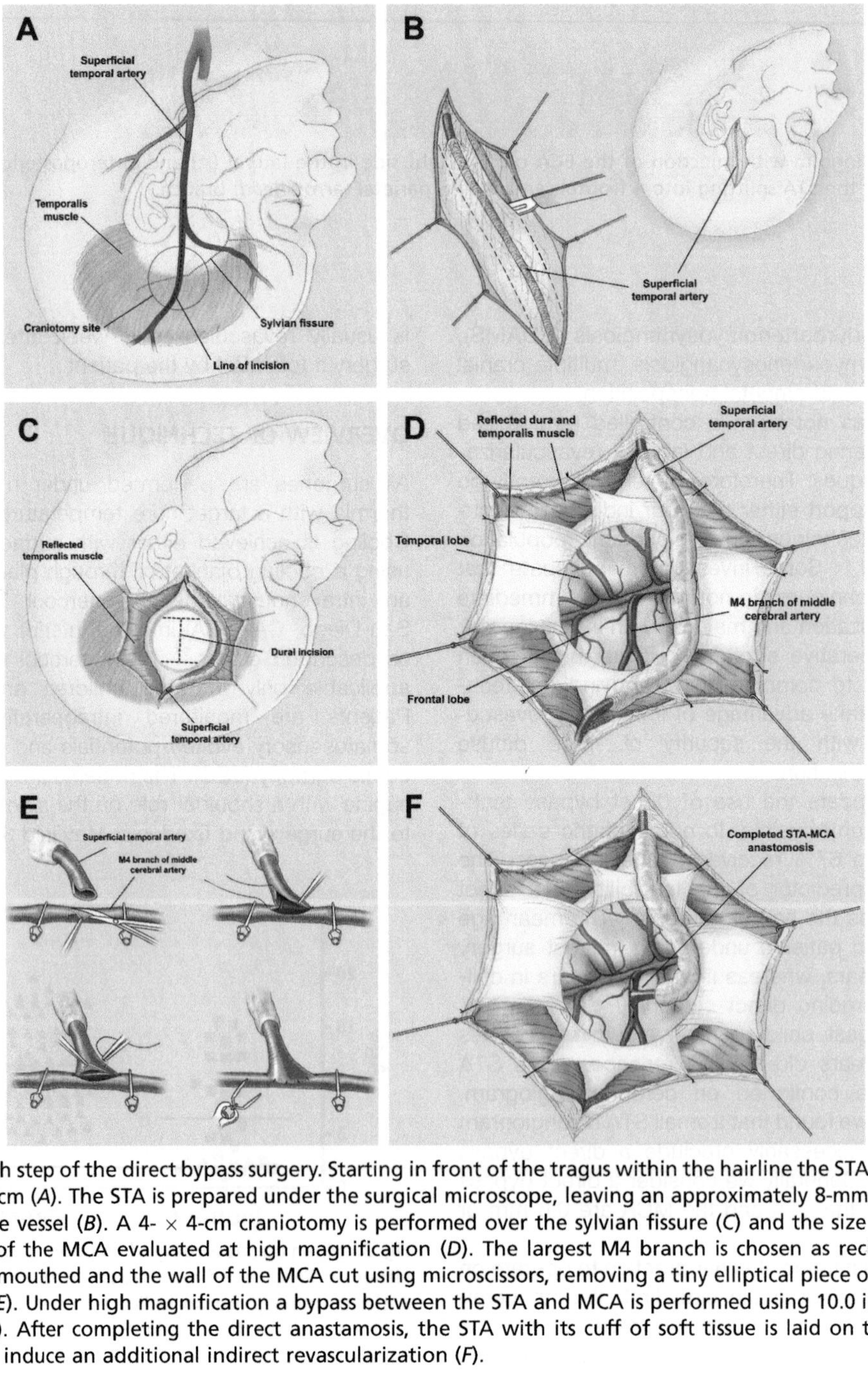

Fig. 4. Each step of the direct bypass surgery. Starting in front of the tragus within the hairline the STA is mapped for 7 to 8 cm (*A*). The STA is prepared under the surgical microscope, leaving an approximately 8-mm tissue cuff around the vessel (*B*). A 4- × 4-cm craniotomy is performed over the sylvian fissure (*C*) and the size of the M4 branches of the MCA evaluated at high magnification (*D*). The largest M4 branch is chosen as recipient. The STA is fishmouthed and the wall of the MCA cut using microscissors, removing a tiny elliptical piece of the superior wall (*E*). Under high magnification a bypass between the STA and MCA is performed using 10.0 interrupted sutures (*E*). After completing the direct anastamosis, the STA with its cuff of soft tissue is laid on the cortical surface to induce an additional indirect revascularization (*F*).

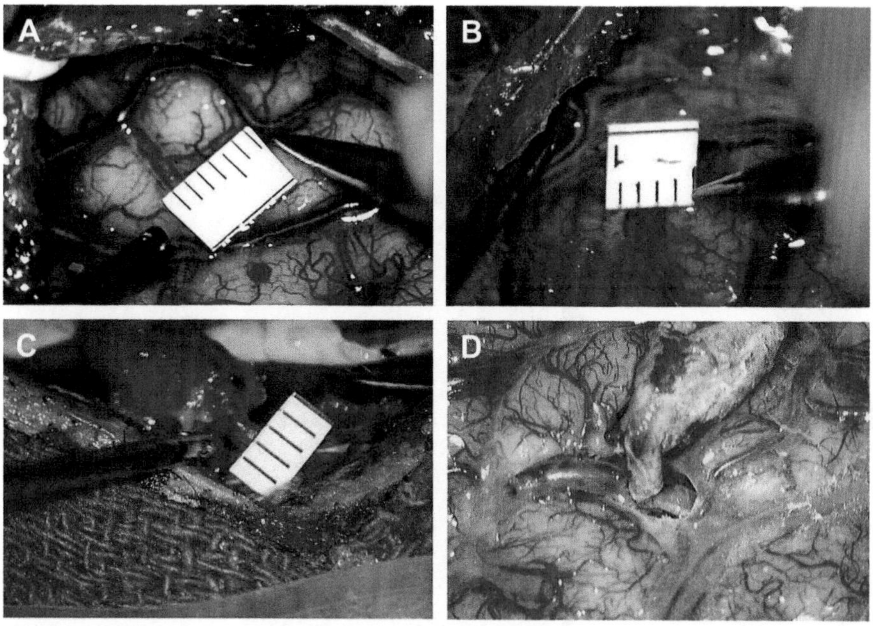

Fig. 5. Intraoperative view of a 1-mm (*A*) and 0.6-mm (*B*) M4 branch of the MCA on the cortical surface. Example of a 1-mm STA at its distal end, prepared for anastomosis (*C*). Completed STA-MCA bypass (*D*).

branch is chosen as recipient. In patients in whom either the STA or the MCA were considered too small (<0.6 mm) or too fragile for a direct bypass, indirect revascularization procedures, such as EDAS, are performed.

The flow within the STA and the MCA are measured with microflow Doppler (Transonic Systems Inc, Ithaca, NY, USA). The STA is fish-mouthed and the wall of the MCA cut using micro-scissors, removing a tiny elliptical piece of the superior wall. Before and during clamping the patient is given thiopental to achieve burst suppression on the EEG. Under high magnification a bypass between the STA and MCA is performed using 10.0 interrupted sutures (see **Figs. 4** and **5**). After completing the direct anastamosis, the STA with its cuff of soft tissue is laid on the cortical surface to induce an additional indirect revascularization (see **Figs. 4** and **5**). Again the flow Doppler is used to measure flow velocities in the proximal and distal MCA as well as the STA.

After surgery patients are kept in the intensive care unit overnight with a tight blood pressure control, usually a mean arterial pressure between 70 and 80 mm Hg for children or 10 mm Hg above their baseline. Aspirin (81 mg) is started the day after surgery. MR imaging including DWI is performed the day after the second surgery to exclude new strokes. Patients are usually discharged 3 to 4 days after surgery.

OUTCOME

The independent use of a direct STA-MCA bypass in pediatric patients with MMD has rarely been reported in the literature. Results of studies performing direct STA-MCA bypasses in children are shown in **Table 1**. Previously, we described the outcomes of direct STA-MCA bypass and STA-MCA + EDAS in a pediatric population.[18] In a group of 12 patients, 21 hemispheres were treated with direct bypass techniques. Concomitant EDAS was applied in 6 hemispheres by using a second branch of the STA, 1 patient underwent MMA-MCA anastomosis plus EDAS, and 1 patient underwent omental transposition. Outcomes in this population included a global reduction in preoperative symptoms and no perioperative strokes. Some patients experienced transient perioperative neurologic symptoms that the investigators attributed to possible impaired autoregulation of the cerebral vasculature. Cerebral blood flow analysis in many of these patients revealed increased flow in 68 of the 76 regions as identified by SPECT. Sakamoto and associates[27] altered the direct bypass technique by including a double STA-MCA anastomoses and EMS. Specifically, the frontal and parietal branches of the STA were harvested as donor vessels for the recipient MCA. The study included 20 pediatric hemispheres, and the combined

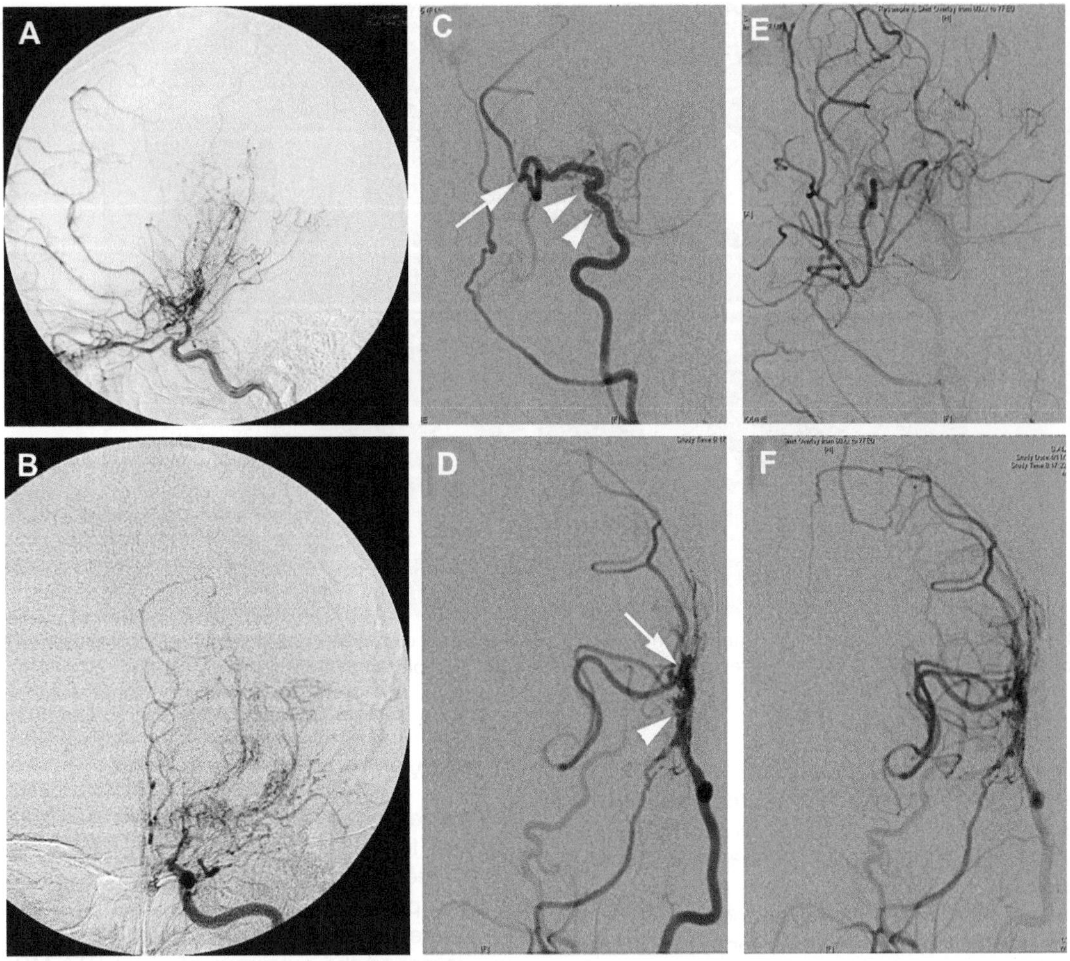

Fig. 6. Angiogram of a patient with severe MMD and completed STA-MCA bypass. The lateral (*A*) and anteroposterior (*B*) ICA injections show occlusion of the supraclinoid segment of the carotid artery with development of moyamoya vessels. Injection of the ECA after bypass surgery shows a robust STA in the lateral (*C*) and anteroposterior (*D*) view with some indirect revascularization (*arrowhead*) proximal to the anastomosis (*arrow*). In the later angiographic phase a robust arterial filling from the graft is noted (*E, F*).

procedure was undertaken in 19. Results from the study showed that of the 38 completed anastomoses, 37 maintained patency on angiography at the 1- to 2-month follow-up. Clinical outcome mirrored radiographically proven success; none of the 10 patients showed any significant ischemic episodes, disease progression, or the development of mental retardation at a mean follow-up of 4 years (range 1–10 years).

In our overall adult and pediatric series we found an excellent long-term patency of the direct bypasses of 98% at a mean angiographic follow-up of 1.5 years.[12] The overall surgical morbidity among pediatric patients was 1.8% per procedure or 3.1% per patient.[12] One patient with mitochondrial encephalopathy with lactic acidosis and strokelike episodes died 10 days after the bypass procedure as a result of multiple strokes, leading to a 1% mortality.[32] There was no statistically significant difference in postoperative morbidity or mortality between children undergoing direct versus indirect revascularization. In the long-term outcome analysis with a mean follow-up time of 4.8 years (median 3 years) no patients suffered a new clinical stroke or hemorrhage among the pediatric population. The combined overall adult and pediatric 5-year risk of recurrent stroke or hemorrhage after bypass surgery was 5.5% in our series.[12]

Table 1
Results of studies on direct STA-MCA bypasses in children

Authors	Year	Country	Intervention	Number of Children (Hemispheres)	Outcome
Matsushima et al[22]	1992	Japan	STA-MCA+EMS or EDAS	16 (20)	Complete resolution of symptoms in 3 of 13 (23%) with EDAS and in 7/7 100% with STA-MCA+EMS (*P*<.01)
Mizoi et al[23]	1996	Japan	STA-MCA+EMS, (+EDAS)	23	Moderate to poor filling with direct bypass compared with good to moderate with indirect method
Suzuki et al[24]	1997	Japan	STA-MCA+EDAS or EMS or BH	36	Frequency of TIAs reduced/resolved within 1 year in 25 of 31 (81%) patients
Ishikawa et al[25]	1997	Japan	STA-MCA+EDAMS or EDAMS	34 (64)	Incidence of postoperative ischemia significantly reduced in the combined group (10%) versus indirect group (56%; *P*<.01)
Iwama et al[26]	1997	Japan	STA-ACA and/or STA-MCA	5	TIAs resolved in 4 patients and reduced in 1 patient
Sakamoto et al[27]	1997	Japan	Bilateral, double STA-MCA+ EMS	10 (19)	All patients were free of significant ischemic episodes, disease progression, and MR
Miyamoto et al[28]	1998	Japan	STA-MCA and/or EMS	113	Resolution of stroke in 110 (97.3%) of 113 patients. Independent lifestyle achieved in 100/113 (88.5%) patients
Golby et al[18]	1999	United States	STA-MCA or STA-MCA+ EDAS or MMA-MCA+EDAS	12 (21)	No perioperative strokes, global reduction of preoperative symptoms, and improved cerebral blood flow
Houkin et al[29]	2000	Japan	STA-MCA or EDAMS	34	Patency of direct bypass verified in 15 sides (53%) versus indirect procedure yielded neovascularization in > 90%
Khan et al[11]	2003	Switzerland	STA-MCA and STA-ACA	19 (35)	No perioperative strokes, stabilization of disease in all patients, and cognitive improvement in 6 of 19 patients
Kim et al[30]	2007	Korea	STA-MCA+EDAMS or EDAS or EDAMS	7 (12)	EDAMS/STA-MCA-EDAMS radiographically superior, all indirect techniques had same clinical outcome
Czabanka et al[31]	2009	Germany	STA-MCA and EMS	10 (20)	Improvement of disease in 14 and stable disease in 6 hemispheres. Moderate to good filling in all EMS at last angiography
Guzman et al[12]	2009	United States	STA-MCA+EDAS or EDAS	96 (168)	No difference in morbidity between 113 direct bypass and 55 indirect revascularization surgeries. Excellent long-term outcome

SUMMARY

Moyamoya is an increasingly recognized cause of stroke in children and adults. Identification of the disease early in its course with prompt institution of therapy is critical to providing the best outcome for patients. Revascularization surgery seems to be effective in preventing stroke in moyamoya, with direct techniques providing durable protection when performed at experienced centers.

REFERENCES

1. Chung B, Wong V. Pediatric stroke among Hong Kong Chinese subjects. Pediatrics 2004;114:e206.
2. Fullerton HJ, Chetkovich DM, Wu YW, et al. Deaths from stroke in US children, 1979 to 1998. Neurology 2002;59:34.
3. Giroud M, Lemesle M, Gouyon JB, et al. Cerebrovascular disease in children under 16 years of age in the city of Dijon, France: a study of incidence and clinical features from 1985 to 1993. J Clin Epidemiol 1995;48:1343.
4. Sainte-Rose C, Oliveira R, Puget S, et al. Multiple bur hole surgery for the treatment of moyamoya disease in children. J Neurosurg 2006;105:437.
5. Hallemeier CL, Rich KM, Grubb RL Jr, et al. Clinical features and outcome in North American adults with moyamoya phenomenon. Stroke 2006;37:1490.
6. Kim SK, Seol HJ, Cho BK, et al. Moyamoya disease among young patients: its aggressive clinical course and the role of active surgical treatment. Neurosurgery 2004;54:840.
7. Scott RM. Moyamoya syndrome: a surgically treatable cause of stroke in the pediatric patient. Clin Neurosurg 2000;47:378.
8. Scott RM. Surgery for moyamoya syndrome? Yes. Arch Neurol 2001;58:128.
9. Scott RM, Smith JL, Robertson RL, et al. Long-term outcome in children with moyamoya syndrome after cranial revascularization by pial synangiosis. J Neurosurg 2004;100:142.
10. Kim SK, Wang KC, Kim IO, et al. Combined encephaloduroarteriosynangiosis and bifrontal encephalogaleo(periosteal)synangiosis in pediatric moyamoya disease. Neurosurgery 2002;50:88.
11. Khan N, Schuknecht B, Boltshauser E, et al. Moyamoya disease and Moyamoya syndrome: experience in Europe; choice of revascularisation procedures. Acta Neurochir (Wien) 2003;145:1061.
12. Guzman R, Lee M, Achrol A, et al. Clinical outcome after 450 revascularization procedures for moyamoya disease. J Neurosurg 2009;11(5):927–35.
13. Fukui M. The Research Committee on Spontaneous Occlusion of the Circle of Willis of the Ministry of Health and Welfare Japan: guidelines for the diagnosis and treatment of spontaneous occlusion of the circle of Willis ('Moyamoya' disease). Clin Neurol Neurosurg 1997;99:S233.
14. Yonekawa Y, Kawano T. Follow-up study of 632 cases in spontaneous occlusion of the circle of Willis registered from 1983 to 1991. In: Yonekawa Y, editor. The Research Committee on Spontaneous Occlusion of the Circle of Willis (Moyamoya Disease) of the Ministry of Health and Welfare, Japan: Annual Report 1991.41, 1992.
15. Kelly ME, Bell-Stephens TE, Marks MP, et al. Progression of unilateral moyamoya disease: a clinical series. Cerebrovasc Dis 2006;22:109.
16. Suzuki J, Takaku A. Cerebrovascular "moyamoya" disease. Disease showing abnormal net-like vessels in base of brain. Arch Neurol 1969;20:288.
17. Steinberg GK, Ogilvy CS, Shuer LM, et al. Comparison of endovascular and surface cooling during unruptured cerebral aneurysm repair. Neurosurgery 2004;55:307.
18. Golby AJ, Marks MP, Thompson RC, et al. Direct and combined revascularization in pediatric moyamoya disease. Neurosurgery 1999;45:50.
19. Karasawa J, Touho H, Ohnishi H, et al. Cerebral revascularization using omental transplantation for childhood moyamoya disease. J Neurosurg 1993;79:192.
20. Veeravagu A, Guzman R, Patil CG, et al. Moyamoya disease in pediatric patients: outcomes of neurosurgical interventions. Neurosurg Focus 2008;24:E16.
21. Wang MY, Steinberg GK. Rapid and near-complete resolution of moyamoya vessels in a patient with moyamoya disease treated with superficial temporal artery-middle cerebral artery bypass. Pediatr Neurosurg 1996;24:145.
22. Matsushima T, Inoue T, Suzuki SO, et al. Surgical treatment of moyamoya disease in pediatric patients–comparison between the results of indirect and direct revascularization procedures. Neurosurgery 1992;31:401.
23. Mizoi K, Kayama T, Yoshimoto T, et al. Indirect revascularization for moyamoya disease: is there a beneficial effect for adult patients? Surg Neurol 1996;45:541.
24. Suzuki Y, Negoro M, Shibuya M, et al. Surgical treatment for pediatric moyamoya disease: use of the superficial temporal artery for both areas supplied by the anterior and middle cerebral arteries. Neurosurgery 1997;40:324.
25. Ishikawa T, Houkin K, Kamiyama H, et al. Effects of surgical revascularization on outcome of patients with pediatric moyamoya disease. Stroke 1997;28:1170.
26. Iwama T, Hashimoto N, Tsukahara T, et al. Superficial temporal artery to anterior cerebral artery direct

anastomosis in patients with moyamoya disease. Clin Neurol Neurosurg 1997;99(Suppl 2):S134.
27. Sakamoto H, Kitano S, Yasui T, et al. Direct extracranial-intracranial bypass for children with Moyamoya disease. Clin Neurol Neurosurg 1997;99:S126.
28. Miyamoto S, Akiyama Y, Nagata I, et al. Long-term outcome after STA-MCA anastomosis for moyamoya disease. Neurosurg Focus 1998;5:e5.
29. Houkin K, Kuroda S, Ishikawa T, et al. Neovascularization (angiogenesis) after revascularization in moyamoya disease. Which technique is most useful for moyamoya disease? Acta Neurochir (Wien) 2000;142:269.
30. Kim DS, Kang SG, Yoo DS, et al. Surgical results in pediatric moyamoya disease: angiographic revascularization and the clinical results. Clin Neurol Neurosurg 2007;109:125.
31. Czabanka M, Vajkoczy P, Schmiedek P, et al. Age-dependent revascularization patterns in the treatment of moyamoya disease in a European patient population. Neurosurg Focus 2009;26:E9.
32. Longo N, Schrijver I, Vogel H, et al. Progressive cerebral vascular degeneration with mitochondrial encephalopathy. Am J Med Genet A 2008;146:361.

Index

Note: Page numbers of article titles are in **boldface** type.

Neurosurg Clin N Am 21 (2010) 575–581
doi:10.1016/S1042-3680(10)00047-1
1042-3680/10/$ – see front matter

D

E

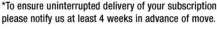

Printed and bound by CPI Group (UK) Ltd, Croydon, CR0 4YY
03/10/2024
01040352-0020